Drawing and cognition

Drawing and cognition

Descriptive and experimental studies of graphic production processes

PETER VAN SOMMERS
Macquarie University

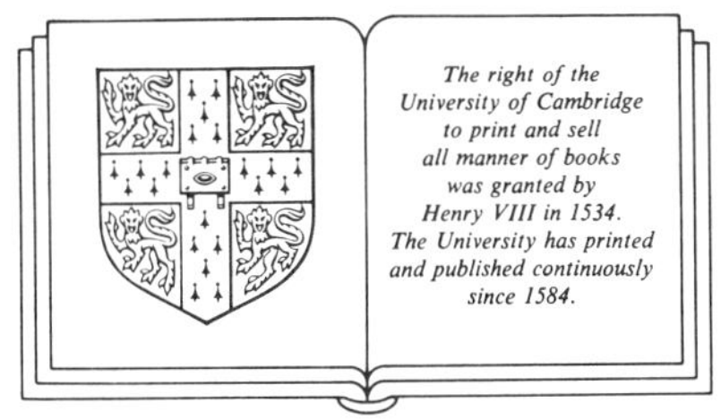

CAMBRIDGE UNIVERSITY PRESS
Cambridge
London New York New Rochelle
Melbourne Sydney

Published by the Press Syndicate of the University of Cambridge
The Pitt Building, Trumpington Street, Cambridge CB2 1RP
32 East 57th Street, New York, NY 10022, USA
296 Beaconsfield Parade, Middle Park, Melbourne 3206, Australia

First published 1984

Printed in the United States of America

Library of Congress Cataloging in Publication Data
van Sommers, Peter.
Drawing and cognition.
Includes bibliographical references and index.
1. Drawing, Psychology of. 2. Drawing ability.
3. Drawing ability in children. I. Title.
BF456.D7V36 1984 153.4 83-7799
ISBN 0 521 25095 1

To Jenny and James

Contents

	Preface	*page* xi
1	Basic executive constraints in drawing	1
	"The multi-storied edifice"	1
	Stroke making	3
	Straight line production	4
	The basis of stroke preferences	7
	Stroke accuracy	12
	Maneuvers for accurate stroke making	16
	A comment on tracing	17
	Working on a vertical surface	17
	Starting locations	17
	Order in stroke making	21
	Script evolution	24
	Western musical notation	27
2	Maintaining paper contact, anchoring, and planning	30
	Paper contact	30
	Geometric constraints affecting order	33
	Drawing hierarchically organized forms	35
	Anchoring and forward planning	37
	Planning for anchoring	42
3	The reproduction of rectilinear figures	52
	The analysis of plane figures	52
	Perceptual preferences: Are there "ideal" triangles?	55
	Distortions in quadrilateral figures	58
	Manipulating starting position and stroke direction	60
	The construction of cubes and prisms	64
	The study of salience	65
	The copying of solids	69

4 The production of curvilinear forms 72
The drawing of arcs 72
Circle production 76
Ellipses 85
Developmental changes 86
Mechanisms of circle production 88

5 The impact of meaning on executive strategies 95
Drawing and speech 95
The expression of action in stroke making 103
Production history and semantic preoccupation 105
Drawing from verbal description 106

6 Simple representational drawing 115
The drawing task and its social setting 115
Formal constraints in representational drawing 117
The facing of objects 120
Drawing in the laboratory 122
Representational contrast 123
Prototypicality and aspect 125
Profiles of detail 126

7 Difficult graphic tasks: A failure in perceptual analysis? 131
Recognition and analysis 131
A study of imagery and drawing competence 135
The spectrum of performances 138
The role of perceptual analysis 158
Good and bad drawers 158

8 Stability and evolution in children's drawings 161
The possible role of stereotypes 161
Surface and structural aspects of objects 163
Conservatism after a time lapse 171
Conservatism and functional knowledge 172
Conservatism and graphic planning 172
Conservatism or evolution 173

9 Innovations, primitives, contour, and space in children's drawings 174
Where do innovations occur in drawings? 174
Collecting repeated drawings 175
Innovation through substitution 180
The question of graphic "primitives" 184
The multiple origins of contours 190

Handling spatial problems 196
Coordination of representational devices 201

10 Children's repeated drawings: How are innovations coded? 204
Consistency of appearance in sequences of drawings 204
Salience and order 211
Types of accretion 212
Connection networks for drawings 215
Variation at the level of microstructure 222
Deliberate variation 226
The source of graphic individuality 227
Happy and persistent graphic accidents 228
Reviewing the variables 231

11 The pragmatics of everyday graphic production 233
Drawing in everyday life 233
Surveying everyday graphic output 238
The charms of doodling 244
Questions of cognitive difficulty 246
Sketches, maps, and plans 246
Orienting maps and plans 249
Time in diagrams 254
Prosodics and thematics 259
On the linguistic analogy 267

References 271
Index 275

Preface

How should this book be characterized? First, it is a monograph on the principles of simple drawing: It takes the reader through those mechanisms and skills that characterize the performance of the child and adult who, without professional training, set out to draw or copy simple (and occasionally not so simple) objects and designs. Second, it is basically empirical rather than theoretical or speculative. It is based on the documentation not only of products, but of processes of production, using video recording and systematic analysis of structure and detail. Third, the philosophy is rationalist. That is, it attempts wherever possible to use the *sense* of why things are done the way they are. I believe we should be most suspicious of the concept of the convention, and in particular the "arbitrary convention" as an explanation of action. Even when drawers fail abysmally to achieve their goals, their efforts are usually orderly and purposeful at many levels.

A note about the characteristics of the subjects. They were all volunteers (or in the case of the small children, were volunteered), and in either case deserve my thanks. Almost all the subjects, with the exception of a group of English left-handers studied in Cambridge (through the good offices of the Cambridge Public Library) and some people whose native scripts and calligraphy were studied (Chinese, Thai, Burmese, Arabic, Hebrew), were part of the Australian population, more specifically the Sydney population. I occasionally encounter some uncertainty about the cultural and educational background this implies, so let me add that like the majority of the current Australian population, most of them have been educated only in the West European tradition, being themselves European immigrants or the descendants of Europeans who occupied Australia at the expense of the indigenous population. They are largely middle-class urban people and so are quite comparable to the sorts of subjects one might recruit from the white middle-class population in England, Canada, or the United States. I have stressed that they are not trained drawers. I did not specifically exclude trained drawers from my samples, but on the few occasions I reviewed the situation I found very few who had done any drafting or were competent artists or sketchers. For this reason I feel safe in referring to their efforts as "vernacular."

A good deal of the data that lie behind these reports was collected by a succession of loyal and resourceful research assistants, notably Liz Grecian, Hilary Cleland, Jenny Case, Jan Milton, Kathy Hossack, and Sue Koenig. Assistance with computing came from John Breen, David Cairns, and June Crawford. Research support came from the Australian Education Grants Committee and Macquarie University Research Committee. I am also in debt to Dr. Alan Baddeley and the MRC Applied Psychology Unit in Cambridge for acting as hosts during much of the writing.

Dr. Penny Jools and three honors students, Neil Sadler, Sharyn Jones, and Robert Stanton, provided data for certain chapters. I am most grateful to Penny Jools and Jacqueline Goodnow for stimulating discussion, and to George Miller and Sylvia Farnham-Diggory for some timely words of encouragement.

1 Basic executive constraints in drawing

"The multi-storied edifice"

One of the classical distinctions in the study of language has been that between its syntagmatic, or horizontal, organization and its paradigmatic, or vertical, structure. The syntagmatic dimension emphasizes the sequential structure of language forms. Its parallel in graphics is the sequence of production. The paradigmatic dimension of language deals with the fact that at any point in the sequence there is available a range of units or segments, the prototypical instance being the choice of word ("I," "you," "she"; "give," "take"; "at," "to," "from"). In drawing we deal with the paradigmatic dimension when, for example, we consider which of a range of standard primitives (lines, circles, dots) are used in portraying parts of an object.

There is, however, another way of viewing the organization of these two systems, which is to consider language and graphics as *layered* systems wherein each action is or can be simultaneously structured or constrained at a great variety of levels. Hence the sound stream of speech carries multiple layers of organization, from the most biologically fixed qualities of the voice through all the phonological, syntactic, semantic, and pragmatic levels. If we choose the convenient starting point in language of the word, we can work down into its phonology, morphology, stress, tempo, the various stable and transient qualities of the voice used in its production; and we can work upward to its function in phrase, clause, sentence, its place in discourse, its social purpose, its multiple social contexts, its relation to gesture and other action. This is what Bolinger (1972) refers to as "layering," and he uses many analogies for it: the various instruments of the orchestra, the waves of different periodicity in the sea, the "multi-storied edifice."

Graphics shares with spoken language this layered quality, and we shall be asking at various points in this book how the "stratigraphy" of the two domains compares. I do not, however, wish to indulge in a lengthy theoretical exploration of the parallel at this point. That is better done when we have in fact begun to peel back the layers one by one. Now it is simply my intention to give notice of the range that a project of this sort must have, a range that extends from skill and perceptual analysis applied by drawers as they produce marks on a page to the broad domain of signification and social and cognitive purpose. When that structure is clearer, it will be proper to ask a further question: whether this rich layering is peculiar to domains like graphics and spoken language, or is a feature of much or most human action.

The principles governing drawing to be dealt with in this book are sometimes mechanical and sometimes cognitive. The studies begin with an exploration of some of the features of execution that are traceable to the anatomy of the drawer in interaction with the furniture and materials of drawing. These are the least ''cognitive'' of all the forces operating, but they are described first because they are almost everywhere evident. They represent the lowest common denominator of executive processes, and so provide the basis for exploring other more cognitive or skill-based principles. Our analytic curiosity is aroused when these principles do *not* predict action. When we cannot explain regularity in a drawing strategy simply in mechanical terms, then we are invited to specify what non-mechanical forces underlie it.

This approach of moving from an established empirical ''beachhead'' applies generally through the whole sequence of studies. When the range of constraints is extended from mechanics to certain applications of the principle of least effort, or a trade-off by subjects between effort and accuracy, or any of the other regularities that constrain simple geometric reproduction, these move from the foreground to become a fresh background against which perceptual or representational regularities can be recognized.

This is not to say that the research was planned in this fashion; in the early stages I was interested in any regularity in the way people compiled drawings. Only when certain principles were uncovered did this process of analysis start to work, and in considering how to go about reporting the principles that govern drawing production, I believed that this movement from basic mechanics, through certain simple skills, plans, and economies to representation and finally to pragmatics was a sensible expository scheme. One significant disadvantage of this approach is the apparent salience it gives to less cognitive matters. For readers who are attracted to this book because of its reference to cognition, a treatment of such things as how mechanical displacement of the drawer's arm may alter stroke making, or how changes in starting position may affect direction of rotation around circles, may seem a little too concrete. But my object has been to be as comprehensive as I can and as true as possible to reality so that it is feasible, at least in theory, to know completely what is going on at successive levels of abstractness in simple drawing.

I might add that even when we are dealing with the most mechanical principles, skill is never completely irrelevant. When we consider the drawing of simple lines, mechanics never *dictate* action; rather, they invite the person who first starts to make marks on paper to move one way rather than another. There has to be a brain that recognizes the pressure of mechanical factors and learns to select one way of working rather than another. The mechanical principles that favor certain actions affect every drawer in much the same way, and every drawer picks up what to do very quickly, so that we might be tempted to see the consistencies as nothing but the tyranny of anatomy and material. But in fact, even at this very basic level, action is in a simple way skilled and rational.

Historically, the whole research program began in a naturalistic way. Rather than setting up hypotheses, I began with observation and analysis. I collected a large body of drawing and copying performances recorded on videotape and analyzed and summarized it in a search for systematic features. I was primarily interested in drawing from life or from memory, but because much of the regularity emerges only when one searches for common features of numerous similar performances, I found it expedient to include a good deal of copying at this early stage, since that provides relatively homogeneous output from which consistencies can be extracted.

Subsequently, the research techniques went off in two different directions: (a) into more challenging drawing tasks and more naturalistic settings, and (b) into a variety of rather more abstract graphic exercises designed to uncover basic principles of operation. Quite a number of these more "experimental" approaches appear in the section dealing with basic graphic articulation.

Stroke making

When one asks a group of untrained adults or children to draw common objects, the vast majority of their strokes are simple lines, arcs, circles, or dots. Relatively few contours are used – that is, lines whose shape is steered and modulated to represent shape. What control there is relates principally to placement, length, orientation, and in the case of arcs and circles, radius of curvature. The general style of production is ballistic: It seems to arise from a predetermined production routine, one or two parameters of which are modulated or calibrated to fit the graphic context.

Are there principles that govern the character of simple stroke making outside representational need? This issue was already being investigated by Goodnow and co-workers (see Goodnow, 1977) when I began looking for executive consistencies in drawing in the early 1970s. There are, however, two justifications for discussing it further. First, the preference for producing certain strokes over others has usually been spoken of in terms of rules analogous to grammatical rules. This view had two sources of support—one theoretical, the other empirical.

The concept of rule enjoyed its most spectacular revival in the context of Chomskian autonomous grammar. Chomsky was most emphatic about the relative arbitrariness of grammatical rules, wishing to show that they possessed a life of their own, so to speak, between the laws of phonology and the field of semantics, with its basis in the structure of the real world. So the concept of rule in psychology carried this connotation of a cultural product – part of a transmitted code. This concept of rule as convention was applied to graphics, and it was supported to a degree by some variability in the application of rules, a variability that could be traced to cultural variations in writing systems. Another feature of this work, not necessarily unrelated to the first, was a certain discreteness of the rules proposed. Rules were tied relatively closely to particular actions, so that there might, for example, be one rule governing vertical movement and another governing horizontal. I should like to support the idea, in line with the general philosophy I mentioned in the preface, that consistencies in such things as stroke direction may be based to some degree on features of the drawer and the medium, and in this sense are not to any great degree cultural products; and second that particular regularities such as horizontal or vertical strokes may be seen as special cases of a more general field of preferred movements.

One problem in trying to establish whether there are basic structural preferences in actions within a representational context is how to neutralize the biases of the subject matter. If one documents the painting strokes made by children, there are bound to be a large number of vertical strokes. This can be traced ultimately not to any drawer-based executive bias, but to a fact of physics: Objects are stable when their centers of gravity fall within their bases; that is, roughly when they are vertical. So if drawers work from a horizontal ground line and represent buildings, tree trunks, fence posts, and so on, there are likely to be many vertical strokes in their productions. One way to circumvent this semantic contamination is to provide a semantically neutral subject matter. We can see this idea in operation in the execution of simple straight lines.

Straight line production

One method I used to neutralize the impact of subject matter bias was to provide subjects with a sheet of paper covered in an apparently random way with short lines of great variety of orientations. There were 56 lines, each 2.5 cm long, and they represented a full spectrum of possible orientations. With the page fixed in a vertical position on the table in front of them, university students were asked simply to trace over all the lines. The performance was videotaped, and the direction in which they moved along each line was documented. The data were collated into a circular plot (Fig. 1.1).

If we imagine the center to be the starting location for each stroke, the radii represent all possible directions of movement. Since a particular line, say a horizontal, could be drawn from left to right or right to left, we can count what proportion of subjects chose one against the other. These proportions are shown as profile around the plot. As can be seen, the subjects were very consistent. With only an occasional exception, all right-handers chose to trace downward to the right rather than upward to the left, and their choices lie in a solid band from about 2 o'clock to 8. The left-handers doing the same task show a profile that is a virtual mirror image of that of the right-handers. So although it is true to say that downward vertical strokes and left-to-right horizontal strokes are favored by the right-handed subjects, these can be seen as special cases of general preference for movement across a wide range of orientations that lie on either side of an axis from 11 o'clock to 5, with left-handers showing an analogous mirror-image preference.

Although this tracing method allows one to detect a preference between any movement and its 180-degree opposite and therefore indicates how a subject might be expected to move when representational need prescribes a line in a particular orientation, it indicates nothing about preferences between, say, a movement toward 3 o'clock and one toward 5. To establish this, we must free the subjects even more completely from task constraints.

Subjects were therefore given a blank sheet of paper and asked to cover it with short lines like those on the tracing sheet, but to do their best to make sure they drew in every possible direction. This instruction was emphasized, and subjects were discouraged from working systematically. The object was to discover whether there was in fact a bias in their stroke production even under the conservative instructions to try to lay down lines in every direction. The outcome for right- and left-handers under these conditions is shown in the second pair of plots in Fig. 1.1. Here the profile represents the proportion of lines laid down by subjects in the various segments of the 360-degree range. The profile reveals that although most lines lay in the broad half circle to the bottom right of the plot, as one might expect from the tracing experiment, subjects showed consistent biases within this that favored neither a horizontal nor a vertical orientation. For right-handers there are peaks toward the top right, the bottom left, and out toward 4-5 o'clock, and again the left-handers showed an outcome that was a mirror image of this.

At the time these data were collected, I was not so sensitive to the inverted versus noninverted distinction brought to prominence by Levy and Reid (1976). *Inversion* refers to the practice, mainly seen in left-handed writers and drawers, of flexing the wrist into a hooked position and working with the pen pointing

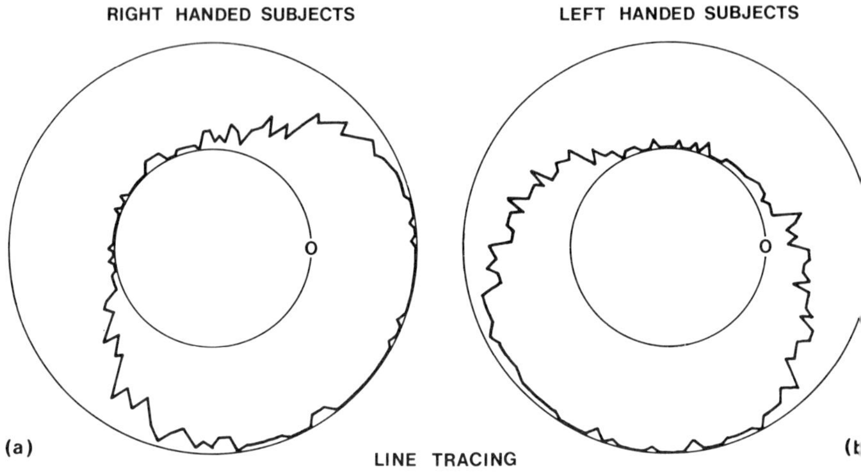

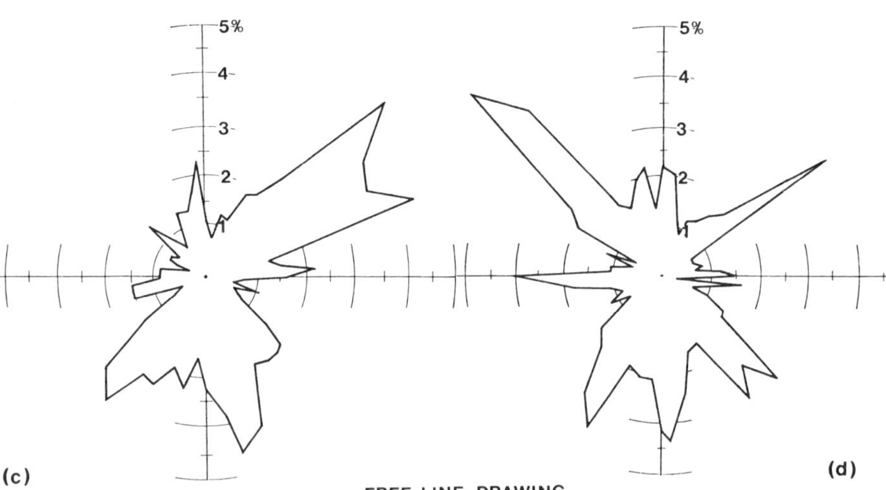

Fig. 1.1. Direction of stroke making in tracing 2.4-cm lines. The lines were arranged at random over a page, and represented all orientations equally. The profile shows the number of subjects tracing in one direction rather than its opposite. The results are from 14 right-handed adults (a) and 14 left-handed (b). Results for 12 right-handed (c) and (d) 12 left-handed adults drawing lines of all orientations on an empty sheet. The departures from random distribution indicate their stroke preference when they are working independently of representational constraints.

toward the body. A left-hander who uses an inverted hand position is more likely to produce movements toward the upper right. Since I included both inverted and noninverted left-handers in my sample, the minor peak toward the upper right is not unexpected.

Herron (1980) has suggested that hand inversion in left-handers can be linked to certain wrist movements, and this is consistent with my impressions. I analyzed the video recording of one right-handed subject who constantly changed hand position while tracing lines. The subject was working rapidly down and across a page of lines whose orientations were randomly distributed. The hand position for each stroke was documented and the outcome plotted in the circular format shown in Fig. 1.2. Here all the line orientations are systematically arranged around the center and the wrist-hand configurations used for various subsets of lines are shown around the periphery. What emerges is an incredibly consistent feat of matching degrees of hand inversion to line orientation, evidently to maximize particular hand movements at the expense of others.

The basis of stroke preferences

What is the basis for this pattern of preference in stroke making? The first evidence comes from impressions of the subjects themselves. I gave a comparable group of right- and left-handed adult subjects a new sheet, now covered with elongated rectangles. At one end of each rectangle was a dark bar (inset, Fig. 1.3), and from this bar the subject had to draw three strokes along the length of the rectangle. After each set of strokes, the subjects were asked to rate the difficulty of making the strokes on a 5-point scale. By orienting the rectangles at random and having them represent again 56 different directions, it was possible to compile a profile of stroke-making difficulty for all possible orientations. (The study was replicated asking for ratings of "easiness" and produced the virtual complement of these values.)

The right-handed subjects reported two principal regions of difficulty – a broad region to the top left and a less prominent region to the right (Fig. 1.3). Again, the left-handers produced data that were horizontally symmetrical to the right, and in both cases these judgments fit two of the larger gaps in the free-line drawing data.

The fact that there is a major peak in the difficulty ratings to the top left, another to the right, but none directly downward raises the question of whether the gap at the bottom of the free-line drawing plot (Fig. 1.1) is a real effect. For right-handers, the avoidance of vertical downward strokes is not nearly as consistent as the selective avoidance of the left-to-right horizontal. Short, left-to-right horizontal lines are often drawn with a slightly shaky, tremulous line, whereas vertical downward movements can be made more confidently. Although

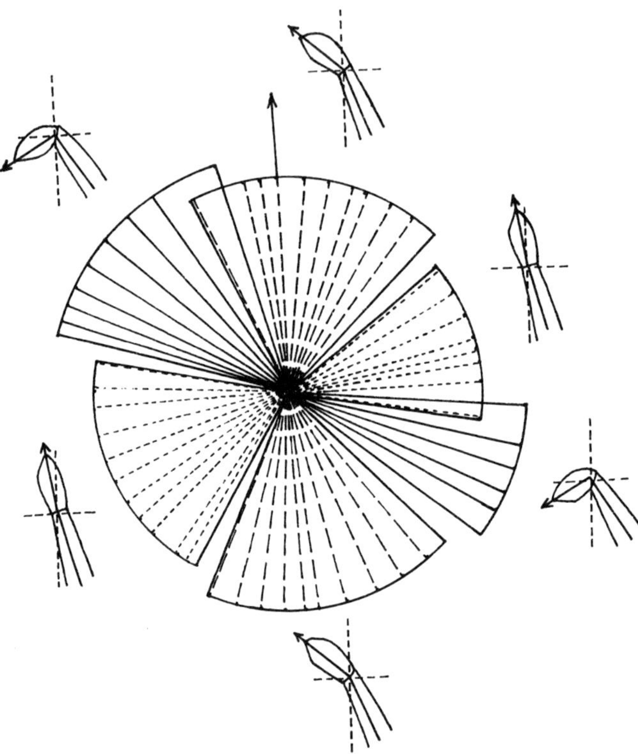

Fig. 1.2. Performance of one right-handed subject tracing lines of every orientation. The traced lines lay at random over the page, and the subject worked quickly down and across the sheet. The hand positions for each stroke were documented from videotapes, and each of 56 directions was plotted with its corresponding hand configuration. This revealed that the subject used a characteristic hand position for each of several segments of the direction plot, switching quickly but accurately to the appropriate position for each succeeding stroke. Line directions sharing a particular hand position are indicated by circle segments. This subject was unusually active in changing hand orientation, but this type of performance is found in both right- and left-handers.

the gap at 6 o'clock in the function may not be as robust as that at 3, it does serve to draw our attention to a possible functional segregation of the movements to the bottom left from those to the bottom right for both right- and left-handers.

A second type of rating asked of the subjects was directed to establishing whether the three main preferred directions were simply three independent movements or were grouped in any way. To do this, a further group of adult subjects was given a set of sheets on which were displayed 120 pairs of dashed lines.

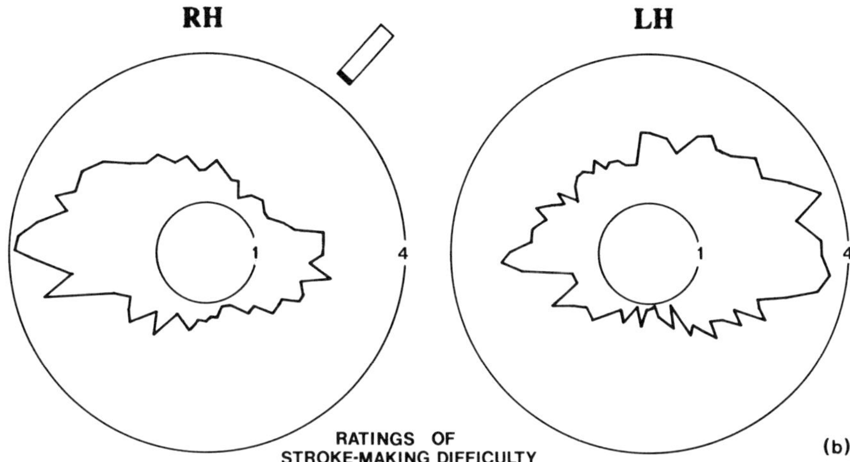

Fig. 1.3. Mean difficulty ratings of subjects drawing lines within elongated rectangles in every orientation. A typical rectangle is shown (insert). Subjects drew from the thickened end of the rectangles and indicated difficulty by numbering from 1 (easiest) to 5 (most difficult.) The right-handers' plot (a) shows a large area of difficult stroke making to top left, a minor peak to the center right. Left-handers show the reverse (b).

Each line was oriented in one of 16 different directions, and the pairs represented each orientation coupled with every other in the order suggested by Ross (1934). Subjects were instructed to draw over the lines in pairs, starting from a specified end, and to indicate with a check mark which line of each pair they found easier to draw. The preferences of each subject were analyzed by a multidimensional scaling procedure (MDPREF, Chang and Carroll, 1968), yielding two strong factors. The first factor combined movements to the top right and those to the bottom left; the second factor corresponds to the region toward 5 o'clock and a weak component in the opposite direction.

What is the likely origin of these groupings? If we look at the video records of the movements, there seems to be a systematic relation between certain hand and finger movements and certain stroke orientations. To explain this, it is helpful to consider the mechanics of the situation. If one holds the forearm in a standard orientation, it is possible to move the whole hand anywhere within a roughly conical space. This has been called the three-dimensional excursion envelope of the hand. It is not entirely symmetrical. Movement up and down is freer than lateral movement, so that a cross-section of the envelope is roughly elliptical. When one writes or draws with the hand resting on a horizontal plane, the intersection of this surface with the excursion envelope restricts it to two dimensions. The wrist movement now produces a fanning path across the paper. The trajectory of this fanning action is determined in part by the orientation of the arm, and in part by the limits of wrist movement to right and left.

When one writes, the orientation of the arm with respect to the paper is actually constrained by another need – that of progressing smoothly across the lines. Right-handers usually rotate the page to the left so that a sweep of the forearm transcribes a path along the lines of the page. The fanning action then cuts obliquely across the lines so that vertical strokes in cursive script commonly lean to the right. The counterclockwise rotation of the paper on the table by right-handed people that allows the hand to sweep across each line actually tends to exaggerate this right inclination, so that writers are forced to "straighten up" their script from an otherwise greatly inclined orientation.

In our studies, the page was always fixed parallel to the edge of the table, and it seems in this case that the fanning action accounts for two of the three peaks in the original plot of preferred movements, top right and bottom left, and the first factor in the scaling study. This view is supported by the fact that the two peaks, like the corresponding high-accuracy points in a copying study to be reported here, do not lie on a straight line. They deviate by 10 degrees, which is consistent with a fanning movement over an arc of 5 cm (roughly two line lengths) with a radius of 12 cm, the typical distance from wrist to pencil tip.

Fanning produces a relatively high-accuracy stroke. Unless they are constrained from doing so, subjects not uncommonly reorient their bodies and arms and rotate the paper to maximize the use of these strokes, particularly that to the top right. This is very likely the basis for much of the busy alteration of hand position shown by the right-hander in Fig. 1.2.

The other factor, that corresponding to the 5 o'clock direction, appears to arise not from wrist movement, but from a flexion-extension movement of the fingers. The large region to the top left that subjects so rarely use is by this account the region of finger *extension*. One common explanation for the dislike of this extension movement is that it involves moving a sloping writing implement point first across the paper, with the risk that it will catch or tear. No doubt in the days of steel nibs this produced difficulties; in classical copperplate script the downward strokes were always heavy and the movements upward faint, even when the upward stroke was a primary element in a letter rather than a linking stroke. But a pencil or modern pen (ballpoint, felt, or nylon) moves relatively freely in all directions, yet the preference persists.

Two other factors are relevant to flexion-extension movements, however. The

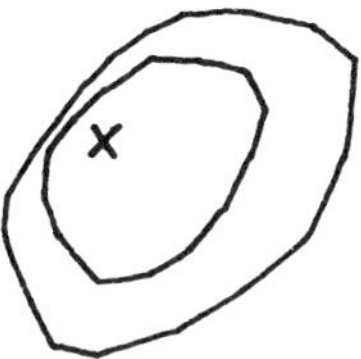

Fig. 1.4. Region covered by lines produced by the relaxed hand and fingers making rotary drawing movements. X indicates the resting position of the pencil before drawing. Ellipses represent the inner and outer envelopes of the region covered by the pencil lines. (Combined data from several right-handed adults.)

first is a competition between pressure to move the pen and pressure to maintain paper contact. In moving a writing implement toward the bottom right, the two forces are consonant; in moving to the top left, they are opposed. Second, when I instructed a group of right-handed subjects to place a pencil at rest on a page and to make a mark, and then asked them to inscribe loose circular spirals around this or to loop out and return while the wrist remained in a standard position, the area over which they moved was an irregular ellipse with the major axis from 1 o'clock to 7, *with the resting point near the upper left boundary* (Fig. 1.4). (The range of movement was just as evident whether the subjects watched their hands or worked with their eyes closed.)

This limitation of scope is an important factor in stroke preference, since to make movements toward 11 o'clock involves extreme finger extension, changes in grip, or whole arm movements. This circumstance becomes important when we consider circle production. The limitation is not absolute, but given this geometry, one might expect consistent aversions to top-left movement to develop quite quickly, especially in those who are not required by their writing systems to develop movements to the top left, which includes writers of almost every modern script. It is worth noting that these preferences are not limited to those who use a pen held in a sloping position. The Chinese brush is held with three fingers and the thumb in a vertical position, but our research has shown that movements upward to the left are likewise relatively restricted.

This account of the articulatory constraints provides a useful first approximation to the situation. Subjects differ in the "openness" of their hands (pronation and supination), which affects particularly the direction of movement to the lower right. They may rotate the hand to a different degree for the fanning action and for finger flexion. Pronation or outward rotation moves the palm away from the paper and releases the fingers from the surface so that they can move more freely. On the other hand, it interferes with upward fanning, which is easier when the palm is rotated downward (supination). Such incompatibilities

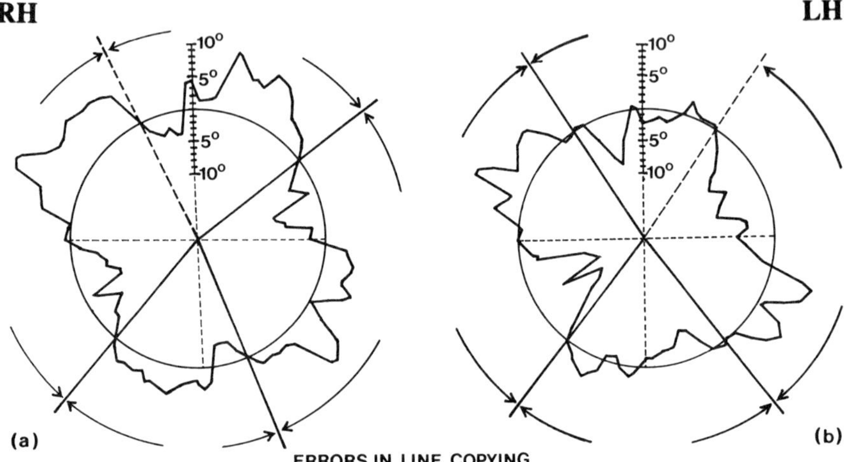

Fig. 1.5. Errors in line copying: (a) right-handers and (b) left-handers (see text for explanation).

may serve to segregate fanning from finger flexion movements, making them to a degree mutually incompatible. This would certainly explain the presence of distinct "lobes" in the stroke preference data and the orthogonality of the first two factors in the scaling study. (We cannot rule out the possibility that these effects are related not only to mechanical properties of the hand, but also involve a difference in central control over the two types of movement – those of hand and those of fingers.)

Stroke accuracy

One further use was made of the random array of lines. Subjects were presented with two sheets. On the first was a set of 56 lines, each with a dot at one end. (The array resembled a scattering of pins over the page.) The subjects were given a second sheet on which only the "heads" of the pins were shown as an array of 56 dots. It was easy to match these dots to the dots at the ends of the lines, and the subjects were asked to copy all the lines onto the second sheet, which was directly before them, starting each line at the corresponding dot. The object of this procedure was to see whether stroke preference affected accuracy of line orientation.

The two plots in Fig. 1.5 show where the greatest inaccuracies occur. The circle represents perfect performance – that is, the exact reproduction of the orientation of lines. Where the profile runs outside this line it indicates that, as a group, the subjects deviated in a clockwise direction from the model. Mean errors in degrees in a counterclockwise direction are indicated when the profile lies *within* the circle.

As one follows the pattern of deviations around the plot, they can be seen to swing successively from clockwise to counterclockwise and back again. Four "crossover" points where copying was most accurate have been marked. That in the upper left quadrant is less significant than the other three, since it lies in a direction subjects normally shun. The other three points of highest accuracy correspond well to the three centers of preferred movement for drawing with the right hand. In other words, subjects attempting to reproduce lines in other than preferred directions tend to make errors in orientation toward a nearby preferred stroke direction. Errors in copying by left-handers show an analogous effect.

At an earlier stage in the inquiry, I had asked some adult right-handed subjects to reproduce a set of crosses, pairs of lines intersecting at various angles (Fig. 1.6). The drawings they produced were superimposed on the models, and the points plotted in Fig. 1.6 show where the ends of the copied lines lay relative to those models. (Each point represents one subject's copy.) The data show that the copies were systematically distorted from the originals. The first interpretation placed on this was that the subjects were somehow "regularizing" the figures, making those crosses with acute angles or very oblique angles more like the perpendicular crosses. The narrow angle between the lines of the first cross, for example, was less acute in the copy. But performances on the lower two designs run quite contrary to this view, since here the lines are made more acute. The issue can be resolved by recording the normal starting position and direction of stroke making. When the various lines are transferred to a circular plot and the median orientation of the copies plotted, the distortions can be accounted for by a movement toward the various preferred stroke directions, as Fig. 1.6(b) shows.

A somewhat freer task produced a similar effect. Subjects were briefly shown a simple line drawing of a tree (Fig. 1.7) and asked to construct one of their own. The sequences of construction varied slightly and were strongly influenced by anchoring constraints, which will be discussed shortly. The main branches and roots were symmetrically arranged, but the directions taken by smaller branches and roots were systematically biased, as Fig. 1.7(d) indicates. (Again the envelope shows the proportion of lines drawn outward in the direction indicated.) Moving one step further out from the laboratory, one finds this fanning movement to be a very important determinant of optional lines in drafting and drawing and a dominant influence in shading. In Porter and Greenstreet's *Manual of Graphic Techniques* (1980), not only is the NE-SW direction of shading and cross-hatching five times more common than the other oblique, but most of the solid objects recede upward to the right. Almost without exception, the formal examples of drawings of solid objects drawn backward from one face utilize the

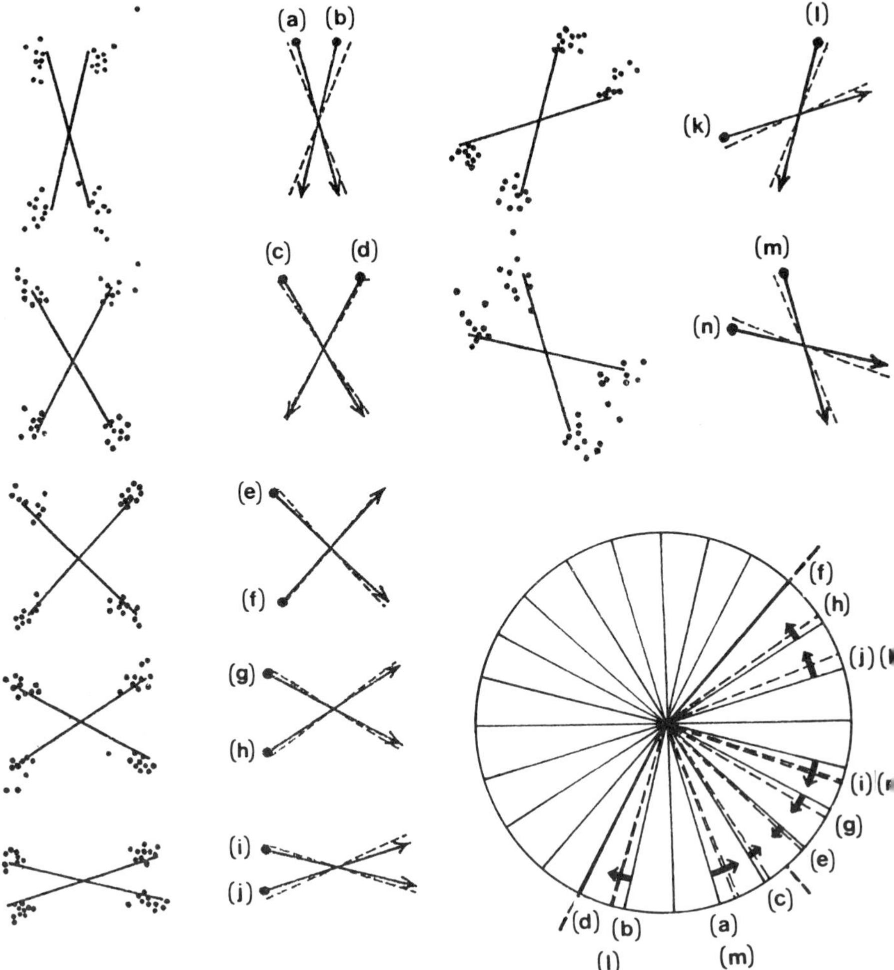

Fig. 1.6. The intersecting lines (crosses) represent the models the subjects were copying. The dots are end points of copies produced by 10 right-handed adults. The same intersecting lines are shown, each with arrowheads indicating the common direction of stroke movement. The dashed lines indicate the median orientation of the copied versions. The circular plot represents direction of movement (from the center). The solid lines represent all the line orientations in the models, each labeled alphabetically. The dashed lines indicate the median orientations of the lines in the copies. Arrows show how each copy has departed from the model in the direction of preferred movements.

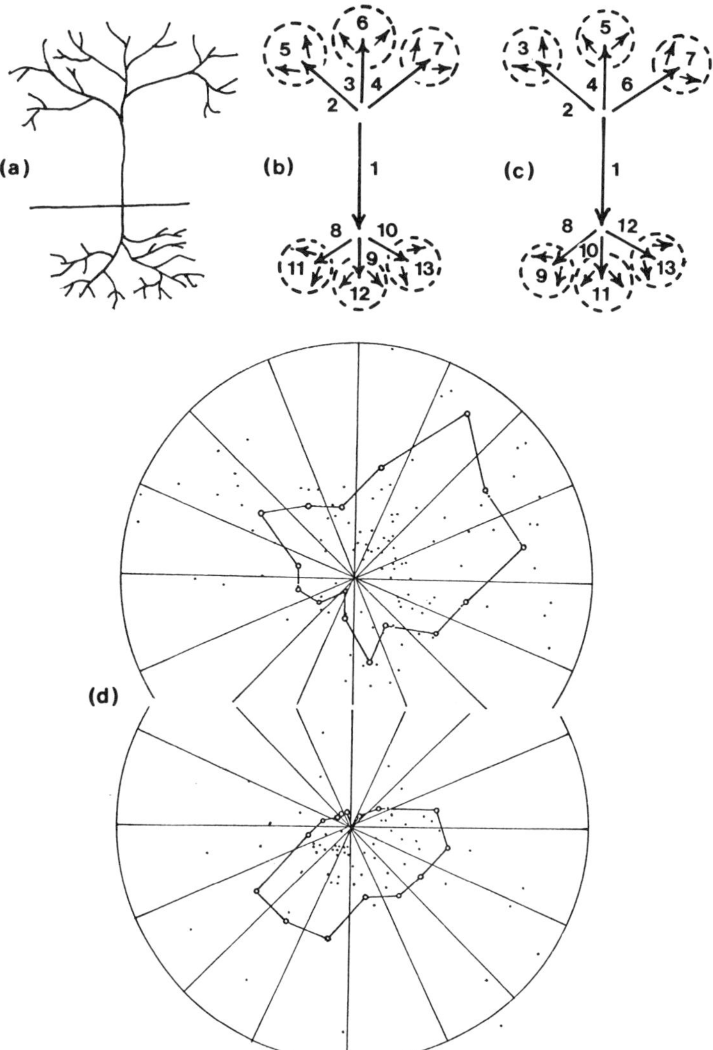

Fig. 1.7. Effects of preferred stroke direction on the drawing of roots and branches of a tree. (a): Tree presented briefly to subjects for reproduction. (b) and (c): Two principal strategies in tree construction. Note successive anchoring at trunk, branches, and roots. (d): Directions and distances of stroke making in constructing branches (top) and roots (bottom). Points represent end points of lines, using center as starting point. Open circles show total number of strokes per segment. Note peaks toward top right (branches) and bottom left (roots).

oblique that runs up toward the top right, even though in the text the choice of right or left is supposed to be made "...in a direction complementing the best angle of view" – that is, on perceptual grounds. Olson (1975) makes the observation that the shading in the sketches of Leonardo da Vinci was the reverse of the normal, and Leonardo was of course the most famous left-handed draftsman.

These preferred directions of movement, which might be called "canonical stroke directions," have important effects in controlling how a great variety of geometric and object drawings are produced – but further discussion of this topic will be deferred to a later chapter.

Maneuvers for accurate stroke making

Those who are themselves involved in serious drawing or who have watched a draftsperson at work may quite reasonably protest that an account in terms of a few basic movements of fingers and wrist is too limited. People who are drawing carefully, and especially those who are drawing large-scale sketches or diagrams freehand, adopt all sorts of maneuvers to escape from the limitations of the hand movements I have been describing. They may move the paper about, often quite radically, and may move themselves around the paper. They may change their forearm orientation repeatedly to optimize certain hand movements, in the fashion shown in Fig. 1.2. When the scale expands so they are trying to produce smooth strokes, say 10 or 20 cm or more in length, they often lock their fingers and wrist and substitute forearm or whole-arm movements for hand movements, pulling or sweeping their hands down or across the paper.

All this does not mean that the style of mechanical analysis I have propounded is irrelevant; quite the contrary. All these maneuvers are aimed at optimizing accuracy and smooth movement by making more universal use of such things as the fanning movement of the wrist or by moving from wrist to forearm, to shoulder, or even to whole trunk to upgrade the size of the mechanical unit to better match the dimensions of the stroke whose trajectory is being controlled. This upgrading of the body part to handle large scale, although important, is not the only justification for deserting finger and wrist movement. One can usefully employ a whole-arm movement to produce a smooth line a centimeter or two long. The drawer is here capitalizing on the limited frequency response of the mechanical system. The point of a pencil held in a locked hand that swings from a fixed pivot at the elbow is not capable of the high-frequency oscillations that can be induced by the fingers, so if smoothness has a high priority, the forearm sweep may be the device to exploit, even over short distances. Of course, the fixity of the system also limits its capacity for self-correction. To achieve accurately placed lines, a certain amount of deliberate rehearsal and calibration may be necessary, like a billiard player or golfer who "sets" the mechanical system, tries a phantom stroke or two, and when it is appropriately adjusted, applies it to the real context, thus combining smoothness with accuracy of placement.

A comment on tracing

The first study of stroke direction involved tracing over lines, and the outcome was consistent with the copying and free-drawing data that followed. Some tracing performances, including working with templates, do not conform to the major drawing constraints. The conformity of simple line tracing is due to the simplicity of the task. When there is a more complex line, visibility becomes more important and the right-handed subjects commonly begin at the bottom right and move up. When one is drawing, the pencil is usually being moved into unoccupied space, and there is no need for visibility ahead of the pencil. But in tracing or following a track, the model has to be left open to view by running the pencil upward away from the forearm or by hooking the hand into an inverted position to reveal the line.

Working on a vertical surface

The earlier reference to patterns of movement of the hand as a basis for preferred stroke directions raises the issue of what happens when drawings are produced by whole-arm movements rather than small wrist and finger movements. The allegation that preferences are related to body geometry and the medium would suggest that there is nothing fixed or universal about them, and that they might very well alter when one writes on a vertical surface. I had all the line copying and tracing material photographed and back-projected it onto a screen. The subjects, university students, stood at comfortable arm's length and produced lines about twice the size of those they drew at a desk. As Fig. 1.8(i) shows, the patterns of performance with the full arm resembled those with the hand, except that the component to the upper right was much less pronounced. As might be expected, the patterns shifted systematically as the area worked moved from directly ahead of the right shoulder toward the left and down, the axis rotating counterclockwise [Fig. 1.8(a) to (h)]. All such demonstrations reinforce the view that these regularities can profitably be studied using methods that minimize the role of representational factors, and that their basis may lie not so much in a series of conventions, but rather in a general theory of articulation.

Starting locations

For theoretical and empirical reasons it may seem unnecessary to consider starting position as something independent of stroke preference. After all, if in drawing

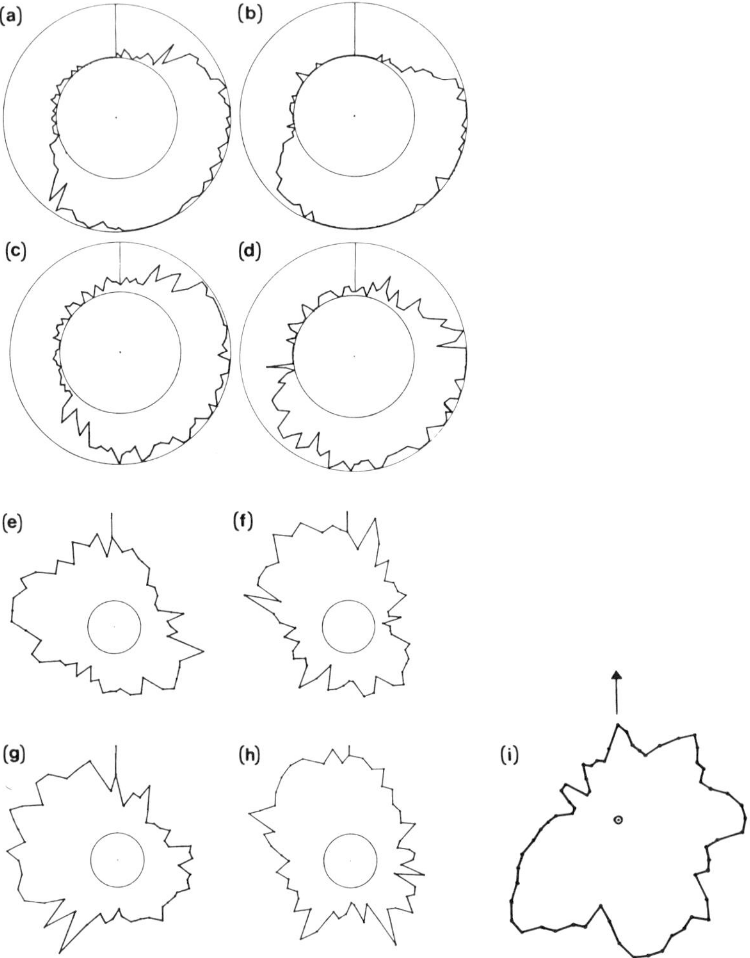

Fig. 1.8. Stroke characteristics of right-handed adults working on vertical wall. (a) to (d): Direction of line tracing. The subjects were tracing over lines at comfortable arm's length in four wall areas corresponding to the four plots. The top right was ahead of their right shoulder, the others to the left and down. (e) to (h): Difficulty ratings of lines drawn in rectangular boxes in all orientations in the same areas. Note in both cases the progressive counterclockwise rotation of the axes of the plots as subjects move left and down. (i): Free line drawing by the same subjects. (The four line drawing plots have been combined after rotating them according to the axes of the tracing plots above.)

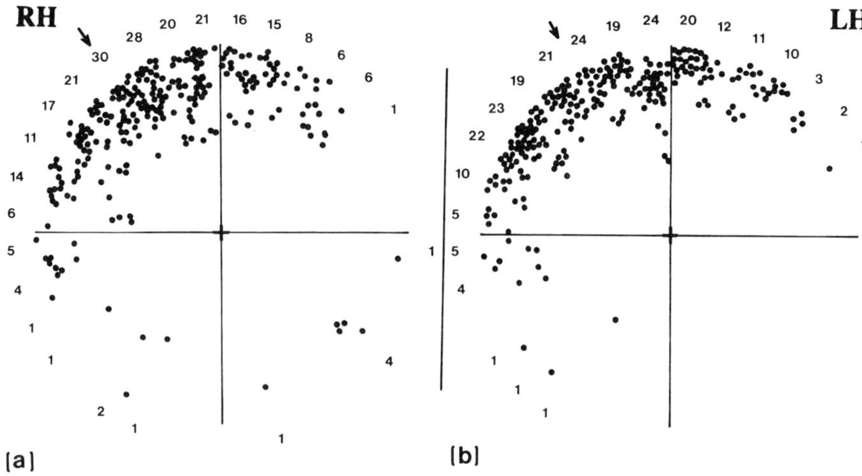

Fig. 1.9. Starting location preferences for right-handed (a) and left-handed (b) adults shown in a dot-tracing task. Each point represents the position of the first dot of a cluster of 10 traced. Each subject completed 20 clusters. Subjects adopted similar starting locations when drawing clusters rather than tracing them. Values at the periphery indicate how many points fell in each 10-degree segment. Note the similarity between right- and left-handers in contrast to stroke-preference data displayed earlier.

a vertical line one moves downward, one inevitably starts at the top. Also, there is a massive amount of evidence that right-handed Western adults favor a starting position near 11 o'clock in all sorts of graphic tasks, and as we have seen the central axis for tracing along lines (in Fig. 1.1) runs from near 11 o'clock toward 5. A parsimonious theory might therefore absorb starting position into stroke-making preference.

This view would be erroneous. It is possible theoretically to define starting position independently of stroke direction – for example, by considering the drawing of clusters of points. When one looks at the evidence from such an experiment, starting position behaves differently from stroke preference both developmentally and in terms of how right- and left-handers behave.

Figure 1.9 shows evidence on this latter point. The subjects, right- and left-handed adults, were shown a cluster of 10 dots covering a circular area 6 cm in diameter and asked to trace the points. Each subject completed 20 different circular clusters. The plots show the distribution of the positions of the *first dot* of each cluster traced by 12 right- and 12 left-handed subjects. The values at the periphery represent the frequency with which the group as a whole began the task in each of 36 segments of the plot. It is clear that the vast majority of all subjects began in the upper left region, centered on 11 o'clock, *irrespective of their handedness*. This is in complete contrast to the stroke-preference data, which showed that right- and left-handers produce mirror-image performances (Fig. 1.1). The same effect occurs when subjects are asked to draw rather than trace a cluster of points: both right- and left-handers begin at the top left.

The independence of starting position from stroke direction preferences is also shown by developmental data. We asked preschool children of different ages to produce a page of random lines. (Some children understood from a simple instruction what was required; in other cases we had to translate the instructions into a description of a pig's straw house that was blown about a field, and the children were asked to represent the straw.) The first three diagrams of Fig. 1.10 show the results for right-handed children ages 3–4, 4–5, and 6–7. There is little change with age; all avoid the upper left region, and although the favored directions do not stand out so clearly, the left- and right-handers show the same mirror-image symmetry we see in adults. (The drawing competence of the youngest children was minimal; they could make almost no recognizable copies of letters, and most knew neither the start nor the proper orientation of pages of simple text.)

Starting location, by contrast, is unstable across a similar age range (Fig. 1.10, bottom). The youngest right-handed children started at the bottom right. In these figures each point within the circle represents the position of the first dot traced in a cluster. Each of the lines around the periphery indicates the median starting position for one child on dot-cluster tracing. Solid lines are for children whose starting locations are highly consistent from cluster to cluster. Dashed lines show those who were consistent but a little more scattered. The youngest group began dot-cluster tracing at a point where their hands approached the page. This was found also to be the location at which they began nongraphic tasks such as moving buttons or counters to and from the center of the page.

As the children matured, the preferred starting position migrated upward and to the left, until by age 6 many have conformed to the adult pattern. It is natural to assume that this change is associated with learning to read and write, but it is possible that there is also an independent discovery being made by each child that graphic work is more straightforward if starting position is consistent with preferred direction of stroke making.

A conflict shows itself in the youngest children between an inferior starting location and downward movement. It is clearly evident when we studied early attempts to copy alphabet letters. When there is a conspicuous linear element that invites a smooth ballistic stroke (E, F, H, I, J, i, j, l), a downward stroke predominates even among children who achieve at best only vague topological equivalence to the original letters. When they embark on more complex strokes (C, S, W, Z), these children do so from a position nearer the body, and upward strokes are at least as common as downward.

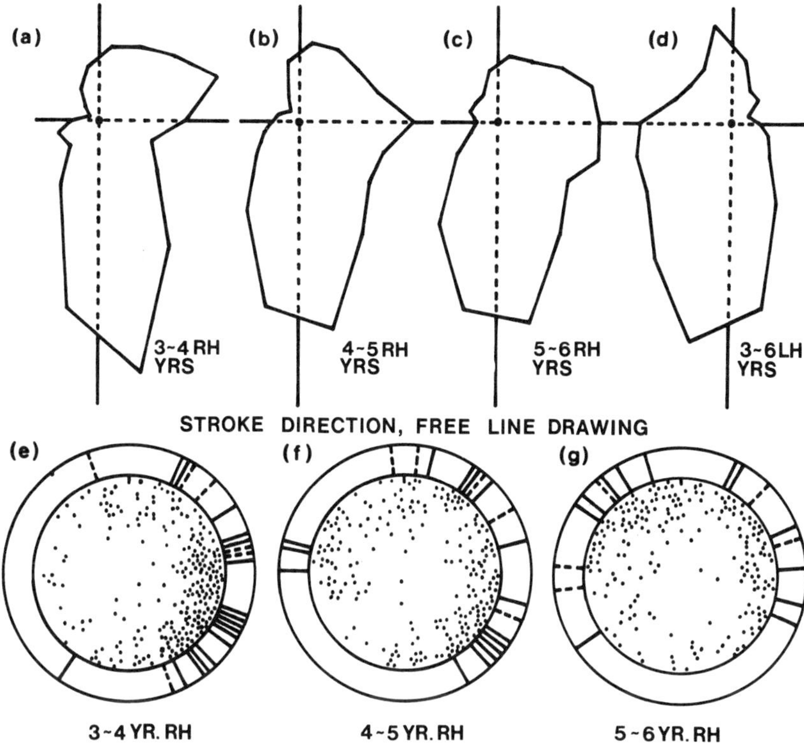

Fig. 1.10. Stroke direction and starting location data for preschool children aged 3 to 6 years. (a) to (c): Right-handed children's free line drawing at the three age levels. Note the relative stability of the performance. All avoid the region to top left. Note also the horizontal symmetry between RH and LH subjects (d). (e) to (g): Dot-cluster tracing by RH children at three age levels. The dot clusters were circular, and each point represents the location of the first point traced by one subject on one cluster of 10 points. Note the concentration toward bottom right in the youngest group and the progressive migration upward and to the left with age. Each line around the periphery represents the median performance of one subject.

Order in stroke making

When a right-handed subject produces a sequence of elements of a similar type, such as a set of short parallel lines, the progression from one to another moves in a consistent direction: 11 o'clock to 5, top to bottom, left to right. This can be seen clearly in the copying of line sets by adults shown in Fig. 1.11. There were four parallel lines in each set, and the sets were in horizontal, vertical, and

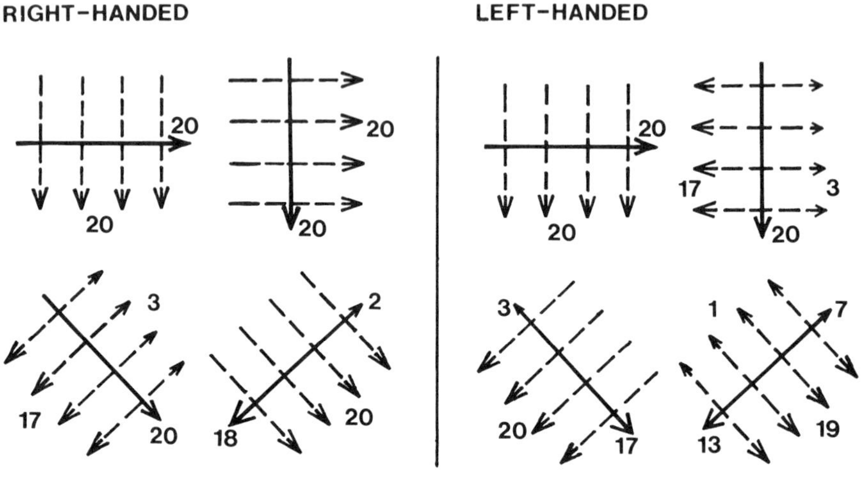

PARALLEL LINE SETS: STROKE DIRECTION (-➤)
ORDER (—➤)

Fig. 1.11. Order of stroke making in copying line sets. There were four parallel lines in each set (shown by dashed lines) oriented horizontally, vertically, and diagonally. They were reproduced by 20 right-handed and 20 left-handed adults. The values near the arrowheads on broken lines indicate the numbers of subjects following that stroke direction. The solid lines represent *order* of line drawing. Note that although stroke direction is a mirror image from right- to left-handers, order, like starting position, is similar for both groups.

two diagonal orientations. The group of right- and left-handed adults performed exactly as one would expect in laying down each individual stroke: The 20 right-handers drew always down, always to the right, always to the bottom right, and were divided when the lines lay more or less at right angles to the 11-to-5 axis. The left-handers were almost as consistent in stroke making toward the left and downward. (These stroke directions are shown as dotted lines in Fig. 1.11.)

When we consider the *order* of compiling these figures, the right-handers move left to right across the set, top to bottom down, 11-to-5 down one diagonal set, and split their order on the other. So far there is nothing to indicate whether order is being controlled by the same principles as stroke direction or arises from starting position. When we look at the order the left-handers follow, however, we see that their *order* is very similar to that of the right-handers: down, left to right, and down to the right. This suggests that ordering of elements in drawing is not determined by stroke direction preference, but from these two constraints: (1) starting position, and (2) proximity of similar elements. So the principle of order for both right- and left-handers is this: Start near 11 o'clock and progress successively through adjacent elements.

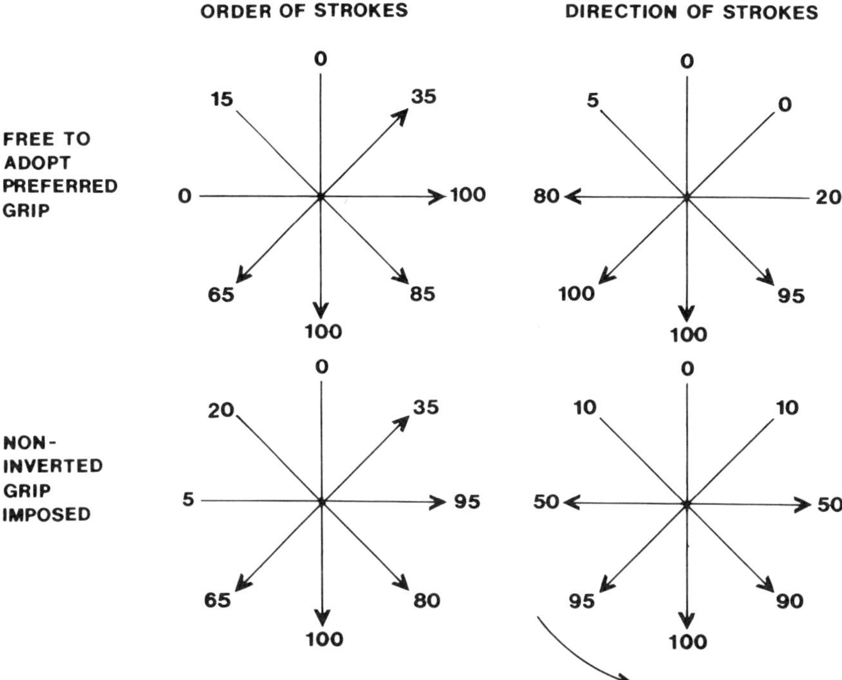

Fig. 1.12. Performances of 20 LH adults on the copying of line sets similar to the dotted lines in Fig. 1.11. Each diagram shows the percentage of strokes made in the order (left) and direction (right) shown by the arrows. The 20 adults copied the line sets under two conditions: free choice of hand position and pencil grip (top) and under instructions to adopt a noninverted ("normal") grip (bottom). Note the stability of order, and the change in stroke direction.

The data shown in Fig. 1.11 for left-handers were collected without placing any restrictions on how the subjects handled their writing implements. Later, however, the same 20 subjects were asked to repeat the task, this time ensuring that the pencil was held in the "normal" (that is, noninverted) position, slanting back toward the left shoulder. This represented a change for at least some of the subjects, who described it as a very awkward maneuver. An analysis of stroke direction and order under these conditions confirms what has been affirmed above: Order remained virtually unchanged, conforming to the right-hand pattern. The axis of preferred stroke direction, on the other hand, showed a net shift. It moved in a counterclockwise direction, following the overall counterclockwise rotation of the pencil from various inverted or semi-inverted positions adopted by some subjects to a consistently "normal" position (Fig. 1.12)

In a later chapter we examine in more detail this sensitivity of stroke making to alterations in the physical relation between drawer and medium. For the moment, our principal interest lies in the support this manipulation affords to the functional separation between stroke direction and order. This view also receives support from the developmental data. When right-handed children of different ages are asked to copy the same parallel line sets their stroke direction remains consistent, but the order of their strokes is labile and irregular, only starting to approximate the adult pattern when they reach 5 or 6 years of age.

Script evolution

If we make a leap from the microhistory of children's development to a speculative reconstruction of the macrohistory of script evolution, we may be able to see how the disjunction of natural starting positions and ease of stroke making can have a broader application.

Most modern scripts have a left-hand start like that of the Latin alphabet (Diringer, 1968), but some important modern scripts begin on the right. To us the most conspicuous examples are Chinese, Arabic, and Hebrew. Traditional Chinese characters are arranged vertically down the page, so the right-to-left progression applies to columns, not to individual characters. As for the characters themselves, they appear to have been produced from the earliest times with strokes that conform to those we have been describing. Tung Tso-pin (1948) commented on the inscriptions produced in the thirteenth century B.C. on tortoise shell for divination purposes. Incisions were cut downward in the shell with a knife and were often made by a "mass production" process whereby each stroke direction for a batch of characters was completed before the shell was rotated to a new position. The cutting followed the delineation of the characters by brush, and Tung Tso-pin observes: "...strokes [of the brush] were made generally from the top downwards and from left-to-right, exactly like modern calligraphy" (1948, p. 127).

In the Chinese case there is no fundamental incompatibility between direction of movement prescribed by strokes and progression from character to character, or at least no more than in Latin script. But in a script like Hebrew there is a conflict, since the letters run horizontally across the page from the right. In spite of this, the predominant strategy of production for each letter conforms to the more convenient actions I have been describing – down and across each letter from left to right – so that to complete a line, one progresses in a kind of "shuffle" two steps to the left, one to the right, across the line.

Arabic script also begins on the right, but there is much more leftward movement within characters and even some upward movement, because ever since its emergence from Kufic, Arabic has been a strongly cursive script with many linked components. Strokes often descend from the top right and progress continuously to the left. The pen, however, does not start individual vertical strokes at the bottom and rise; rising strokes are always the product of continuity upward from linked right-to-left horizontal movements. Lines of Arabic script have a tendency to depart from the horizontal and to drop downward. As a result, many of the otherwise horizontal right-to-left movements are not in fact strictly directed out to the left, but run downward toward 7 or 8 o'clock. This trend becomes exaggerated as the script is more rapidly or carelessly produced.

I have collected samples of various script productions from informants who wrote Hebrew, Arabic, and so on as their native script, and subjected them to a summarizing process that reveals the overall direction of movement. This was achieved by videotaping the writing and marking the direction of movement within each character. The individual letters or letter groups were then enlarged to approximately 20 times their original dimensions; then a line was carefully inscribed down the center of each stroke and marked off at short (5 mm) intervals. The coordinates of all these points were next entered into a computer by means of a digitizing pad. The vectors through each succeeding pair of points were calculated, and these vectors combined for each stroke, each character, and ultimately for each alphabet or other script sample.

The outcome is displayed in the form of a polar plot very similar in principle to those shown in Fig. 1.1. The 360-degree circuit is divided into 36 segments of 10 degrees each, with a line in each indicating what proportion of the hand movements used to produce the character or group of characters was in that direction. The letter "l" produced as a downward vertical stroke would be represented as a single vector down from 6 o'clock, and a perfect circle would yield a plot like a sun, with equal values in all segments. A sample of these plots for various script samples is shown in Fig. 1.13.

The whole situation is thus more unified than it may at first appear. Preferred movements are most evident in scripts in which starting position has moved to the left or the top. In a script like Hebrew, with separate characters, line starting does not dominate character production as much as it does with a cursive script like Arabic, and even in Arabic preferred stroke directions play a part whenever there is an unlinked vertical stroke or when the style is more lax and the movement runs down to the left.

I do not wish to imply that ease of production and resolution of the conflict between directional ease and "natural" starting position are the only driving forces in script evolution. It is a truism for any communicative system that its properties evolve as a compromise between economy of production effort in the sender and economy of perceptual effort in the receiver. I mentioned earlier that the fanning movement runs obliquely across the lines of a page, predisposing writers to strongly right-sloping script. But legibility is maximal for characters that are perpendicular to the lines, so the final outcome will result from the intersection of at least four forces: the two executive constraints I have described,

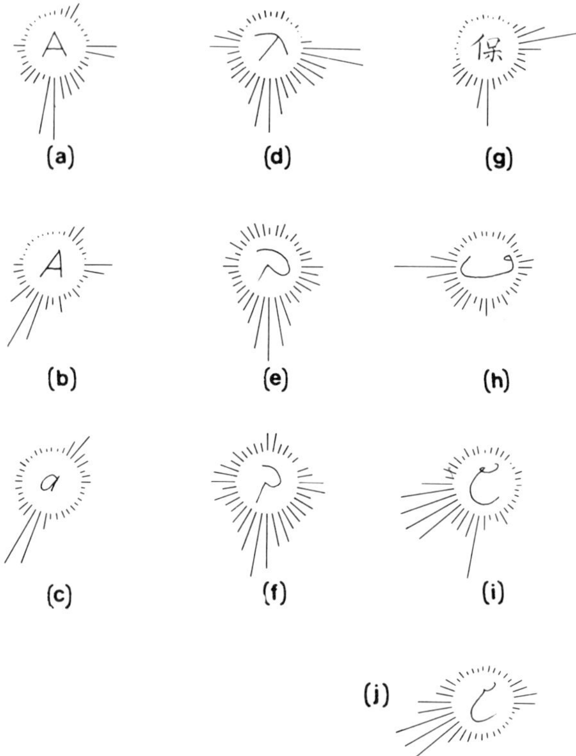

Fig. 1.13. Polar plots of average direction of pen or brush movements in the production of alphabets or other typical characters in various scripts. All characters were produced by native born and educated users of the scripts. The length of each vector is proportional to the amount of movement in the direction indicated. Each plot is a summary of a number of characters. The single character in the center of each plot provides one example of the characters summarized.
(a): Latin alphabet of upright capital letters (A, B, C).
(b): Latin alphabet of sloping capital letters (*A, B, C*).
(c): Latin lowercase ("script print") alphabet in sloping position (*a, b, c*).
(d): Square Hebrew alphabet.
(e): Contemporary Hebrew cursive style.
(f): Hebrew cursive alphabet produced rapidly.
(g): Summary of direction of movement in 13 common Chinese characters produced by three native-born Chinese informants working with a brush.
(h): Contemporary Arabic alphabet produced formally.
(i): Arabic cursive alphabet written slowly.
(j): Arabic cursive alphabet written rapidly.
Note that in the Arabic alphabet there is a strong component of movement to the lower left, reflecting the impact of the right-to-left progression, but that as the script becomes less formal and is produced at speed, the movements move toward an axis from top right to bottom left, not so dissimilar from the sloping lowercase Latin alphabet (c).

the degree of cursive linking, and a legibility factor. This conforms to the view taken by analysts of cuneiform script, which evolved toward a small set of stylus movements that were easy to make, but at the same time contrastive (André-Leicknam, 1982). This principle of contrast is a central issue in graphics, and can be seen in the evolution of another symbol system – namely, musical notation.

Western musical notation

I see the development of European musical notation as another example of competing graphic forces, except that the competition is not between two different executive constraints like movement and starting position, but between executive principles (shaping the symbols to suit ease of production) and symbolic processes. I will describe the pressures on symbol form of this second type in terms of the need to establish *representational contrast*, a notion that will be developed in more detail later in the book. When executive constraints and symbolic needs are in conflict, there are various possible outcomes, two of which we will encounter: either symbolic representation will exclude graphic convenience altogether, or the exclusion will be only partial, so that in the case of a binary contrast one element may be consistent with graphic convenience and the other not. In such cases, one can perhaps expect graphic convenience to prevail with the symbol that is most often written.

The main source of information used in this brief analysis comes from the examples and description in Bent, Hiley, Bent, and Chew (1980). The earliest European musical notations illustrated in their review come from Germany in the tenth century and France in the eleventh. These consisted simply of sequences of dots and dashes or clusters of small marks placed above or to one side of text to indicate either rhythm or melody. Because the code carried relatively simple information, the orientation of strokes could be dictated to a large degree by graphic convenience, and the strokes sloped down to the left.

In the thirteenth century a more sophisticated notation was developed that combined pitch and duration information, the so-called Franconian system (named after Franco of Cologne). The significant event from our point of view was the departure from the principle of one note symbol for one pitch, so that a single long mark showed the position on a stave of the first and second of a pair of pitches. These were represented by a long horizontal rectangle or a parallelogram sloping upward or downward from the left (Fig. 1.14). All the remaining single notes were short and were drawn as squares with a flat pen tip, presumably to contrast with the slope of the double-note oblique lines that indicated a shift in pitch. In other words, the scribe lost the prerogative of choosing a graphically convenient sloping form for the single notes because slope was absorbed into the system of contrasts representing musical values.

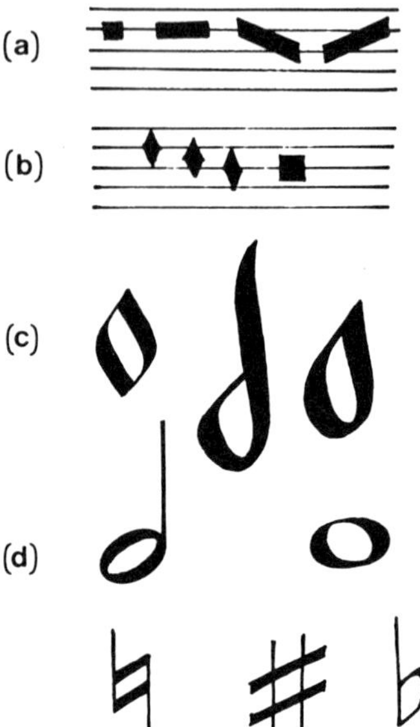

Fig. 1.14. Approximate form of Western musical notation mentioned in the text. (a): Franconian notation, including conjunct oblique marks indicating a change of pitch. (b): Italian diamond shaped note heads and square notes equivalent to a minim. (c): Open note heads of fifteenth- and sixteenth-century European notation. (d): Modern minim, semibreve, and accidentals.

In the examples of fourteenth-century Italian notation, long strokes representing two notes did not seem to be common, and the shape of the majority of note heads shifted to a narrow diamond equivalent in value to our crotchets or quavers. This shape, like the Franconian notes, seems to have been constructed as a solid ink mark made with a flat pen tip, now drawn down to the right with a flexion movement of the fingers. That relatively convenient (and common) diamond shape was contrasted with a less frequent (and less convenient) square note of double the metrical value.

The final major development from a graphic point of view was to produce note heads as outlines, filled or open, and here natural stroke preferences showed themselves again. Some symbols were made as a continuous line from stem to note head. Various note-head shapes clearly show the impact of canonical movements. There was a transition period when diamond-shaped marks were drawn in outline, and then various semirounded forms evolved. As we will see, within mainstream drawing practice and in script, many "round" forms are not drawn as perfect circles but are faceted, and this seems to have been the rule in musical notation. The shapes that emerged included a lozenge shape with the sides descending to the right drawn more thickly, pear-shaped notes (rather more like a teardrop), and finally the ellipse with the axis sloping down to the left that has become the standard form in modern musical typography.

What appears to have happened is that the systems of musical notation continued to carry a large volume of information, as they did in the Franconian system, but the reason this did not "squeeze out" graphic convenience was that the semiotic function of representing note duration shifted away almost entirely from modulations to the outline shape of the head of the note to whether it was stemmed or unstemmed, filled or open, dotted or undotted, with or without flags – which in turn could be single or multiple. As a consequence, note-head shape was largely free to reflect graphic convenience again. Other musical symbols, such as the accidentals (sharp, flat, natural), are not individually information-rich, and certain components within them are also able to follow the fanning movement – top right/bottom left.

There are two illuminating exceptions: The modern semibreve and the minim both have open oval heads. The two notes are contrasted by the presence or absence of a stem, and also in the orientation of the axis of the note head, with the more frequent shorter minim being made with the fanning movement down to the left and the less frequent semibreve being constructed more horizontally, with thicker flexion movements. Second, the "beam" that connects quavers, and so on to one another has to conform to the pitch contour, as the old Franconian oblique mark did. It therefore does not have a standard orientation, but is horizontal or rises or falls according to representational need.

Now that there has emerged a new generation of avant garde personally creative notation, it is interesting to speculate whether the unconscious bias of hand movements involved in creating musical instructions may subtly affect the form of the music itself, because many of the scores have moved into a less codified form, one where there is a more direct semantic link between physical score construction and performance.

2 Maintaining paper contact, anchoring, and planning

Paper contact

When subjects reproduce simple geometric forms, the majority of strokes conform to the preferred stroke direction. One important source of exceptions arises from a tendency to keep contact with the paper as the pencil moves from one linear element to another. Subjects not uncommonly turn a corner without lifting off and may then be compelled to proceed in a normally nonpreferred direction. This practice is sometimes called *threading*, and is of course the factor that in writing distinguishes cursive script from lettering. We have seen that such stroke continuity has been a significant force in script evolution, and accounts for the very fundamental difference between the execution of Hebrew and Arabic script.

Before I describe some of the factors that favor or discourage continued paper contact, it should be noted that the medium we used does not itself limit continuity. When traditional draftspeople used pens and brushes that needed continual replenishment with ink, there was an upper limit on stroke length that had to be integrated into the structure of the drawing performance. Since all our subjects worked with pencil or nylon-tipped pens, this was not an issue.

The analysis of a large number of rectilinear figures shows that drawers are very systematic in determining whether they will lift off or continue. If they have not continued around a corner, it is because they are going to relocate at another point on the figure. They virtually never lift off and then continue from the same point. It is possible to force subjects to break contact by asking them to reproduce figures with gaps at all the vertices. Under such circumstances, where no threading is possible, movement in the nonpreferred direction completely disappears. Unless they can continue in a congenial direction after breaking paper contact, subjects always relocate.

Empirical inquiry shows that certain characteristics of figures favor maintaining paper contact:

1. Small figures are more often constructed with continuous lines than are large figures.

Table 2.1. *When subjects draw rectangles they may maintain paper contact at one or more corners. The top row indicates what percentage of rectangles are drawn by adult RH subjects in a single stroke, the second row in two strokes, and so on. Columns indicate whether the figures were constructed of continuous or broken lines. Breaking lines promotes "threading."*

No. of strokes to complete rectangle	Form of lines		
	Continuous ———	Dashes – – – –	Dots .....
1	13	40	45
2	29	35	50
3	29	30	5
4	13	5	0

2. The more sides there are to be produced in a figure, the less threading there is per corner.
3. If subjects have to produce a series of similar figures, threading becomes more common as the series progresses.
4. There is more threading when figures are traced rather than copied or drawn.
5. Threading is more common when figures are produced from broken lines (dotted or dashed) than normal lines. (Table 2.1 shows the consistent relation between how many corners of a quadrilateral are threaded and the type of line used.)
6. Threading is more common around open (oblique) angles than acute, so that paper contact is much less common when an acute angle leads into a nonpreferred stroke direction than when the same stroke emerges from a right angle.
7. Certain right-angle transitions are more often constructed continuously. In drawing a square, for example, two angles are likely candidates for threading, the bottom left and top right, and of these the top right is much more commonly threaded. (In a typical sample of squares, the top right was threaded on 92 percent of occasions, the bottom left, on 57 percent.) Hence the most usual sequence for a right-handed drawer producing a square or rectangle is a vertical on the left, a linked stroke across the top and down on the right, and a final stroke across the bottom. This is also the prescribed sequence for producing the important rectangular radical *k'ou* or *kuchi* in Chinese and Japanese calligraphy.

There is a logic to these facts. The principal motive for threading is economy: It reduces the number of executive commands while maintaining accuracy at line intersections without requiring separate locational control. We have noted the increase in threading when forms are made repetitively and fast. It is increasingly evident in lettering when that is done rapidly or more routinely, and the existence of cursive script itself testifies to this view. Subjects choose to package a number of movements within a single hand placement, even if they have to move in nonpreferred directions. This is doubtless why there is more continuous contact with small figures: All the movements fall easily within the scope of a single placement. Likewise, the farther one moves around a form, the greater the possibility of awkward transitions. Discontinuous lines may favor continuity because the interruptions allow small relocations of the hand. (The other possibility is that a central process is involved. Perhaps the same machinery is used for interrupting lines as for lifting up and relocating the pencil, so that its use for one purpose reduces its availability for the other.)

The difference between top right and bottom left transitions in drawing squares seems to demand a more specific explanation. It may be due to a difference in articulatory ease: It is easier to drop down after a horizontal stroke than to move horizontally after the fingers have flexed on a downstroke.

Continuous paper contact plays a part in graphic production at an early age. Penny Jools made some data available to me on the production routines of children in the age range 3.6 to 5 years, and in them almost all the principles I have been describing were present. There was almost universal threading around simple right angles even when this carried the strokes upward or to the left. As the figures became more complex, threading systematically declined. There was less on figures resembling three sides of a square and less still for rectangles; and within these figures, maintaining paper contact was more common for some right-angle transitions than others. In particular, the top right transition was threaded substantially more often than the bottom left, as is found with adults. In reproducing triangles, children showed less threading on acute angles (58 percent) than right angles (72 percent) even when both led in similar stroke directions. All these findings support the idea that threading principles arise from basic features of the medium and the drawer and show up almost as soon as the child begins to display competence in handling a pencil.

Continuous paper contact has an important role in the production of more complex figures by adults. A figure such as a stepped pyramid or a staircase can be organized as a stack of adjacent regions or as a frame or envelope with interior detail added. The tendency to maintain paper contact may be one of the factors that biases drawers toward delineating objects with a continuous frame. If this is true, we are dealing with a case of an articulatory principle beginning to affect broader aspects of graphic planning. This would not be a unique case of peripheral factors affecting central programs, for we will be dealing later with a number of instances of constraints arising from physical execution feeding back to more abstract levels of command.

So far I have emphasized the effect that paper contact has on departures from normally preferred stroke directions, but of course it can also alter stroke order. Indeed under certain conditions this may be its only effect – as when, for example, a symmetrical triangle is drawn sitting on its base. If it is built from three independent strokes, the favored order will be left, right, bottom. If paper contact is maintained at the end of the first stroke, direction of movement along the sides will be unaltered, but the order will of course become left, bottom, right. In this way, paper contact makes an independent contribution to stroke order.

Geometric constraints affecting order

We now turn to a constellation of additional principles that interact and compete with those forces controlling order in stroke making we have already discussed. Order or sequence is of course affected by a very wide spectrum of factors – geometric, semantic, and pragmatic – but those to be dealt with now are simply those geometric and perceptual factors that invite subjects to depart from a standard order of construction for relatively abstract subject matter. The overall principle says that other things being equal, subjects will group components on the basis of four geometric factors: proximity, similarity, symmetry, and collinearity.

Proximity is of course the primary influence that converts starting position into standard order. Subjects producing parallel line sets or dot clusters, as in Fig. 2.1(a) and (b), invariably move to the nearest element, or the element along the trajectory they are following, with obvious economies of effort and decision. In the case of equally spaced lines, it might also appear that this stepwise progression makes it easier to control the relative sizes of intervals between the elements. But in some situations, this is not the case. A common counterexample is entering marks on a clockface or any other regular radial figure, where subjects are particularly sensitive to mislocations at 12, 3, 6, and 9 o'clock and frequently enter these first, filling the gaps later. This also applies to linear arrangements where the end components must be accurately located or space segmented into a precise number of intervals.

Fig. 2.1(c) to (e) demonstrates departures from normal order based on similarity of size, form, orientation, or inclusion in closed figures. In Fig. 2.1(d), there is competition between the horizontals as horizontals and the rectangular form in the center. In Fig. 2.1(e), a perceptual unity based on proximity of the two center lines combines with anchoring constraints and collinearity to overdetermine the order of construction shown by the arrow.

Symmetry effects are shown in the stool, Fig. 2.1(g), and table, Fig. 2.1 (h), although in the case of the table it is not clear whether an additional representational force prescribes that the "front" legs be drawn as a pair before the back. Fig. 2.1(i) and (j) show the same effect of collinearity we saw in (e): For geometric (and perhaps semantic) reasons, drawers follow the trajectory of the interrupted lines. Of course, just as semantic forces can reinforce continuity

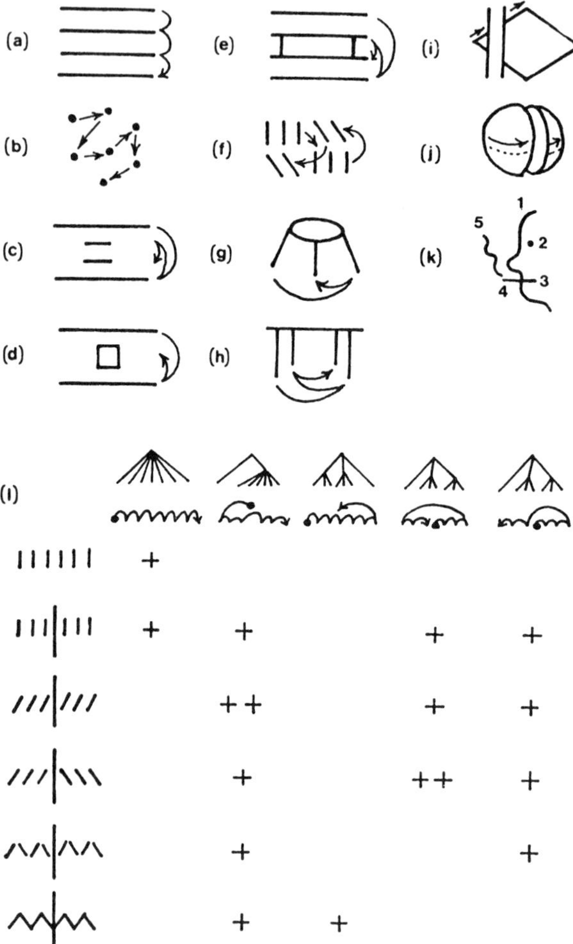

Fig. 2.1. Principles of order based on geometric grouping. (a) and (b) illustrate simple orders based on conventional starting position combined with proximity. (c) is grouped by similarity of size, (d) and (e) by form. (f) shows grouping by similarity of orientation. (g) and (h) show grouping of symmetrical elements, (i) and (j) illustrate collinearity. The final figure (k) indicates a departure from geometric ordering based on a semantic organization that contradicts it. The matrix (l) shows which ordering strategies were commonly applied to the six designs on the left. Each column represents a different perceptual-representational structure shown in tree diagrams and arrows showing sequence; + marks commonly used strategies. Note, for example, that in producing design 5 subjects tended to move *out* from the center line, presumably to achieve symmetrical spacing. The final design was the only one in which the center line was regularly drawn last so that it could be located accurately on the freely drawn zigzag.

of this sort, they may equally well interfere with it, as we see in the case of the mouth and cigarette, Fig. 2.1(k), where a geometrically continuous line is normally constructed in two parts for representational reasons.

Finally, in the matrix at the bottom of Fig. 2.2 are six designs that in all but one case comprise a longer vertical line in the context of two groups of shorter lines. The arrows at the top of the matrix show possible orders of construction, and along with tree diagrams suggest the perceptual and representational organization that seems to underlie the executive routine. The first, and left-to-right sweep, is dominated by proximity; the remainder segregate the components on the basis of similarity. The left-to-right strategy may continue when components differ only in size, but size plus differences in orientation cause segregation. When the smaller lines themselves differ in orientation, production is further biased. The final two rows in the matrix show how the process of geometric subdivision may be subverted. In row 5 complete segregation by orientation would demand a painstaking subdivision of space if all the right-sloping lines were drawn as a unit, and the task of guiding that zigzag to have it intersect the vertical appropriately pushes subjects to a reversal of order.

Drawing hierarchically organized forms

The question of order and similarity has been dealt with here in the context of simple abstract designs, where similarity is defined in terms of single lines or other elementary units. Within naturalistic drawings of houses, vehicles, furniture, and so on, there will be more complex units such as wheels, windows, and table legs, and it seems a logical step to extend the principles of grouping by similarity to such items. After all, drawers tend to draw the wheels of a car, train, or bicycle, or the legs of chairs and tables, successively. In so doing, they often used a standard routine comprising several strokes. So it seems reasonable to extend the principle of similarity affecting executive order to the repetition of these larger "semantic" units drawn in a standard manner.

In Chapter 1, I showed how stroke direction preferences affected the geometry of tree branches and roots. The tree the drawers reproduced comprised two hierarchies, one proceeding upward from trunk to limbs, branches, and twigs, (perhaps also to leaves), and a similar if not so deep hierarchy of roots below. Subjects took two different approaches to the ordering of their drawings: either they dealt with each level in the hierarchy completely and then proceeded to the next (drawing all limbs before branches, all branches before twigs, and so on), or they moved upward from node to node along one limb, branch, twig, and then repeated this. The same sort of choice faces subjects drawing the human figure: whether to draw arms, then hands, then fingers, or to proceed to draw arm, hand, fingers on one side, and then do the same on the other.

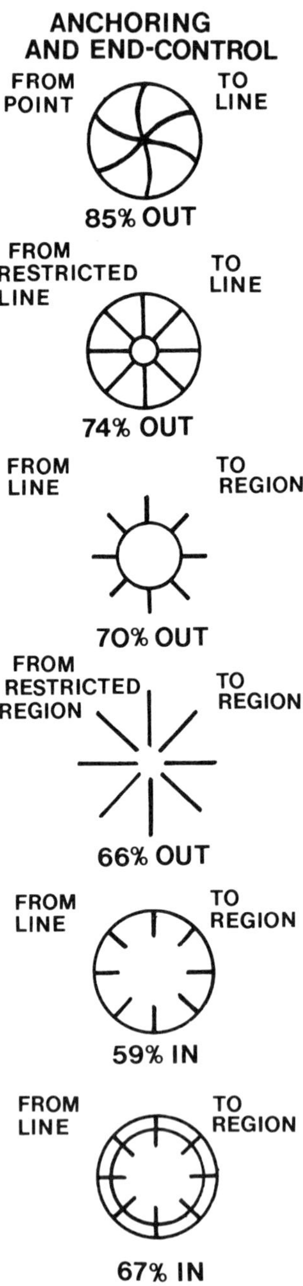

Fig. 2.2. Six designs, each incorporating radial strokes. The location of the endings of the radials is indicated on each, and below the designs are the percentages of radial strokes drawn outward or inward for that figure.

This description of the way drawers handle hierarchical material with repeated identical elements shows that in fact the idea of a *subroutine* (of an arm, for example), rather than being a case of order governed by similarity, is in one sense just the reverse. Order based on similarity prescribes movement across all identical items at one level in the hierarchy; subroutines represent a movement up the hierarchy, and order within the subroutine is based on connectivity, adjacency, and/or semantic unity. Of course once the subroutine is established, it must by definition be repeated, and quite commonly it will be repeated without any other drawing acts intervening. Overall, then, the handling of a hierarchy with multiple units at each level (a very common organization in graphic material) may be dominated by geometric similarity in the strict sense, or it may be produced through an alternation between orders based on proximity and semantics at the microlevel and similarity operations at the more global level of the subroutine.

In my experience, subroutines usually preserve their internal order within a single drawing, but they may not do so when a similar form is produced on another occasion. Two wheels on a bicycle may be drawn in the order rim, hub, spokes on one occasion, but in a different order by the same person on another day. This is not to say that the basic representational form changes. Subjects may preserve the means of representation while varying the order or production from one occasion to another. In such cases we need to distinguish the production sequence (the subroutine) from the graphic *schema*, a concept that implies a regularization of form without necessarily involving a regularization of execution. So it is possible in theory, and it occasionally happens in practice, that a drawer will move from one item to another, window to window on a house, flower to flower on a tree, person to person in a crowd, using a standard schema and grouping the execution of these visually similar units together in the overall sequence, but varying the microstructure of execution within each unit. This possibility calls for some principle of grouping by similarity, but it will be something quite different from the narrow concept of similarity in execution based on geometry from which we began.

Next we deal with the final executive constraint at the geometric level – that governing the anchoring of one stroke to another within drawings. It too can influence the order of compilation of a drawing. Once it has been described, we will be in a position to show how these several constraints taken together can be used to give a relatively comprehensive account of many graphic performances.

Anchoring and forward planning

Drawing as a skill represents a unity in our minds because of its special communicative and expressive significance in culture. But many of the principles that govern its execution do not enjoy any unique status on account of this; they are often simply general features that apply to any controlled movement where a degree of accuracy is required. *Anchoring*, or more generally *end control* of lines, provides an example of such a general aspect of skill. It reflects a balance between control effort and the obtrusiveness of miscalculation. Its significance is broader than this, however, since it provides the background for important aspects of graphic planning as well as controlling immediate action.

Anchoring in radial figures

My attention was drawn to anchoring or end control of lines in the very early stages of these inquiries in reviewing the stroke-direction preferences of adult subjects drawing a series of objects and designs incorporating radial lines: suns, wheels, beach balls, and so on (Fig. 2.2). The most obvious phenomenon one encounters in designs incorporating both circles and radials is that the circles are almost invariably drawn first and the radials anchored to them. But I should like to discuss first a more subtle systematic difference across these figures – a variation in the number of radial lines that were drawn inward toward the center or outward. This bias in the direction of radial strokes turns out to be a good point of departure because it reflects the direct operation of anchoring constraints on stroke making, whereas the other effect, the drawing of substrate (circles) before attachments (radials), involves advanced planning for anchoring, an indirect effect that will be considered later.

Generally radial lines are drawn from a starting position near the upper part of a figure, but the order is somewhat variable. In 70 percent of cases, right-handed adults progress in a regular sequence, usually in a clockwise direction, conforming to the proximity principle. Fig. 2.3 shows some of the typical orders subjects followed, many of them involving a movement from one side of the array to the other in a series of collinear movements, or zigzagging across horizontal pairs to preserve symmetry. The sequence is seldom haphazard, and this ordering represents the first level of regularity in these performances.

The second force is, as one might expect, preferred stroke direction, which of course prescribes that lines be reproduced in a direction parallel to or on either side of the 11-to-5 axis. This meant that a summary of the stroke making, independent of order, showed the radials to the upper left moving in toward the center of the figure and those on the bottom right moving out, so that it was possible in most cases (43 of 49 drawings) to draw the boundary between inward and outward movement for each type of figure very clearly. As might be expected, these boundaries were roughly perpendicular to the 11-to-5 axis. Note that as subjects followed their own particular principle of order, they simultaneously and independently conformed to stroke direction. For example, subjects laying

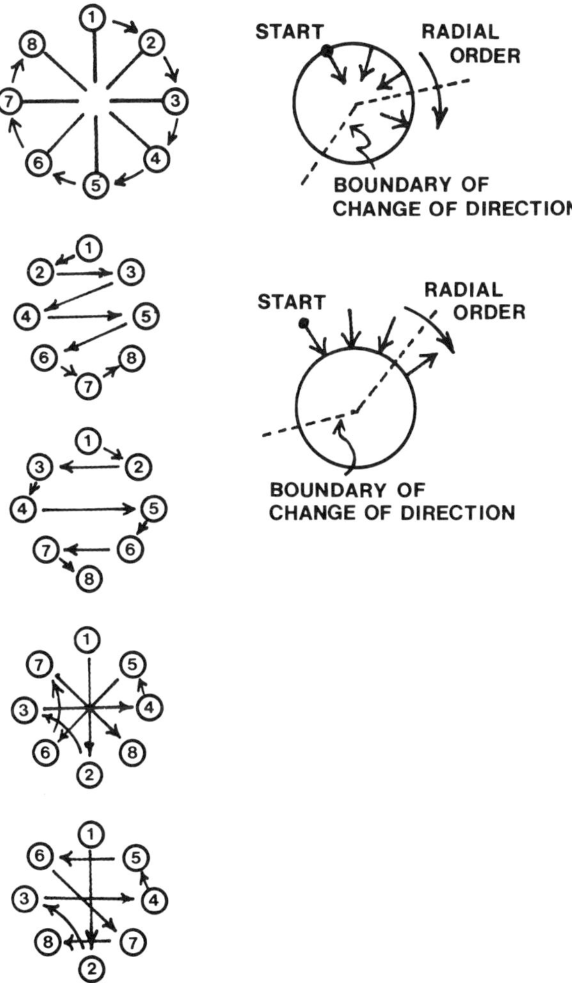

Fig. 2.3. Typical orders of construction adopted by right-handed adults producing radial lines. Principles of proximity, collinearity, symmetry, and mixtures of these govern the performances. The diagrams to the right show how drawers change from inward to outward movement at different points according to whether the radials are internal or external to a circle. Subjects do not seem aware that they behave so systematically.

down radials by rotating from a top-center position changed stroke direction from inward to outward at about 2 o'clock and then reverted again at about 8.

Third, if one counts the number of strokes in the inward versus the outward region, these vary from figure to figure across the group, which have in fact been ordered in Fig. 2.2 from those that are predominantly outward (beach ball) to wheel-like figures that have most radials drawn inward. What this means in practice is that the boundaries between inward and outward movement, although generally perpendicular to the 11-to-5 axis, divide each figure unequally. This bias, which subjects observe just as automatically and unconsciously as stroke direction preferences, reflects anchoring constraints. In other words, subjects who are rotating around clockwise from a top-center position making radials on a "sun" design will convert from inward to outward movement earlier than they might if they were drawing a circle with short inward-facing radial lines, and likewise will revert later on the opposite side of the design.

The basis of anchoring or end-control preferences lies in a balance between perceptual and motor elements in the performance. Subjects appear to apply an unconscious calculus to the various configurations before them. Their performances can be understood by postulating two interacting factors: first, an estimate of the detectability of error at the end points of the lines in the figure they are producing; and second, a general judgment about the relative ease of controlling the writing instrument at rest at the beginning of a stroke, moving, or coming to a stop.

We can identify several types of end location in the designs of Fig. 2.2. The three major categories are at points (or multiple intersections), at T intersections on lines, or in space. From the point of view of detectability of error, these are in descending order of priority. It is easier to see a small miscalculation at a defined point or at a complex intersection such as that which forms at the center of a beach ball than on a line where displacement along the line is seldom critical, or within a region of open space where small discrepancies in any direction may go unnoticed. Furthermore, if the extent of the line or the size of the region is large, less control need be exercised than if they are short or restricted. It is therefore possible to classify all the end locations of lines in the designs of Fig. 2.2 according to the taxonomy I have described: After one or two strokes have been laid down in the interior of the beach ball, subsequent lines run from the point of their intersection to an extended line (segment of the circumference). The wheel-like figure with the small central circle involves strokes from restricted (inner) to liberal (outer) line sections, the sun from liberal lines to open space, the radials from restricted region to open region and so on.

The other item in the calculation involves control to achieve accuracy. It is easier to control a stationary pencil than a moving one, especially if one wishes to exploit smooth ballistic movements, and it is easier to locate the pencil at the start than when it is terminating a stroke. So the subject will "anchor" the line by starting at the location at which an error would be more easily detectable according to the priorities set out above.

As with all other graphic constraints, anchoring principles have no monopoly on determining action, although they are very potent. In the case of all the designs of Fig. 2.2, they are in cooperation or conflict with preferred stroke direction and probably with a general inertia about changing a production routine. (A small minority of subjects will simply continue with either inward or outward strokes right around a figure.) The net results of these interactions of anchoring constraints and stroke direction are indicated by the percentages of inward or outward movements shown in Fig. 2.2. These values will be seen to correspond precisely to the relative positions of the two ends of the radials in each design.

The term *end control* is rather more awkward than *anchoring*, but it is more comprehensive. Anchoring involves the attachment of a new stroke to an existing substrate (usually at a T intersection, but also at ends of lines), but as we saw in the case of the cluster of radial lines, even where there is no contact between strokes exactly the same principles may apply, and anchoring, though the most common, must nonetheless be seen as a special case of general end control.

Anchoring is a ubiquitous constraint. If one had to name one substantive organizing principle in vernacular graphics that is most salient and universal, it is the fact that drawers, both adults and children, almost never build up their drawings except by accretion – the attachment of elements and regions to existing structures. Occasionally there will be an inclusion (like facial features or textural marks), but most strokes will be attached to those present, and the attachment process usually means that the new elements are laid down by anchoring them to those present. This tendency cannot be ascribed entirely to pure graphic forces. After all, most objects in the world are coherent (otherwise under the force of gravity they would convert themselves into piles!). Although drawers could in theory build up their drawings as separate elements that are united late in the executive process, neither the nature of the physical world nor their own control processes encourage them to do so.

Drawers show evidence that even when they do not anchor, they prefer to keep their aggregations under control. Even when our focus is on contents, for example, we tend to draw containers first. Food on a plate is drawn plate–food; utensils on a table, table-utensils; writing on a page, page–writing; and so on. When enclosures or substrates are drawn later they are often included as an afterthought (fence around a house), rather than as part of the original plan. This seems to represent a *frame : topic*, or *given : new* ordering, combining perhaps with graphic motivation. Just as a hat rack is best drawn before the hats, the plate or the table provides an important organizing structure within which to locate the food or the utensils, both conceptually and graphically.

End control in tracing

When people are tracing, the anchoring constraints may not apply so strictly, or rather they apply to what is visible in the model as well as or in place of the lines in the tracing itself. In tracing, it is quite usual to draw a line and have another intersect with its end en passant, a thing rarely done in drawing. In drawing a comb, one invariably produces the back and adds teeth. In tracing, one might well draw the teeth first, aligning them with the visible back in the model. Careful inspection of tracings sometimes shows small gaps at such intersections that result from this ordering, a phenomenon rare in drawings, where the subsidiary or "branch" lines begin on the main stroke.

Planning for anchoring

Earlier I mentioned that the drawing of the disc of the conventional sun before the rays is a universal practice, but that this move is *planning* for anchoring, and not anchoring itself. If subjects draw rectangles with two extended sides, these sides are drawn first. Most asymmetrical Latin capital letters are built with a downstroke on the left and elements are anchored to them, which seems to represent this same process of anticipation enshrined in a traditional symbol system.

If these processes were reversed and we drew the sun's rays or the wheel's spokes first and the circle second, two costs would be sustained. First, the radials would have to be positioned in space in anticipation of the insertion of the circle, and so located with respect to an imaginary line that had to be re-created for each stroke; and when the ring of radials was complete, the circle would have to be guided through their end points and at the same time drawn smoothly and symmetrically. It is practical rationality that dictates the substrate-plus-anchoring strategy, and this anticipation of the consequences of various graphic options is in some ways a more significant fact than executive processes like anchoring itself.

We will deal now with some examples of simple planning for anchoring and then move to more complex cases. The first example (Fig. 2.4) I have called "grape clusters." These can be described semantically as successively overlapping discs, topologically as regions accreted to one another, or geometrically as a network of successively intersecting arcs. When we think of them representationally, we might say that someone constructing them is likely to work front to back or from intact to occluded. Geometrically, we can say that they can be built by laying down the crossbar of every T junction before the stem. Whichever interpretation we choose, the effect is the same: If we rotate the cluster so that the intact circle moves closer to or farther from 11 o'clock, the order of con-

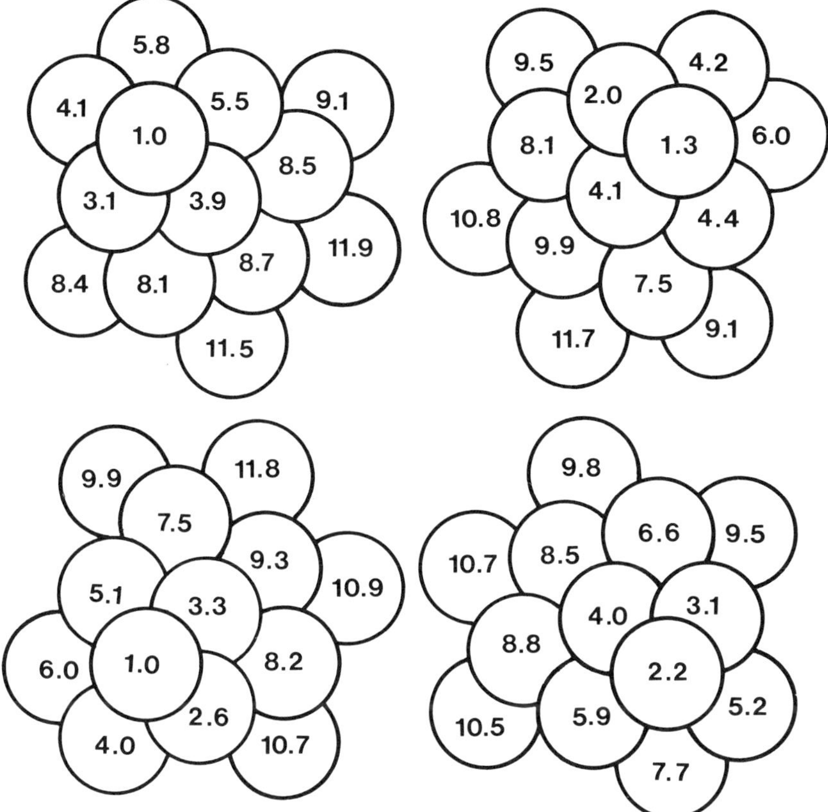

Fig. 2.4. Grape cluster. The value in each region is the mean of the order in which right-handed subjects drew the boundaries. Rotation of the cluster to bring the intact circle toward or away from 11 o'clock never displaces it from first rank. The progression can be seen as a "front-to-back" perceptual ordering, but probably owes much to an executive constraint: the systematic avoidance of the complex control processes required when the stems of T junctions are constructed before cross elements.

struction hardly alters. As the values in Fig. 2.4 show, subjects (both right- and left-handed adults) begin at the intact circle in all orientations and progress in an almost perfectly consistent way through the hierarchy of successive intersections, thus avoiding the dual load of anticipating the location of future end points and intercepting end points of completed arcs with moving lines.

Avoidance of close forward control and backward dependency is evident in the construction of figures that do not have the perceptual "depth" of the grape

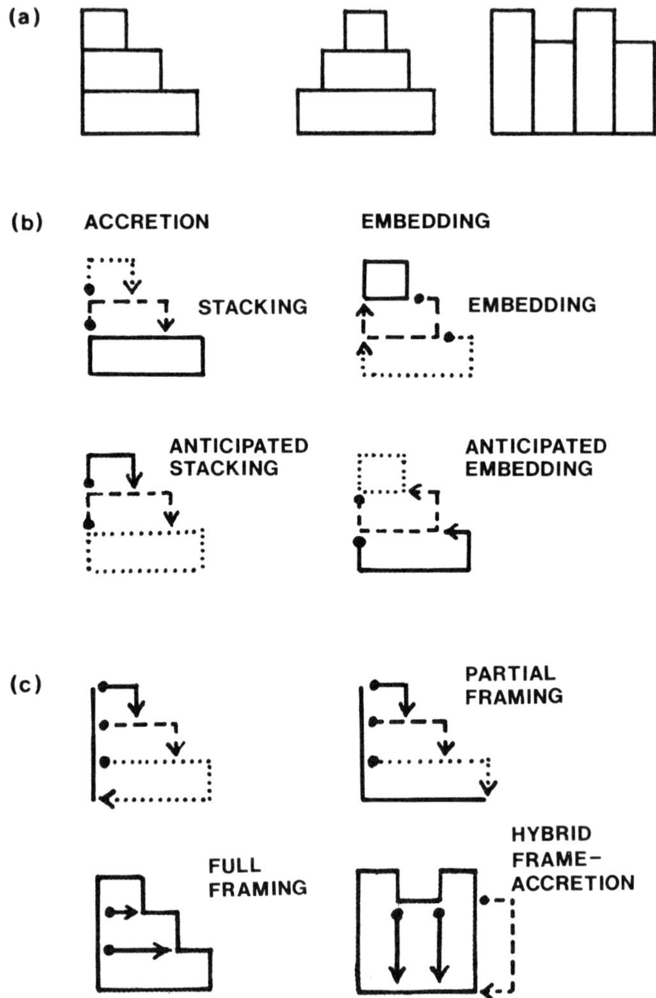

Fig. 2.5. (a): "Stairs," "pyramid," and "ramparts" comprising regions with shared boundaries. (b): Four basic procedures for their production. (c): Framing and partial framing procedures. The order of construction is indicated by the quality of line in these diagrams. Solid lines indicate first drawn lines, followed by dashed and dotted. Arrow heads indicate direction.

clusters. Fig. 2.5(a) shows what I have called "stairs," "pyramids," and "ramparts." Each comprises juxtaposed rectangular regions, and each was presented in a variety of orientations. Naturally, subjects do not build these figures by juxtaposing complete rectangles; for the most part, they construct them region by region. Under such circumstances, there must be some deletion of boundaries. An alternative is to treat the design partly or wholly as a single unit enclosed in a complex frame, with the shared boundaries represented as added internal lines. We have already identified this as a possible example of the constraint of continuous paper contact, but it is probably as much a product of perceptual organization as a construction routine designed to minimize executive commands, especially since occasionally a frame is used that is itself built with discontinuous strokes.

Fig. 2.5(b) shows a review of all the common strategies for building up these figures, using the "stairs" as an example. On the left are the accretion strategies that build the figures from one region after another. This can be done by "stacking" – that is, having a large intact unit with a number of three-sided rectangles accreted to it – or it can have each smaller intact rectangle embedded in the broken boundary of a larger. These two forms – stacking and embedding – can themselves be produced by two different procedures: by starting with the intact rectangle and stacking onto it or embedding around it, or by starting with one of the open rectangles and moving toward the intact. I call these procedures "anticipated stacking" or "anticipated embedding." They involve the deletion of sides or parts of sides in anticipation of the next unit being added or inserted. All these strategies occurred in my data, with the exception of anticipated embedding.

Making a large rectangle and stacking smaller open-sided regions on it is obviously the simplest solution, but subjects use other solutions when simple stacking contravenes starting position constraints. In other words, as one rotates these figures around so that the largest region is remote from 11 o'clock, subjects must abandon normal order or use anticipated stacking or progressive embedding. Anticipated embedding – that is, producing successive components with a gap in one side – is as awkward as it is unnecessary in this situation; it could occur only when subjects are progressing from large regions to small. Since the common boundaries in these figures are straight, simple accretion (stacking) can be used. (The anticipated embedding procedure is awkward because of the judgment it demands concerning gap size and the alignment of each succeeding rectangle within the gap.)

Anticipated embedding or gap forming and filling is not uncommon in adult representational drawing, even though it is virtually nonexistent in this context. It typically occurs when there is a large region with smaller regions penetrating through the boundary. Drawers are then faced with two unattractive alternatives: leaving gaps in anticipation of embedding, or locating the embedded units in open space and building around them.

To digress for a moment, it is perhaps worth asking what representational tasks in the real world call for embedding. The most common cases are associated

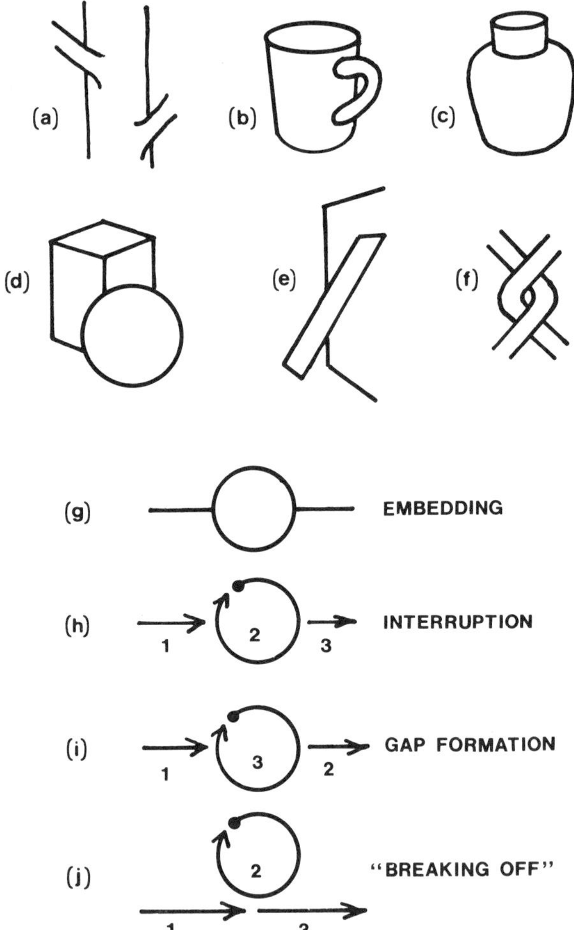

Fig. 2.6(a), (b), (c): Embedding arising from excrescences on objects. (d), (e): Embedding from front-to-back occlusion. (f): Mutual embedding. (g) to (j): Distinction between embedding as a static structural description and the procedures of interruption and gap formation (anticipated embedding) that realize structural embedding. "Breaking off" is an example of one routine inserted in another without structural embedding. Arrows indicate stroke direction. Numbers represent order of construction.

with depth. Either an excrescence on a larger object (like a tree branch on a trunk or a handle on a vessel) is aligned so that it cuts across the object's rear boundary, or one object partially occludes another so that their common boundary is not simply a segment of a straight line or smooth arc (Fig. 2.6). Most of these instances can be handled by a front-to-back strategy, so that simple embedding rather than gap creation is used. The exceptions are cases in which the occluded object has to be placed first because it is needed to direct the alignment of the embedded (front) objects, or as in Fig. 2.6(f), where mutual occlusion occurs. We will be examining mutual occlusion in a little more detail when we discuss difficult graphic tasks.

So far we have been discussing strategies used to draw the unframed staircase figure. They also apply when, as often happens, one side or the side and bottom of the figure are constructed first as a "partial frame," and the balance is built up by accretion or embedding, as in Fig. 2.5(c). Likewise, the pyramid when oriented base down will induce subjects to reverse order and stack upward, to maintain order and embed, or occasionally to maintain order and drop down with anticipated stacking, leaving each successive rectangle with an open side to be filled with the next boundary. The final strategy is, of course, to coalesce the regions, draw a full frame, and insert divisions. With regular figures like the pyramid it is not such an attractive alternative, presumably because of all the remote alignments required. The ramparts figure is chiefly of interest because, unless framing is used, embedding is unavoidable, since the small and large rectangles alternate. (The first step down can be accreted; the next step up must then be embedded.) Subjects not uncommonly coalesce regions to avoid embedding.

By tracking individual subjects from design to design through a series, one can see the development of their graphic reasoning. Subjects may adopt a hybrid strategy at the first attempt. They may start with an intact rectangle, discover that embedding is required, and then move to anticipated stacking – but on the next figure, the approach is likely to be unified and consistent.

All these devices and principles are found in ordinary object drawing. Subjects stack, embed, and frame, but always the pressure is against having to exercise the control needed for anticipated embedding.

Definition of embedding

This might be an appropriate time to draw attention to two levels at which we can talk about embedding – the structural and the procedural. The term is, of course, borrowed from linguistics, where one can speak of one clause or proposition embedded in another:

1. "The fact (that there was no money) was overlooked."

When someone pronounces this in real time, the bracketed (complement) clause is delivered during an interruption in the main clause. It is less common (but quite legitimate) to extrapose the clause:

2. "The fact was overlooked (that there was no money)."

In this sentence, the two phrases of the main clause are delivered together, and the complement follows. We still identify the extraposed clause as an embedded clause structurally, although it is not enclosed in the main clause in real time.

The equivalent situation in drawing would be to identify embedding structurally as in Fig. 2.6(g), and then specify the two strategies of production: interruption, Fig. 2.6(h), and anticipated embedding or gapping, Fig. 2.6(i). There is a third possibility in graphics, that a drawer may interrupt a sequence to carry out a piece of construction that is not structurally embedded, as in Fig. 2.6(j). In language, this would be regarded as a minor aberration in grammatical terms, as when someone might say:

3. ''The whole idea – I didn't think of it – strikes me as strange.''

Here the term ''embedding'' would be used only in a lay sense. It might be simpler to speak of it as ''breaking off.'' The upshot of this is that ''anticipated embedding,'' like most of the other things we have talked about, is a procedural term, one way to produce a structurally embedded design.

Later I will document the performances of children drawing the same motif repeatedly at intervals of a few weeks, and all these procedures will be found in their performances – interruption, gap formation, and ''breaking off.'' Interruption and gap formation are unambiguously marked by the presence of structural embedding, but breaking off, where a child stops working on a unit or chunk and attends to a nearby routine before returning, may have no structural parallel within the finished drawing and may be pure history. Often we feel intuitively that a child has interrupted a unit, putting an incomplete sequence ''on ice'' while something else is attended to. But it would be useful to have a firm definition of what a ''unit,'' ''chunk,'' or ''sequence'' is when there is no geometry to guide us. Fortunately, the history of sequential drawing helps us here because we can often see a routine established and repeated, and when later another action is inserted into it, we can more safely say that ''breaking off'' or procedural embedding has occurred.

Asymmetrical conformity

I should like now to return to a number of designs (Fig. 2.7) that extend further the idea of anticipation or planning. The first example I gave of planning was the anticipation of anchoring: Draw the substrate before the attachments. This can be extended as a principle to any situation in which one part of a drawing depends on or conforms to another, but in which one ordering is quite different from another in terms of the control load it incurs. I coined the rather clumsy term ''asymmetrical conformity'' to refer to these cases, the asymmetry characterizing the two contrasting paths through the task.

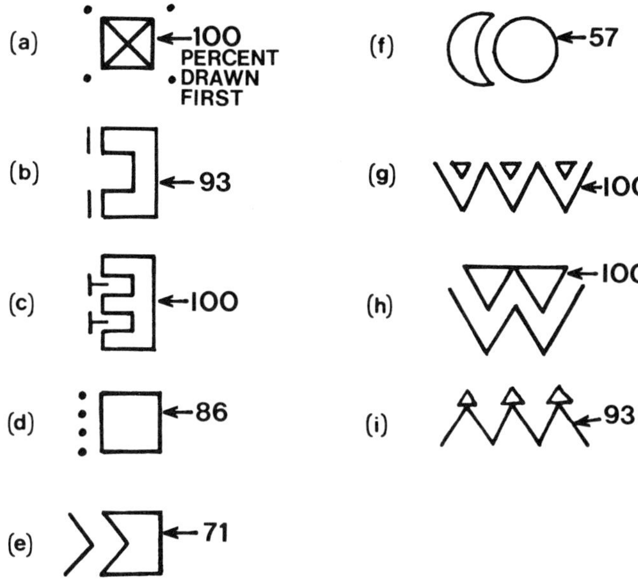

Fig. 2.7. An asymmetry in demands for tight graphic control according to order of execution makes it likely that normal starting position preference will be overridden in these figures.

In each of the designs of Fig. 2.7, the normal 11-to-5 progression has been overridden because of the dependency of some element at the top left on the remainder of the design. Inspection suggests that, in general, the first drawn of the two interrelated components is simply more complex than the second. But this takes a static view of the situation. If we consider simple anchoring at the intersection of a T, neither the crossbar nor the stem is in itself more complex or demanding. Rather, the decision to anchor or intersect involves an assessment of courses of action. Were subjects to draw the "dependent" elements first in the designs of Fig. 2.7, they would be faced with a more disadvantageous complex of requirements – segmenting space, arranging juxtapositions, adjusting proportions – and it is this load that increases when the components drawn later are complex.

The same basic balance applies between the expenditure of control effort and the detectable consequences of error as was described for anchoring, which is in a sense the prototype of asymmetrical conformity. (The two courses of action to be compared are the two stroke directions.) In these new designs, however, the elements are more diverse and depend on judgments not only of what is difficult, but which of a number of relationships is visually most important. Subjects who recognize that in Fig. 2.7(f) the inner boundary of the crescent is parallel to the left side of the circle and try to preserve this in their reproductions will very likely decide to begin with the circle and make the crescent follow its curvature. This reflects a tacit recognition that an initial miscalculation of the crescent's inner curvature (drawn without the circle as a guide) will compromise either the parallelism or, more important, the diameter or shape of the circle. This simple case is instructive because it shows how these asymmetrical paired relations readily extend themselves into chains of consequences, since in this instance the inner surface of the crescent itself depends on the outer. A drawer who proceeds left to right has to control the outer curvature in order to allow the inner to conform to the circle and at the same time have appropriate width across the crescent itself.

One formula might simply say, "Be accurate in the production of each element in a reproduction." The fact is that copying, like imitation in language, is not a matter of item-by-item matching of perception to action, but a translation process, extracting relationships and using available skills to reconstruct them. Even in reproducing a figure as simple as a crescent or an arc, one has available a motor program that has to be calibrated to the needs of the case. What I am drawing attention to is how consequences extend forward through a sequence. A slight flattening or shortening of the crescent's outer arc means that unless the crescent is to be too narrow, the inner arc will be flattened, and that flattening in turn means that either the channel between crescent and circle will not have parallel sides, or the circle will be too large or distorted in shape. Naturally there will be differences among subjects in how many and which relationships they detect and to which they assign priority. But the evidence of systematic choice contravening the principle of order indicates that analysis is going on at some depth – enough to recognize the pitfalls of excessive risk of error or excessive control and to guide the drawer to a less risky or laborious line of action.

The principle is not restricted to geometric forms. In representational drawing one does not normally draw a spade and then the digger, a basket and then a balloon, whiskers and then a chin. One does not draw parallel lines to indicate the sea and then delineate the coast. If I draw a profile head I begin with the face not simply because I am more interested in it, but because when I draw it first I can concentrate on its form and proportions with some leeway with regard to size, whereas if I have already drawn the back of the head, I have assigned a depth to the face to which I must now conform. It is better to offload the precise control of depth to execution of the boundary of the back of the head, where there are few competing form constraints that must simultaneously be honored.

Much of this analysis is necessarily inferential, but the method of placing normal ordering constraints in competition with candidate asymmetries allows one to map the three domains of factors relevant to this issue: (1) priorities about error, its importance and detectability; (2) estimates of cost in control relative to skill; and (3) the depth of analysis, the capacity to recognize and compute the equations that allow us implicitly to decide which course of action to take.

3 The reproduction of rectilinear figures

There are two ways in which to draw a simple horizontal line – from left to right and from right to left. When lines are combined together in closed figures such as triangles, rectangles, and rhombuses, the number of possible construction sequences rises steeply. For example, if we ignore whether or not the drawing instrument is raised from the paper at the corners, there are 48 ways to draw a triangle; if we include the option of raising the pencil, the number of possible courses of action rises to 192. The corresponding values for quadrilaterals are much higher.

There is, furthermore, a great variety of proportions and orientations of figures like triangles, so any attempt to provide a comprehensive formula for specifying how the figures are produced by subjects may seem unattainable. Fortunately subjects do not exploit more than a tiny fraction of the courses of action available, and the principles governing their approaches are quite general, so it is possible to utilize the same methods of analysis and emerge with the same laws not only across all types of triangles in all their orientations, but across all other rectilinear figures, including solids.

The analysis of plane figures

The original attack on the problem was to collect copying performances on a great variety of abstract forms exploiting differences not only in basic geometry and orientation, but in the type of line used (plain, interrupted, oscillating) and the various combinations of forms – concentric, overlapping, and so on. The first step in data condensation was simply to list all the action sequences for each design. Immediately a certain consistency across subjects became evident, so it was feasible to condense the data into a series of flowcharts, each column of which represented a stroke, either single or threaded.

Fig. 3.1(a) shows a set of right-angle triangles, the same form in eight different orientations. Fig. 3.1(b) shows a typical flowchart generated for the triangle marked X in Fig. 3.1(a). The numbers represent the number of subjects (of a

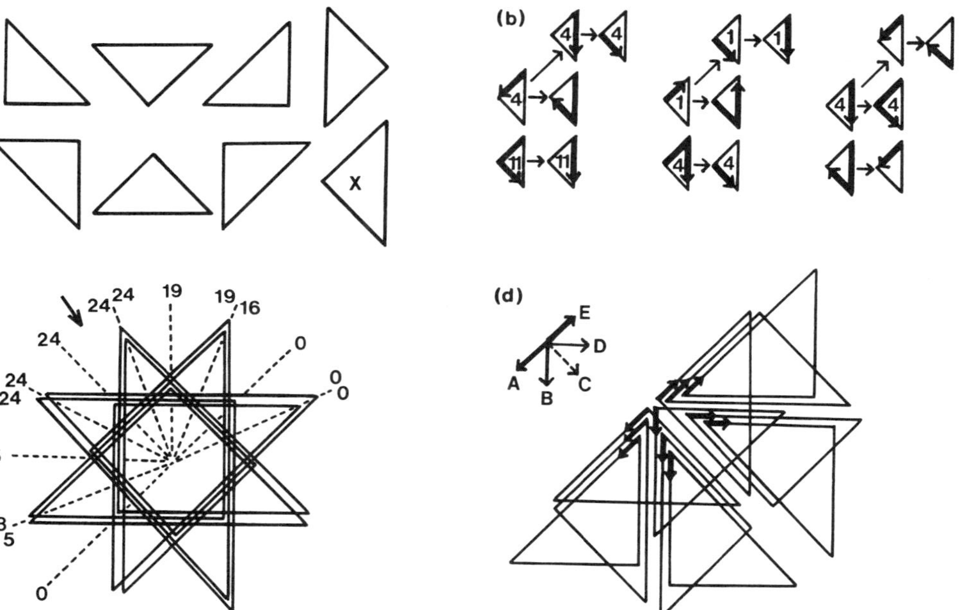

Fig. 3.1. (a): Right-angled triangle in eight orientations. The triangle marked x is the subject of the flowchart (b). All orientations are included in the data in the lower figures. (b): Three flowcharts showing sequences, stroke by stroke, for right-handed adults. The number of subjects following each path is indicated by the values within the triangles. (c): Starting position: all eight triangles are superimposed at their centers, and the number of subjects starting at each vertex is shown. (d): The same triangles are now superimposed at their starting positions rather than at their centers. Arrows indicate along which of the two sides emanating from a starting position the majority of subjects chose to move. Movements to top right and bottom left are favored over all others.

total of 24) who adopted this sequence. It can be seen that only 5 pathways of the 192 possible are utilized, and almost half the subjects adopted one strategy, that at the bottom left. At the time this analysis was conducted, the studies reported earlier on preferred stroke direction, and so on, had not been carried out, but an inspection of a number of flowcharts of this sort made it obvious that the consistencies of approach lay in two factors: (1) which vertex subjects were choosing as their starting location, and (2) which strokes they favored at successive points.

In order to specify economically the preference for starting position for figures such as the right-angled triangles, I found it useful to superimpose all eight orientations at their centers [Fig. 3.1(c)], and at each vertex of each orientation to plot a value showing the number of subjects who began their drawing at that point. What emerges is the very orderly distribution shown, with the vertices closest to the top left (11 o'clock) being most frequently chosen. For those triangles oriented with one vertex close to 11 o'clock, the selection of that vertex as a starting location was unanimous across subjects. When the *side* of a triangle lay adjacent to 11 o'clock, as in Fig. 3.1(b), subjects distributed themselves between the two vertices, with a preference to that closer to 11 o'clock. As I mentioned earlier, this preference for an 11 o'clock starting position prevails over a wide range of subject matter. It is found not only in copying, but in creating simple designs, drawing common objects from memory, drawing imaginary village plans, representing cubes and prisms, coalescing solids and geometric forms, drawing solids that had been divided into sections, drawing objects superimposed on one another, and so on.

The next step in the condensation of the subjects' performances was to examine their direction of movement from the chosen starting position. This was achieved by a device a little different from that in Fig. 3.1(c). Rather than superimposing them about their centers I placed the triangles so that all the vertices used as starting locations fell on or close to the same point; see Fig. 3.1(d). For each vertex there are two possible directions of movement, and a count was made to identify which was preferred. The preferences are shown in the form of arrows in Fig. 3.1(d). It can be seen that there is a hierarchy of preference, with the movement toward the top right and bottom left favored over all others. In triangles of this shape, the preference for some movements over others overrides the length of the side being constructed. In some other figures (such as elongated rectangles), lengthier sides tend to attract earlier strokes.

An analysis of a similar type carried out for left-handed adults can be condensed in a similar way. As might be expected, the pattern of stroke direction preferences differs from the right-handers, and does so in a predictable way, being generally a mirror image of those of the right-handers. The center of the starting position data also differed, and this requires a little exploration. The center for the starting position data for left-handers lay not at 11 o'clock, but slightly to the right of 12. It should be noted that this represents a movement away from the starting position left-handers favor when they are drawing or tracing dot clusters rather than reproducing line figures. (As we saw in Chapter 1, left-handed adults favor the same 11 o'clock start as right-handers on dot production tasks.) The shift toward the right in their starting position in producing triangles is probably due to the conflict that exists in left-handers between adopting their ''pure'' starting preference and starting at a location that allows them to exploit their major hand movements. The 12 o'clock start seems to represent a compromise between the 11 o'clock starting location and an average stroke commencement near 1 o'clock.

The only other element needed to complete the specification of strategies of production of triangles was the paper contact constraint. The continuation through from line to line was governed by the familiar pressures: the direction of continuation and the acuteness of angle. Reduced size, faster production, irregular outlines, and locating triangles one within another or within other geometric forms all alter order and direction of stroke making, and these effects can all be attributed to the constraint maintaining paper contact. Any context that reduces size or interrupts strokes promotes continuous movement around corners.

Some consistent distortions of shape of triangles occurred, and it seemed reasonable initially to attribute these to a drift toward preferred stroke direction. Although the effect when it occurs is sometimes congruent with stroke preferences it is not consistent, and it is possible that there is some as yet unexplored tendency to produce some perceptually ''ideal'' triangular prototype.

Perceptual preferences: Are there ''ideal'' triangles?

To see whether there are independent perceptual forces that might contribute to these graphic distortions, I undertook an inquiry among a separate group of adult subjects. This began by generating a suitable set of 40 triangles of different shapes and orientations derived from two basic forms: the equilateral and a right-angled isosceles triangle. The equilateral was rotated through four positions, with one side down, up, to left, and to right. It was then expanded a little or shortened to produce isosceles triangles, one ''taller'' and three ''shorter,'' yielding 20 forms, as in Figure 3.2(a). The right-angled triangle was also rotated into four positions, with the right angle at each corner of an imaginary square, and in each orientation the ratio of lengths of sides adjacent to the right angle was varied from 1:1 to 2:1 in each direction, producing five figures in each orientation, as in Fig. 3.2(b). These 40 triangles were then arranged in columns in a quasi-random order, 18 to a page, and beneath each was a horizontal 5-point scale labeled at the left ''Poorly shaped,'' and at the right ''Well shaped.'' Fifteen right-handed adults rated all 40 triangles.

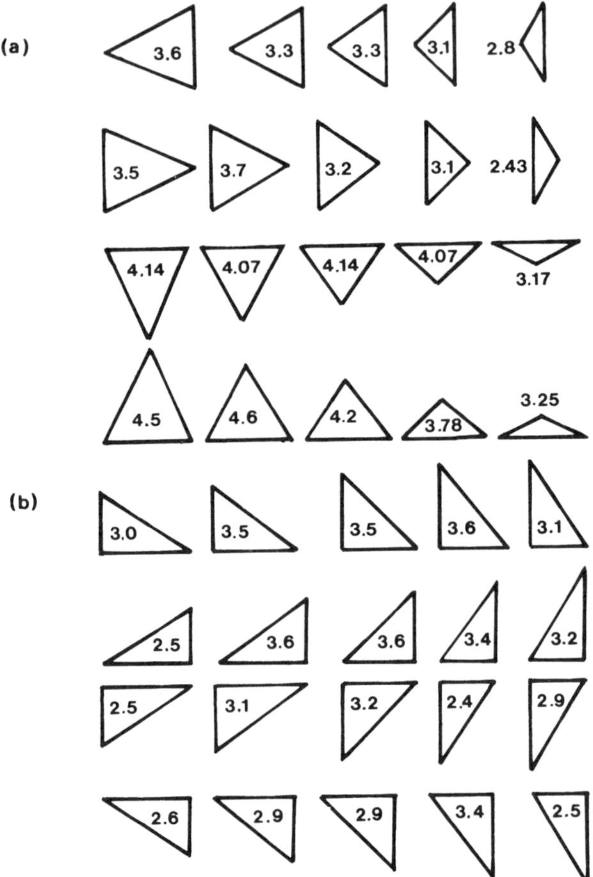

Fig. 3.2. (a): Four families of triangles based on an equilateral in four orientations. The height is increased (left) or decreased (right). (b): Four families of right-angled triangles in four orientations. The center triangle is isosceles, and the ratios of perpendicular sides increase progressively to left and right. These forms were presented to subjects in a quasi-random order for ratings of good or poor shape. The values are the mean ratings of their judgments. A rating of 1 represents "poorly shaped," a rating of 5, "well-shaped." The data are from 15 right-handed adults. These values were used to order the triangles in Fig. 3.3.

Overall, the results were very systematic (Fig. 3.3). Subjects gave strong first preference to the equilateral triangle sitting on its base and high ratings to its close relatives. Next were the same triangles upside down, so that the first eight most preferred triangles were isosceles triangles with bases down or up. Next were equilaterals or near equilaterals facing left or right. As a class, all these

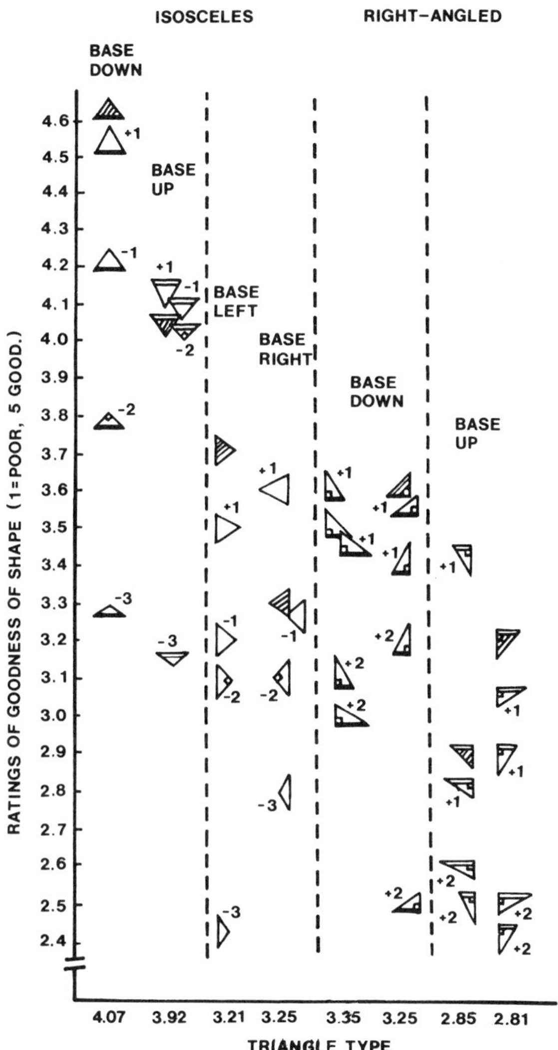

Fig. 3.3. Average rankings from 15 right-handed adults giving their preference for the shape of triangles. The vertical scale shows mean ranking (5 is "well-shaped," 1 is "poorly shaped"). The triangles are arranged in columns according to type and orientation. Dark lines mark "base-down" figures, double lines show "base-up." The shaded triangles are those in the middle of the series shown in Fig. 3.2. Values beside triangles in the left half of the figure indicate changes in height, −3 being the shortest. Values on the right show ratios of perpendicular sides. Values at the bottom of each column show the mean rankings for all the triangles in the column, higher values indicating stronger preference.

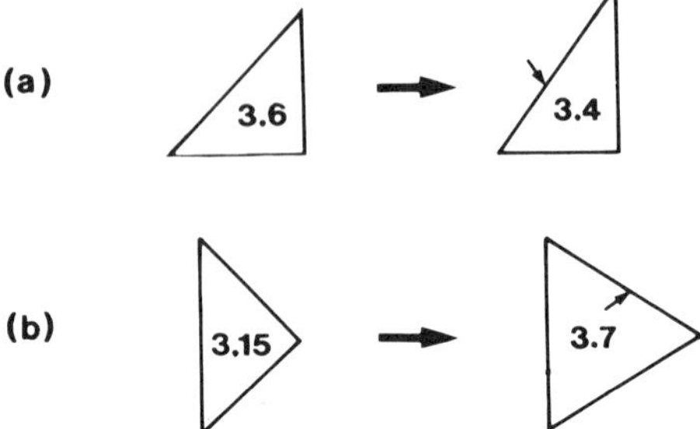

Fig. 3.4. The triangles on the left were models, those on the right were the distorted copies produced by subjects. The values within the triangles are mean ratings of well-formedness of corresponding forms in the study of visual preferences. The distortion in triangle (a) is consistent with stroke direction preferences, that in (b) corresponds to a relatively strong visual preference.

equilaterals and related isosceles triangles were favored most when they were generously proportioned. Ratings fell regularly from "well shaped" to "poorly shaped" as their height decreased and the two base angles became more acute. Of the other class, the right-angled triangles, those with a horizontal side as a base and a vertex up were strongly favored over those with a horizontal at the top. Finally, those in the center of the range – isosceles right-angled triangles – were favored most, and those with unequal sides and one strongly acute angle were considered poorly shaped. To summarize, subjects favored symmetrical, "base-down," generously proportioned figures and gave low ratings to those with base up, base left or right, unequal sides, and one or more acute angles.

When these perceptual preferences are applied to the distortions observed in drawing triangles, the situation is at least partially resolved. The distortion in the top triangle of Fig. 3.4 is consistent with stroke direction; that in the second triangle conforms to one of the strong visual preferences. The intrusion of perceptual forces in the form of shape preferences in these cases is not dramatic, but it illustrates in principle the need to examine forces that interact with formal executive biases. The analysis of rectangle and parallelogram production reveals a similar situation.

Distortions in quadrilateral figures

The same method of data reduction that has been described for triangles – videotaping, transcription of sequence and direction, flowchart production and superimposition of related forms – was applied to rectangles and parallelograms, with very similar results. There were, however, one or two additional phenomena not accounted for by the major constraints.

In the copying studies, there were 36 rectangles of different proportions, sizes, and types. Again, the number of theoretically possible routines for producing a rectangle is very large (3,072 if we allow variation in leaving the paper surface at corners), whereas the actual number of routines followed is quite small: Three-quarters of all performances followed one of three courses of action, and 12 routines were enough virtually to encompass them all. Next, all the principles governing threading apply – size, position in a series of figures, broken outlines, and so on. If two sides of a rectangle are extended beyond the corners, the standard procedure is completely overridden. The extended sides are always drawn first as a pair and according to the normal principles of order, and the nonextended sides added between them. This accords with the anchoring principles described earlier. Whether the extended lines are longer or shorter, widely spaced or close, straight or undulating makes no difference; anchoring to the extended sides is dominant.

We have already noted that the long sides of elongated rectangles attract early attention, and when they are very long, they are often drawn as a pair. This may simply be in line with another general principle we have explored, the grouping of similar units within figures, although it is very likely that subjects are struck by the parallelism of the long sides and move first to portray it, perhaps using a special stroke position in the process. When rectangles are arranged concentrically, subjects usually work from outer to inner. When they overlap one another, the normal principle of order does not necessarily control their construction; rather, subjects adapt their strategies to ensure that the first line drawn in each successive square is that which cuts across its already constructed neighbor. This is a manifestation of the general strategy that minimizes problematic prejudgments: It is easier to arrange the intersection between the two overlapping figures at the outset than to begin at a remote boundary and try to anticipate correct positioning.

When we turn to parallelograms, we encounter other variants on the basic theme based on perceptual effects that operate at different points in the construction process. The parallelograms in question had two horizontal sides and sloped to the right and to the left. Preferred direction would certainly favor initial movement down a left-sloping side, but performances favored the upper horizontal. There are probably two reasons for this – one perceptual, the other associated with accuracy of orientation. Although the parallelograms were virtually rhomboid – that is, they had four almost equal sides – subjects exaggerated the horizontal sides, making them a third longer on the average than the oblique sides. In other words, subjects seemed to treat the length of side as though it were the length of the whole figure. (A rhombus in this orientation does look more rectangular than square.) Having thus distorted the figure perceptually, they then treated it as they would any elongated figure, drawing the "long" sides first. (In line with this view, a proportion of subjects drew the two horizontals as a pair.) Furthermore, the horizontality of the figure is very salient, and subjects may well have judged it wise to establish this before completing the sloping sides, which do not have to be oriented so carefully.

As well as being extended horizontally, parallelograms are also drawn more "upright" than the models, with an error of about 10 degrees. This cannot be attributed to preference for certain stroke directions; it may well be a compensation for the misjudgment in length of the initial horizontal. In other words, the horizontal length seems correct when it is drawn alone, but subjects may well realize as they move to extend the figure to right or left that the whole figure will now be too elongated unless the sloping sides are made more vertical.

These matters, although in one sense quite local or idiosyncratic, serve to illustrate two general points. First, that this level of analysis in terms of formal constraints and perceptual biases seems to be able to account for most regularities in subjects' performances; and second, that although their performances are to some degree distorted by motor or perceptual biases, the subjects appear to apply a consistent practical logic to their actions even when they are working on incorrect premises.

Manipulating starting position and stroke direction

Before we proceed to the next stage in complexity in figure construction, the reproduction of solid figures, I should like to address a question about the nature of the relation between simple graphic predispositions and their bases, using some of the tasks we have already described. The general theme so far is that there is a logic to simple drawing performance, that stroke making and sequencing have a basis in mechanical and economic forces. Showing that they are understandable in these terms does not remove all the ambiguities about their psychological status, however. How immediately are starting and movement preferences tied to mechanics? Do mechanical forces operate directly, or have they been absorbed into a system of convention before being translated into action?

I can perhaps make this issue at the same time clearer and considerably more general by reference to another pairing of forces and conventions—namely, social forces and social conventions. The first example concerns greetings and farewells, which seem to represent conventional behavior par excellence. Goffman (1955) treats them as social interactions that give guarantees that personal relations from one encounter to another will or have remained constant. Length of farewells and greetings is usually a function of the duration of the separation and the closeness of the relationship. It seems rational that as time of separation or expected separation increases, farewells and greetings should get longer rather than shorter, and it is this "naturalness" that predisposes us to regard the conduct as rational rather than arbitrary and purely conventional. But even granted that it is reasonable, this does not necessarily answer the question of whether or not the individual subject is a party to the reason and uses it in generating farewells and greetings. Brown and Levinson (1978) raise the same issue in discussing the rational basis of polite requests: Is it possible to establish the pattern of needs to which politeness forms pander? Even if it is possible, it is a separate question whether or not each individual adopting and using those forms has re-created the logic of that relation, and in the case of ritual it is not unlikely that subjects simply reproduce forms without even a tacit knowledge of their function.

When subjects use their language system generatively in new contexts, as they do in the domain of greetings or the pragmatics of politeness, this is circumstantial evidence that they are not just acting conventionally, but have encompassed the basic rational relationship between the system of language and the external domain of need to which it relates. But it *is* possible to use arbitrary conventions generatively, and it is useful to be able to show that when the structure of the outside world changes, individuals alter their attack in a way that shows they are in a deep sense responsive to the links between their actions and the purposes they serve. We have shown that some of the elementary principles governing simple graphic execution are related in a rational way to the structure of the drawer's body and the drawing medium, and that these principles operate widely and can be applied to a great variety of subject matter. Could they nonetheless be conventions – apt rules applied generatively?

The early demonstration of significant changes that show up when a subject draws at a wall rather than on a desk supports the view that in each drawer there is a direct link between physical configuration and performance. The very early appearance of many of the constraints in young children points in the same direction. The following simple manipulation of the physical substrate of drawing is a further test of this view, and it allows us to identify whether all or any of the constraints of starting position, order, and direction have a conventional status. If one had to guess, the 11 o'clock starting position, since it alters developmentally and has been supported by the technology of our writing system, would seem to be most likely to lack a practical link to the physical context of drawing.

The method we developed to manipulate the physical context involved changing the configuration of the arm with respect to the drawing surface. When a subject sits at a table whose surface is almost at the level of her elbows when her upper arms are in the normal vertical resting position, the elbows themselves may be held relatively close to the body while drawing. If the hand then makes contact with the table surface directly in front of the body, the forearm points roughly in the direction of 11 o'clock, as Fig. 3.5(a) shows. If the orientation

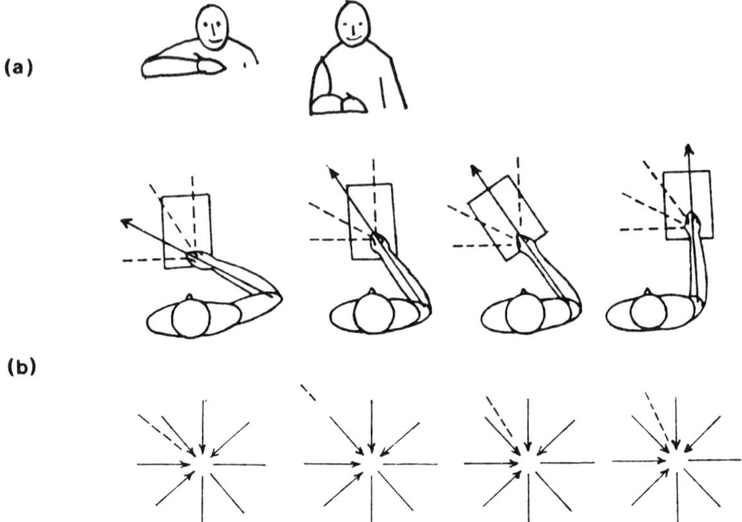

Fig. 3.5. (a): Manipulations to change the relation between arm and drawing area. Rotating the paper 20 degrees or moving it to the right moves the axis of the arm clockwise. Raising the arm to chest or shoulder level rotates it counterclockwise. (b): Effects of rotation on drawing of a set of radiating lines. The dashed line shows the axis of inward or outward movement in producing the lines.

of the forearm and hand does in fact relate directly to stroke direction, order, and starting, these should be susceptible to change by manipulating the resting angle of the forearm with respect to the paper. This was achieved first by rotating the paper through 20 degrees to the left. A second method was to displace the drawing hand to the right. The latter is most easily achieved simply by keeping the paper upright and moving it 30 cm to a position ahead of the drawer's right shoulder so that the hand points directly toward the top of the page. If the drawing surface is raised to shoulder height, on the other hand, the elbow is forced out from the body and the forearm points much farther to the left, toward 10 o'clock. Thus we have four maneuvers, two pointing the arm toward 12, one (the normal position) toward 11, and the last toward 10.

The first task involved the drawing of a set of eight lines radiating from a point, one of the radial designs shown in the section on anchoring (Chapter 2). Figure 3.5(b) shows how, as the forearm direction rotated from left to right, the axis of inward and outward strokes also swung clockwise, suggesting some direct link between body geometry and stroke direction. The same outcome is produced when subjects draw elongated rectangles in various orientations. Fig. 3.6(a) and (b) show the normal pattern of starting positions and stroke directions for the

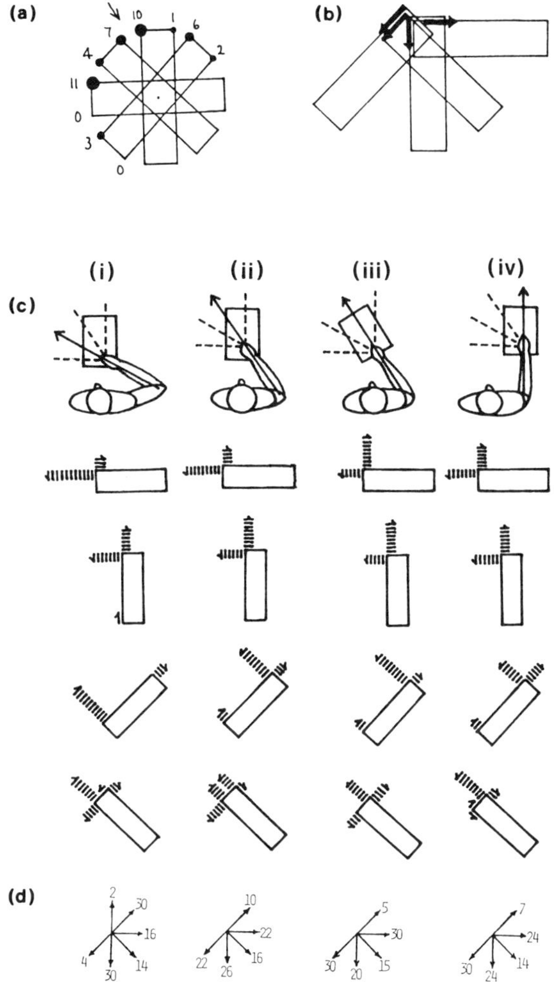

Fig. 3.6. (a): Normal starting position choices for 11 adult right-handed subjects copying elongated rectangles in four orientations. (The rectangles have been superimposed at their centers.) (b): Normal preferred direction of stroke making. (The rectangles have been superimposed at their starting locations.) (c): Effects of altering the position of the forearm and hand with respect to the vertical paper axis. The first column indicates the starting position and direction of first stroke movement when the arm is raised to shoulder height, pointing the arm toward 10 o'clock. Column (ii) shows the normal position, arm pointing to 11 o'clock. The last two columns show the effect of rotating the paper 20 degrees to the left or moving it to the right of the body so that the forearm points toward 12 o'clock. Both starting position and stroke direction alter. (d): Charts summarize stroke direction data for each position.

conventional drawing position, using the device of superimposing the four figures. Starting positions are close to 11 o'clock; line direction follows the usual hierarchy of preferences, although it is affected by the long sides of the figure. Fig. 3.6(c) shows how the two measures were affected by the movement of the axis of the arm produced by the changes in paper position and orientation and by the raising of the writing surface. The small lines at the corners of the rectangles indicate where the drawing started, and they extend along one side or another to indicate the direction of the first stroke. The effects on starting position in the first two rows of Fig. 3.6(c) are not dramatic because changes in arm orientation cannot be expected to affect a figure with one vertex close to the 11 o'clock position, although there are some stroke direction changes. When either the short or the long sides of the figure are approximately at right angles to the 11-to-5 axis, there are substantial changes both in direction of movement *and* in starting position, which migrates clockwise as the direction of the forearm moves from 10 toward 12 o'clock.

As we saw in the case of triangles drawn by left-handers, starting positions and stroke directions are not independent in drawing figures of this sort. In order to make certain strokes, starting position must change. So to clarify whether the physical change is indeed translated into changes in both major constraints, a separate group of 20 subjects was given the dot-cluster task, tracing six clusters in each of the four positions. The outcome seems to indicate that starting position, when measured in this way without contamination by stroke direction effects, does *not* vary with physical orientation of the arm. The departures from the standard drawing position caused some slight increase in variability, but there was no systematic swing of the median starting location as arm orientation changed.

This outcome confirms the guess made earlier that there is a different relation between stroke preference and starting location on the one hand, and the physical situation of the drawer on the other. Unless starting location is driven by stroke direction preference, it seems to be conventional. This does not mean it is "irrational." For right-handers, 11 o'clock is a more sensible starting location than any other, since it allows all the natural stroke directions to be accomplished easily. But it appears to have been formalized by experience.

The construction of cubes and prisms

The principles so far described permit us now to extend the inquiry from the representation of plane figures (squares, rectangles) to solid figures. In order to do this comprehensively, it was necessary to generate a collection of representations of solids of varying dimensions and orientations, beginning with a cube and extending it in one dimension or another to form an elongated prism (or ''bar'') and contracting it to form a shortened prism or ''slab.'' From a single cube it is possible to produce three slabs or bars by changing the length of one or other of its dimensions. Further, the cube itself can be rotated so that we are looking down on it, looking up from underneath, or viewing it from one side or the other; in each position there are corresponding shortened or extended prisms. So by taking a single cube, rotating it, and extending or contracting it, we generate a ''family'' of solids comprising 4 cubes, 12 ''bars,'' and 12 ''slabs.'' Fig. 3.7(a) shows one of these families.

The original cube with one face upward (bottom center) can not only be rotated on the paper surface, but it can be tilted forward or back in space to reveal more or less of the upper surface. In these new orientations it can again be rotated, expanded, and contracted to form further families of prisms. The family in Fig. 3.7(a) has the upper face at 60 degrees. Another family was generated with the upper face narrowed to 45 degrees and a third and fourth facing directly at the subject. Strictly speaking, these latter forms with one square face are anomalous, since if one face is facing directly at the viewer, the other faces are not visible. But since this is a shape commonly drawn by both trained and untrained drafts-people, two families were generated, one with the square face in a ''diamond'' position, the other with the square face sitting horizontally, as in Fig. 3.7(b) right.

Using 4 cube positions, each in 4 orientations and each with slabs and bars, we finally have 112 figures, representing the raw material for two related studies. In neither case were the forms presented in the organized fashion in which they were generated. They were printed in two columns down a page, with 8 solids to a column. Their order was systematically rearranged to give an impression of a random succession of all the various figure types. Fig. 3.7(c) shows a typical sheet arranged for copying by a right-handed subject.

The study of salience

Subjects were given a complete set of seven sheets, the order of sheets being varied from subject to subject. The subject was first asked to make judgments about the appearance of the figures on the first three or four sheets of the set, and later was asked to copy the balance in the empty columns provided on each page. The instructions for the first task were designed to establish how the subjects organized the figures in their minds, and in particular which face seemed most salient. These were the instructions:

Pick out what you think is the most important face for each block. You might call it the ''primary'' or ''dominant'' face of the block. It isn't necessarily the largest. It may or may not be. Call it the ''first face,'' put 1 on it, 2 on the next,

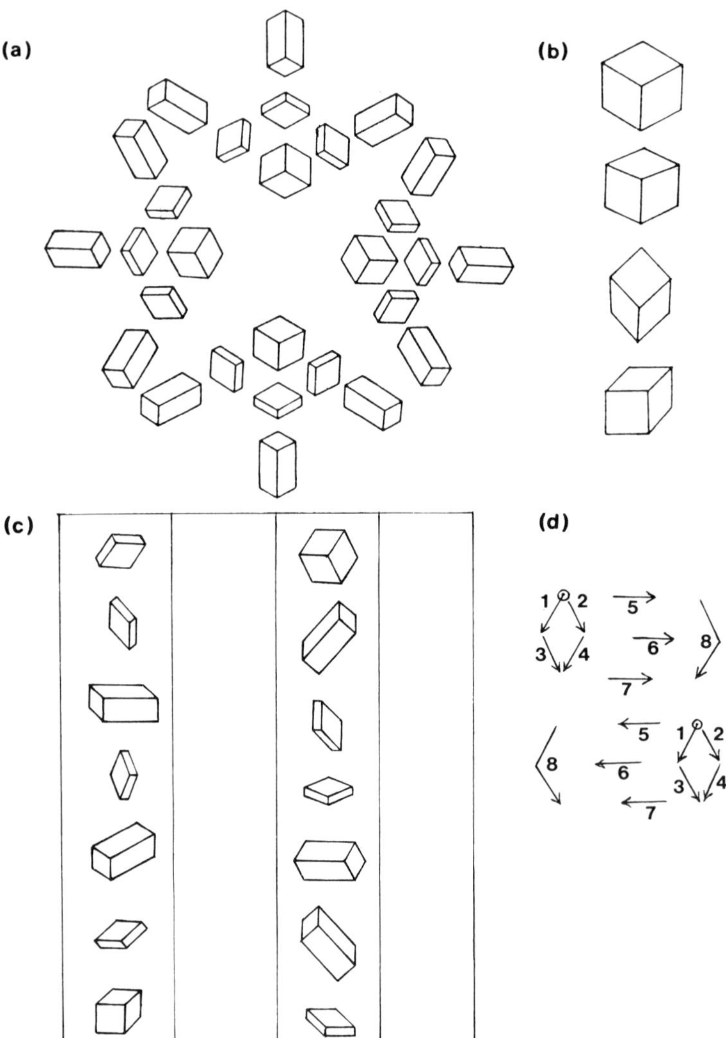

Fig. 3.7. Materials for studies of copying and perceptual judgments involving cubes, "slabs" and "bars." (a): One of four families of solids. This family is generated from a cube with all faces at 60 degrees from the viewer, the so-called isometric projection. The cube is rotated into four positions and expanded and contracted to form slabs and bars in each. Three other families of the same size were generated based on other positions of the cube in space (b). Typical sheet with solids in quasi-random order (c). Two typical copying sequences (d).

3 on the last. Just look at each block in turn for a few seconds and make a judgment.

When this task was completed for the first half of the sheets and subjects began copying the balance, all their movements were videotaped to document how they tackled the reproduction task.

One object of this dual exercise was to establish if and how judgments of salience of faces of solids might affect construction strategies. Preliminary observations with other subjects copying and drawing from models and from memory had suggested that the majority of subjects approach the representation of cubes and related solid figures in a relatively standard fashion, constructing one face as a rectilinear closed figure according to the principles of starting position, stroke direction, continuity, and so on already described for squares and parallelograms. They then move out from three corners of this "primary" face with three parallel lines, sometimes against the direction of normally preferred movement, and complete the figure with one or two strokes that conform to preferred movement. Fig. 3.7(d) shows two examples. The upper sequence, with the primary face to the left, allows lines flowing out from it to move in preferred direction; the lower sequence, with the primary face to the right, shows an overall right-to-left ordering and nonpreferred stroke direction.

If, as these examples suggest, the overall strategy is affected by an initial decision to build a figure around one face, then a knowledge of the principles of allocating priority to faces is needed. The instructions above were designed to elicit priorities based on perceptual judgments relatively independent of any intention to draw, and it always preceded the copying phase or any mention of copying.

The outcome of the rating task is displayed in Fig. 3.8, which shows two families (45 and 90 degrees). Twelve or 13 judgments were available for each face. These were averaged and mapped into 7 equal categories. In the figures, each category is visualized by a step in the density of shading. Light shading represents frequent high priorities, dark represents low ratings of "salience." The variable that dominates salience is area, with independent contributions from acuteness of internal angles and orientation. The area variable in this case refers to the actual area of the region on the paper, not the size of the face on the corresponding real solid. As the face of a "slab" is turned progressively toward us and its area as a region increases, its "primacy" rating goes up. Next, we regularly find that some small faces on "bars" are rated higher than one of the larger sides. (This is easy to see in the bars at 10, 2, 4, and 7 o'clock in the 45-degree family.) This typically occurs when the large side in question takes the form of a rather oblique parallelogram. The main effect of orientation (rotation in the picture plane) is to increase the salience of upper faces, and to a lesser

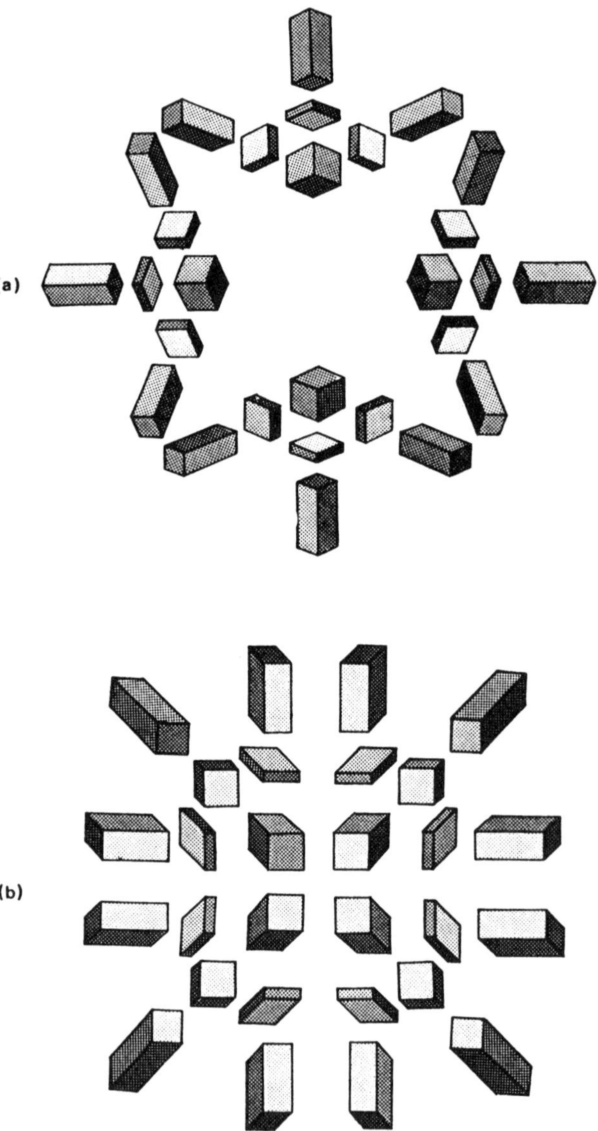

Fig. 3.8. Outcome of judgments of salience of faces of two families of prisms, 45 degrees (a) and 90 degrees (b). The seven gray levels indicate subjects' judgments. They run from most often rated "primary" (light) to least often (dark). Ratings emerge as a function of area of region on the page, acuteness of angles, and orientation to top and top-left.

extent those that face to the left. (This can readily be seen by comparing the top 45-degree cube with its partner at 6 o'clock.)

The copying of solids

Subjects performing this task are extremely consistent, so that the results for related families of solids are comparable down to extremely fine distinctions. This applies also to the drawing data (Fig. 3.9). Copying of solids is dominated not by area, but by orientation. The faces oriented toward 11 o'clock are strongly favored, so that the gray scale used to portray order of construction imparts to each family of prisms the appearance of solids bathed with light coming from the top left. The graphic performance is also affected to a less marked extent by the factors that promote salience. More open (larger-area) regions are preferred over small-area regions. Larger sides with acute angles are left until smaller but squarer faces are drawn. This can be seen in the "bar" at 1 o'clock on both arrays; the small face that is not facing towards 11 o'clock is nonetheless drawn before the lower larger face. This is not because drawers prefer to construct end faces early, because in many other cases where both large faces are toward us and do not contain acute angles, the small end face is drawn last.

The actual drawing procedure that lies behind these regularities has already been described: One face is drawn first, following normal stroke preferences, and lines project out from it to make a complete second face or to construct three parallel edges followed by the final boundary. The first procedure is more common with cubes and the second with "bars," presumably because of the salience of the long parallel edges. These basic strategies for constructing solids are found in representation drawing of many kinds. When subjects were asked to reproduce a drawing of a stack of cubes and other prisms, they adopted the same basic approach for each (and in those cases where prisms occluded one another, they built them in a front-to-back order).

The only important exception to this strategy occurs when one face of a solid is highly distinctive by virtue of its shape. So, for example, a cylinder with a round face to the right will commonly be built up from there. This is not necessarily a perceptual effect. As we saw in the section on anchoring, construction in the opposite order would require that the round face be inserted into a pair of lines representing the long sides of the cylinder. Since this would involve a more highly controlled performance, many subjects prefer to work backwards toward the normally favored starting location. What characterizes rectilinear solids such as cubes as opposed to objects like cylinders is the fact that all the alternative construction strategies are equivalent from a control point of view, and starting position therefore dominates the approach. This characteristic face-by-face analysis and top-left-down synthesis often has significant

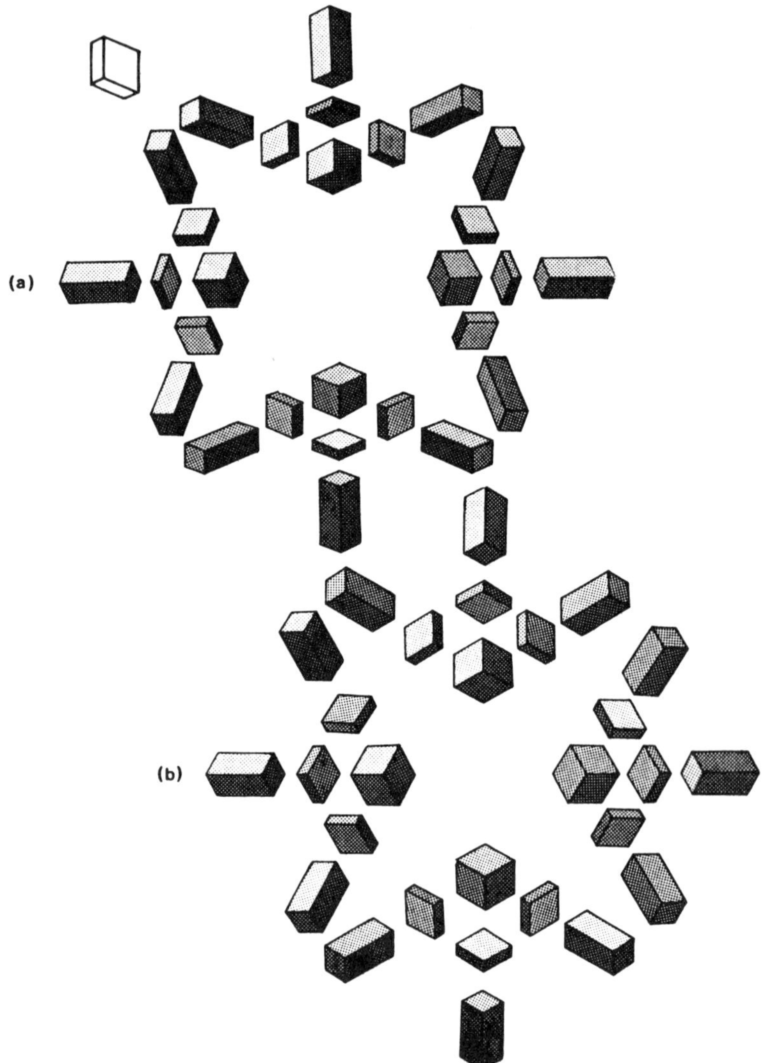

Fig. 3.9. Outcome of copying performance for two families of prisms, 45 degrees (a) and 60 degrees (b). The insert shows the form in which prisms were copied. The seven gray levels indicate the order in which the three faces of the various prisms were drawn on the average by the 12 right-handed adult subjects. Light indicates early construction, dark indicates late. The outcome is strongly dominated by which face is closest to 11 o'clock, combined with the area and angle variables associated with salience.

consequences for the location of anomalies within subjects' drawings of simple solids.

We have almost reached the end of the exploration and analysis of the formal or geometric aspects of vernacular drawing. Before extending the discussion to deal with various problems of meaning and representation in simple drawing, one further phenomenon needs to be dealt with: the construction of curved elements.

4 The production of curvilinear forms

Chapter 1 revealed that particular actions can often be shown by analysis to be special cases of more general principles of action. For example, a right-to-left horizontal movement or a top-to-bottom vertical movement can be located within a spectrum of preferred stroke directions, and may not in such a context be of special significance. And certain features of action that seem at first to be unified can be shown to be functionally differentiable – for example, fanning movements may be distinguished from finger flexion movements, and starting position can be shown to have different properties from stroke preferences. Third, the analysis may simply be descriptive, or it can be pursued to the practical logic that makes sense of the generalities and distinctions. I cannot promise that the analysis of the production of curvilinear forms will clarify all the issues, but it does have some of the features I have reviewed: There are some useful general principles and one or two unexpected disjunctions in the data, and I have tried to make sense of the concrete underpinnings of the structure that emerges.

The drawing of arcs

Geometrically we define arcs as portions of circles, and so it is somewhat surprising to discover that arc production is not only divergent from circle production, but is in fact quite its antithesis. I have analyzed the production of arcs of two lengths: 90 degrees (quarter circles) and 180 degrees (half circles). I will begin with results from right-handed adults. The subjects copied arcs in the context of other simple geometric forms. There were eight different 90-degree arcs and four of 180 degrees, usually drawn in isolation but also as pairs or as arcs within circles. (The construction was basically similar in either case.) Fig. 4.1(a) and (b) show in condensed form the orientation of the various arcs, and the diagrams at right show the percentages of subjects drawing the arcs in one direction or another.

The outcome is easily summarized. Arcs of both sizes are constructed in a direction similar to straight lines through their end points; in other words, right-

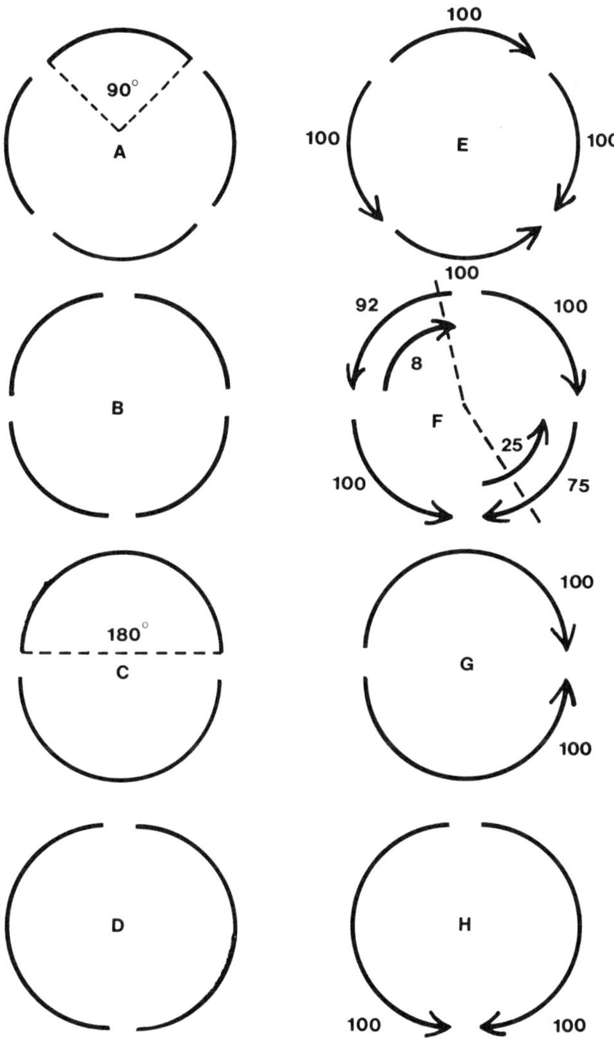

Fig. 4.1. (a) and (b): Quarter-circle (90-degree) arcs. (c) and (d): Half-circle (180-degree) arcs copied by 12 right-handed adults. All arcs had a radius of 1.25 cm and were presented in vertical columns mixed with other figures. (e) to (h): Percentages of subjects producing the arcs in the direction indicated. The dashed line in (f) shows the axis that typifies the right-handers' performance.

handed subjects began at that end of the arc closest to 11 o'clock, and the 11-to-5 axis segregates the clockwise from the counterclockwise strokes. The only variability across the subjects was in the construction of the 90-degree arc running from 12 o'clock to 3 and its opposite, that from 9 o'clock to 6. These arcs cut across the 11-to-5 axis. A minority of drawers constructed them upward to the right, just as some draw straight lines of this orientation upward. Since for right-handed adult subjects starting position and stroke preferences are consonant, we cannot use these results to specify which controls arc production.

Left-handed arc production

I have collected data from two groups of left-handed adults. The first group of 17 subjects, tested in Sydney, was not screened for hand inversion; that is, the tendency of some left-handers to hook their hands over their drawings. The second group of 43 left-handed English adults studied in Cambridge included no subjects who inverted their hands in this fashion. (It was my original intention to compare inverted and noninverted left-handed subjects, but the sample of 45 people, drawn from borrowers at the Cambridge Public Library, included only two who wrote and drew with an inverted left hand. One was a Canadian, the other Japanese! It isn't clear whether this indicates tyranny or tolerance in the English school system with respect to left-handed writing practices.) The data in Fig. 4.2 are from this larger group of noninverted left-handed adults drawing eight different half circles and eight quarter circles.

The outcome is rather more complex than for the right-handers. I have segregated a set of quarter and half circles in Fig. 4.2(g) to (k) where virtually all subjects conform to the same pattern, drawing arcs from their upper ends. The group was divided in its treatment of the other arcs, those that were concave upward and downward, shown in Fig. 4.2(l) and (m). The majority drew the upper arcs from the right. Right-handers always draw theirs from the left end, so this pattern implicates preferred stroke direction rather than preferred starting position – which, it will be recalled, is to the left for both right- and left-handers. The *lower* arcs, however, are divided almost equally between a right-to-left movement (consistent with stroke direction) and left-to-right (consistent with a start on the left). Possibly the fact that the dish-shaped arc has one end closer to 11 o'clock than its concave downward partner encourages left-to-right movement.

These 43 left-handed adults completed a number of other graphic tasks, including tracing dot clusters. It was therefore feasible to relate variations in preferred starting position to arc construction. Since, as expected, the great majority of left-handers began dot clusters on the left, the correlations were always rather weak; but there is a significant positive association between the

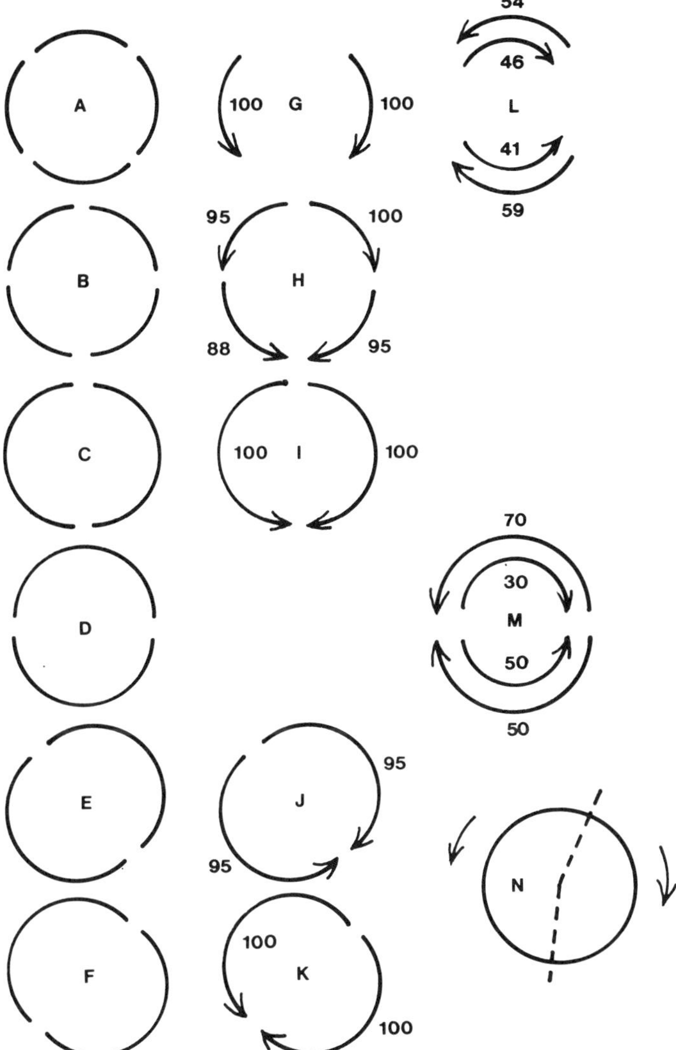

Fig. 4.2. Arcs copied by 43 left-handed adults. (a) and (b): The eight 90-degree arcs. (c) to (f): The eight half circles. (g) to (m): Percentages of subjects constructing arcs in the directions indicated. The arcs in the concave upward and concave downward orientations, (l) and (m), produced a mixed outcome. Stroke direction (right-to-left) preferences dominated the upper arcs; the lower were split more equally between starting on left or drawing from the right. (n) shows the axis that characterizes left-hand performance.

direction in which arcs were drawn and the bias in starting position. On the other hand, a small minority of people in the group drew lines from left to right, and almost all these also drew arcs in that direction. These two conjunctions, combined with the splitting of the subjects in mode of production of these two arcs, argue for the joint involvement of stroke preference and starting position in arc production. If we attempt to draw a line across the circular plots that corresponds to the 11-to-5 axis for left-handers, it will be roughly vertical, as in Fig. 4.2(n), but with a bias to the right expressing the slightly stronger influence of stroke direction in these performances.

Circle production

The almost universal direction of rotation in drawing circles among adult right-handers in all our Australian and English samples was counterclockwise. In one of the earlier copying studies of the series, there were 17 different figures incorporating circles. These included plain and dashed circles, circles with irregular outlines, circles with radial extensions inside and out, concentric circles, and circles embedded in or otherwise combined with rectangular forms. The ratio of counterclockwise to clockwise rotation across all these figures was 546:21.

Left-handed subjects tend to draw circles in the opposite direction, although the bias is not so strong. The Cambridge noninverted left-handers favored clockwise to counterclockwise movement 52:32; an earlier unclassified group of left-handed adults in Australia favored this movement 580:109. About two-thirds clockwise rotation seems a fairly representative proportion. The tendency for right-handers to draw circles in a counterclockwise direction is not developmentally stable. Thomassen and Teulings (1979) review some developmental studies, including that of Blau (1977), who showed a progressive switch from clockwise to counterclockwise continuing to the age of 12 to 16 years, with a majority producing counterclockwise circles at 7 to 8 years. Haworth (1970) found the changeover a little earlier, with the majority of normal right-handers rotating counterclockwise by the age of 6, and 94 percent doing so at 8 years. Ilg and Ames (1964) found a similar transition, with girls a little in advance of boys. Goodnow et al. (1973) attributed the change to writing tuition in the Latin alphabet, since they did not find the same shift in children learning Hebrew script. Bender's (1958) work with alexic children is consistent with this, since they continued to move clockwise with the right hand and counterclockwise with the left, and when Thomassen and Teulings asked adult subjects to make circular scribbles or to draw circles very fast, they tended to follow the same pattern. Thomassen and Teulings make the suggestion that these movements are the natural "nonfigurative" motor movements on which figurative movements are imposed.

What could be the nature of this imposition? One possibility is that it is a new generally applicable graphic habit or routine for circle production. I wish to dispute this, for there is evidence to show that under certain circumstances, both in the experimental situation and in normal drawing practice, both right- and left-handed adults will drop the "habit" and consistently adopt the opposite rotation. They do not do this because they have deserted the "figurative mode." The adult right-handers' clockwise rotations are just as controlled as their counterclockwise movements and just as consistent, and the left-handers' performances are likewise controlled and systematically variable in direction.

Starting position and rotation

First we should look at data showing "natural" or context-free circle production. By this I do not mean scribble, but rather circles produced free of any graphic context that might bias production and without any special instructions about where to commence. Fig. 4.3 shows the percentage of circles of 2.5 cm diameter started within the various 22.5-degree segments of the circle's circumference and their direction of rotation for Australian and English right- and left-handed adult subjects.

Although there is some spread of starting positions, all but 3 of the almost 200 circles commenced in the upper half of their circumference, and for both right- and left-handers the most popular starting position was within the two narrow segments around 12 o'clock. If there is a bias, it is for the left-handers to spread to the left of top center and the right-handers to spread to the right, an effect we will see in a more pronounced way in the production of ellipses (Fig. 4.8). Next, *all* the right-handers rotated counterclockwise, while the left-handers split in the fashion I have already documented, a little over 60 percent clockwise. The left-handers were also considerably more variable in their starting location. (This variation in starting position and rotation was largely between subjects. Each of the 43 left-handers constructed two plain circles at different points in the testing program. Of them, 77 percent rotated in the same direction on both circles, and 80 percent adopted starting positions on the two circles within 60 degrees of one another.)

Some minor effects

There are one or two less salient effects I might mention before discussing the main issue, the link between starting position and rotation. First, starting position does vary slightly according to the size of the circle. As circles get smaller, the right-handers' starting position migrates progressively to the left, although the effect is not great and 12 o'clock remains in all cases the modal starting point.

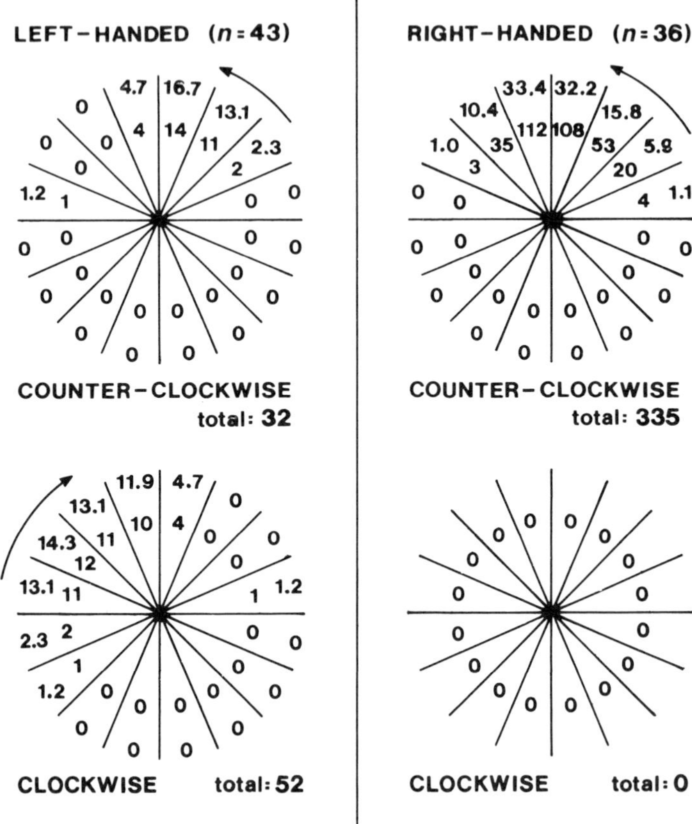

Fig. 4.3. Starting position and direction of rotation for right- and left-handed adults drawing circles. The inner values are numbers of free-standing circles whose start lay within the segment, the outer values are the same data expressed as percentages of all drawings of circles by the group, irrespective of direction. The left-handers comprised 43 English adults, none of whom inverted their hands while copying, the right-handers (n = 36) were Australian adults. All circles were 2.5 to 3 cm in diameter. Left-handers copied on the page to the left of the model, right-handers to the right. All worked with moderate speed.

Whether a circle is smooth or oscillates back and forth as it rotates also biases starting position, so irregular circles, like their smaller and smoother cousins, tend to have starting positions closer to 11 o'clock than to 12. The rare cases of clockwise rotation by right-handers were associated with irregular circle production, and this is probably linked to the shift in starting location. Increasing speed of circle production by a modest amount had negligible effects on performance.

This is contrary to the experience of Thomassen and Teulings (1979), who reported that rapid execution produced a reversal in rotation. It occurred to me that I might get a similar outcome if I asked people to produce rapid circular scribbles, so I devised a study with 24 right-handed adult subjects in which they believed themselves to be testing ballpoint pens, pencils and so on. They were asked to make rapid rotary scribbles down a column with each of the pens, just as one does when trying to get a dry ballpoint pen to make a mark. Of the 69 spirals, 63 rotated counterclockwise. Note, however, that when they repeated the exercise moving upward, two-thirds of the spirals were in the opposite direction. Although this task was conceived of as "nonfigurative," it in fact shows all the characteristics of normal circle production, as we will see.

Concentric circles were all drawn counterclockwise by right-handers with one exception: Half the subjects, when confronted with a smooth circle surrounded by an irregular or dashed outer circle, drew the latter from near the top in a reverse direction, just as they start the sequence of radial lines of a stylized sun near the top and move clockwise around the disc even though they use a counterclockwise stroke for the disc itself. (The reasons are obscure. I can only add that young children who draw the sun's disc clockwise from a low starting point commonly start the radial strokes near the bottom and progress counterclockwise!)

My speculation about the popularity of 12 o'clock as a starting location for circles (rather than the usual 11 o'clock) is that it fixes the upper limit of the circle in space at the outset rather than having it be defined by the moving line at a later stage in construction. This would be consistent with the change in starting location associated with decreases in size, because as the circle is reduced in diameter to 1.0 cm or less, its location in space will hardly vary much with changes in where drawing begins. It is also consistent with the pronounced difference in starting position between left- and right-handers drawing ellipses.

Starting and rotating

The left-handers whose data are displayed in Fig. 4.3 were tested relatively late in the research program. By that time we had completed a number of studies with right-handed adults and children that explored the relation between starting position and rotation. Nonetheless, we can use the left-handers' data as a convenient instance because its greater variability makes the critical association very clear. Fig. 4.3 shows that the starting positions for clockwise rotation by the left-handers lie largely in the quadrant from 9 o'clock to 12, whereas the starting positions for counterclockwise movement are largely to the right of top center. This situation is quite general among left-handers. With another large group of Australian left-handed university students (not classified with respect to hand inversion), I found that of the 700 circles they produced, the 580 that rotated clockwise began on the average to the left of 11 o'clock and the 109 that rotated counterclockwise had their median to the right of 1 o'clock.

We do not immediately see a relationship of this sort for the right-handers simply because they show so little variation in where they start. For this reason, a number of maneuvers were adopted to induce the right-handers to depart from their normal starting position. The first tactic was to give subjects circles to copy whose circumference was interrupted at one point or another by a small gap. Even without any instruction beyond being told to copy these figures, the subjects universally adopted one or other side of the gap as a starting point for their circular stroke. (Nobody began at the top and made the circle in two strokes.) Whether they rotated in one direction or the other was found to depend on where the gap was located, as shown in Fig. 4.4(a). Here it can be seen that for right-handed adults, the 11-to-5 axis is critical. When the gap and hence the start lay *above* that axis, rotation was counterclockwise; when the gap was *below* the axis, it was clockwise. This is not a "trend," but a very strong effect shown by almost all subjects at almost all gap positions. *What this outcome suggests is that the "normal" counterclockwise rotation is not a primary effect, but a special case of a more general relationship between rotation and starting position, with starting position driving rotation.*

As I have said, the result is extremely robust and consistent. Nor is it an artifact of the procedure of drawing from a gap. The gap was used simply to induce a change in starting position without an explicit instruction. The effect was replicated first by substituting a dot for the gap and instructing the subjects to draw from that, as in Fig. 4.4(b), and then by asking subjects simply to cover a page with freely drawn circles, starting each at a different point on the circumference, as in Fig. 4.4(c). The subjects, 22 right-handers, found it difficult to obey the latter instruction; their starting locations were still biased toward the upper region. Nonetheless, over a sample of 600 circles, 70 percent of the counterclockwise rotations began above the 11-to-5 axis, and 78 percent of clockwise rotations started below it. *The outcome is as anomalous as it is striking. The initial movement in all these cases is precisely the opposite of preferred movement along straight lines or around arcs.* Subjects are regularly moving upward toward the top left, not away from it.

We can expand the generality of the effect not only from the standard circle drawn from its characteristic starting location to all circles drawn from all possible starting positions, but also to closed figures other than circles. The effect is found in ellipses and in a variety of closed rectilinear figures, including squares, rectangles, and triangles, as Fig. 4.5(a) to (d) show. When right-handed subjects were asked to copy a square with a gap in its left side or in its base, they moved clockwise to the top-left corner, again making strokes opposite to their normal

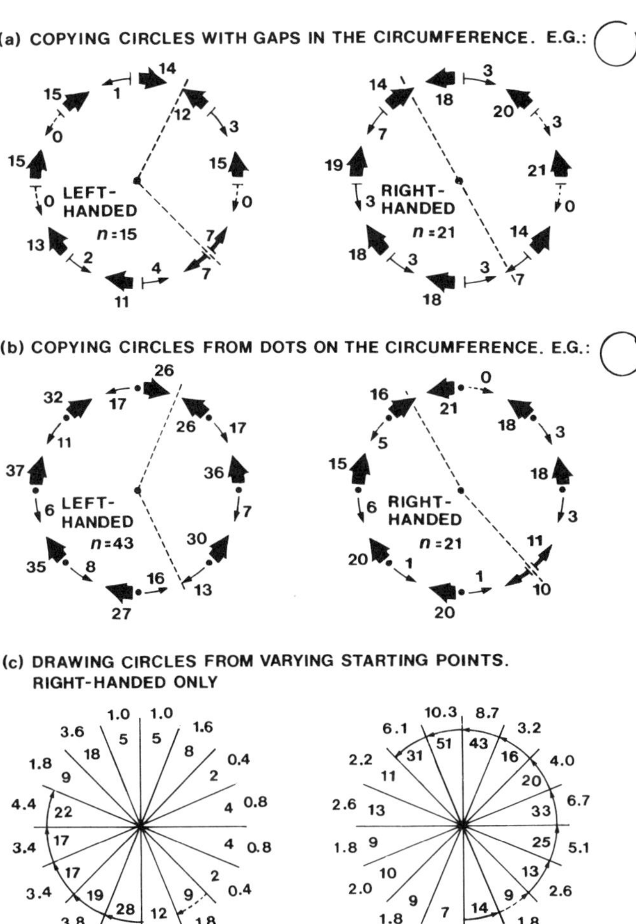

Fig. 4.4. (a): Left- and right-handed subjects copying circles from small gaps at one point or another on their circumference. An example of such a circle is shown at the top right of the figure. Dark arrows indicate in which direction the majority of rotations were made. The left-handers were the Cambridge sample, the right-handers Australian adults. (b): Similar data showing direction of rotation from a dot on the circumference of a circle. Note that in (a) and (b) there is a straight boundary dividing the two directions of rotation for right-handers and a discontinuous boundary for the left-handers. (c): Australian right-handed adults (n = 21) instructed to draw circles from a variety of starting points. Clockwise and counterclockwise rotations are plotted separately. Inner values show actual numbers of circles, outer values are percentages of all circles drawn. Arrows indicate the direction of the majority of movements.

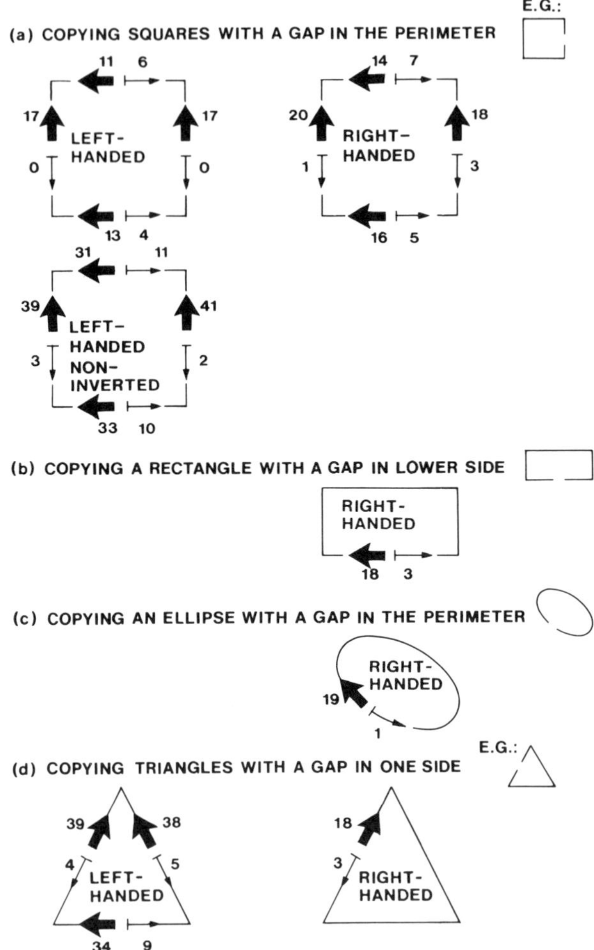

Fig. 4.5. (a): Two samples of left-handed adults and one of right-handers copying squares each of which had a gap in one or other of the four sides. The upper sample of left-handers (n = 17) was not screened for hand inversion. None of the lower groups (n = 43) inverted their hands. There were 21 subjects in the right-handed group. The heavier arrows indicate the predominant direction of movement from each gap. The fact that the left-handers most often move to the left on the horizontal strokes is not consistent with their circle production, but seems to reflect their right-to-left stroke preference. (b) and (c): Right-handed adults (n = 21) copying a rectangle and an ellipse with a broken boundary. (d): Left- and right-handed adults copying triangles with a broken boundary. (Left-handers, n = 43; right-handers, n = 21). The figures on the right illustrate the appearance of the copied forms, which were 2.5 cm across.

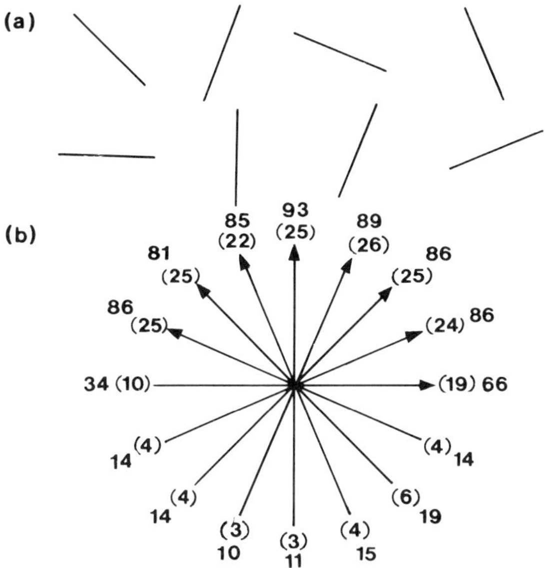

Fig. 4.6.(a): The array of eight lines presented to subjects, each to be copied starting from its center. The lines were 2.5 cm in length, and half the subjects had them presented in reverse order. (b) Performance of 31 right-handed adults. The values indicate how often a line in that orientation was drawn first in the direction indicated. Inner values are totals, outer values are percentages moving in the direction shown rather than the reverse. Arrows indicate the most common initial direction of movement.

stroke preferences. Breaks in the upper or the right side also produced leftward or upward initial movement.

The next extension was to see if this applied even to single straight lines, and indeed it did (Fig. 4.6). When another group of 31 right-handed adults were given simple straight lines 3 cm long in eight different orientations and asked to copy the lines, starting each in the center, 80 percent of them drew *upward* with the initial stoke. (Needless to say, the subjects were given no clue about the object of this bizarre exercise, let alone what the investigator expected. The instructions allowed them to move downward from the center and then upward or downward to complete the second half of the line. Those few who did move downward in their initial stroke all completed the figure with an upward stroke, probably because of the end control involved in the alternative maneuver.)

Endogenous deviations from standard practice

Before tackling the question of why we find these systematic relations, which as we will see is a thorny issue, let me mention the relevance of the phenomenon to normal drawing practice. I have described the most common practices of right- and left-handed adults raised on Latin script, that of starting circles near top center and moving right or left depending on handedness. This is the approach used for most free-standing circles, the letters "O" and "Q" and the numeral zero. The structure of a drawing and the microhistory of its production, however, can induce "endogenous" or uncontrived departures from this pattern.

One such case is the drawing of a loop from an existing element in a drawing. For example, if subjects draw a conventional flower with center disc and circular petals, they invariably begin with the circular disc, adding the petals in various orders (often clockwise from top right, as with the radial lines of the sun figure). Some subjects begin with one direction of rotation on the first petal and continue this subroutine for the entire series, but most frequently the petals to the upper right will be drawn clockwise and those to the lower left counterclockwise as in Fig. 4.7(a). This effect can be traced to the anchoring constraint that invites the drawer to begin each round petal at the edge of the disc to which it is attached. Since each successive petal is making contact with the disc at a different point on its own circumference, the anchoring principle prescribes a systematic variation of starting positions on each petal. Combined with the constraint I have been describing linking start with rotation, it leads to the outcome shown in Fig. 4.7(a). Again it is independent of where the sequence of petal drawing itself commences, so subjects will change from one rotation to the other and back again at whatever points the geometry and the constructional principle prescribe.

Early letter construction

When he was an Honours student at the University of New South Wales, Neil Sadler (1971) examined the production strategies of first-grade Australian children who had recently learned to print the lowercase Latin alphabet. He was pursuing the problem of letter reversals, and the relevant letters from our point of view are the highly confusable "p," "g," "b," and "d." All four letters are commonly formed by both children and adults from an initial downstroke with a circle or arc added. In most cases, the young children drew the curve clockwise for "p" and counterclockwise for "g," but "b" and "d" were both split between clockwise and counterclockwise rotation. Two forces are operating in constructing all four letters: (1) anchoring the circle or loop to the end point of the initial stroke, and (2) moving around the circle or loop in accordance with the start-rotation principle. For "p" and "g," the two forces are congruent and the results uniform. For "b" and "d," they are opposed and the results divided, as shown in Fig. 4.7(b). One should expect this sort of variation wherever contextual forces cause changes from normal starting location, so "typical"

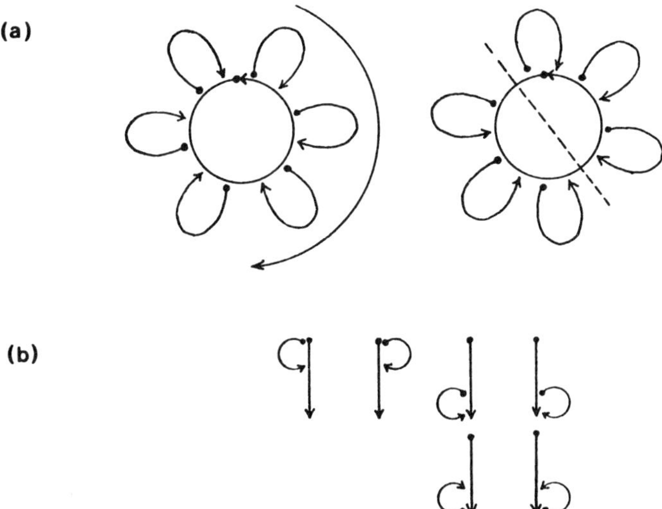

Fig. 4.7.(a): Production routines for drawing a flower with round petals. In both cases, the subjects (right-handed adults) began with the circular disc drawn counterclockwise from top center. The first petal was placed at the top left, anchored to the disc, and as a consequence began its rotation at the bottom left. Rotation was therefore clockwise. Subjects like those on the left continued with this routine in a continuous sweep around the disc. Subjects on the right adopted the common practice of reversing rotation as the anchoring brought the starting position close to the 11- to 5-o'clock axis. (b): The circular element in letters "q" and "p" are produced with counterclockwise and clockwise rotation for two reasons: because they are anchored to the top of the vertical and because of the start-rotate association. The letters "d" and "b" are produced in different ways by different children because anchoring and the start-rotate principle are in conflict.

rotation can be depended on to show itself only when drawers can select a starting position freely.

Ellipses

The production of ellipses is similar to circle production, but with one exception: The "ends" of ellipses, the regions of shortest radius of curvature, tend to attract starting positions away from top center, and the more eccentric ("elongated") the ellipses are, the stronger is the tendency for the starting point to migrate toward the ends (Fig. 4.8). There is also a tendency for a line that begins near one end of a narrow ellipse to move along the flat side rather than around the end, and this produces some minor departures from the start-rotation principle,

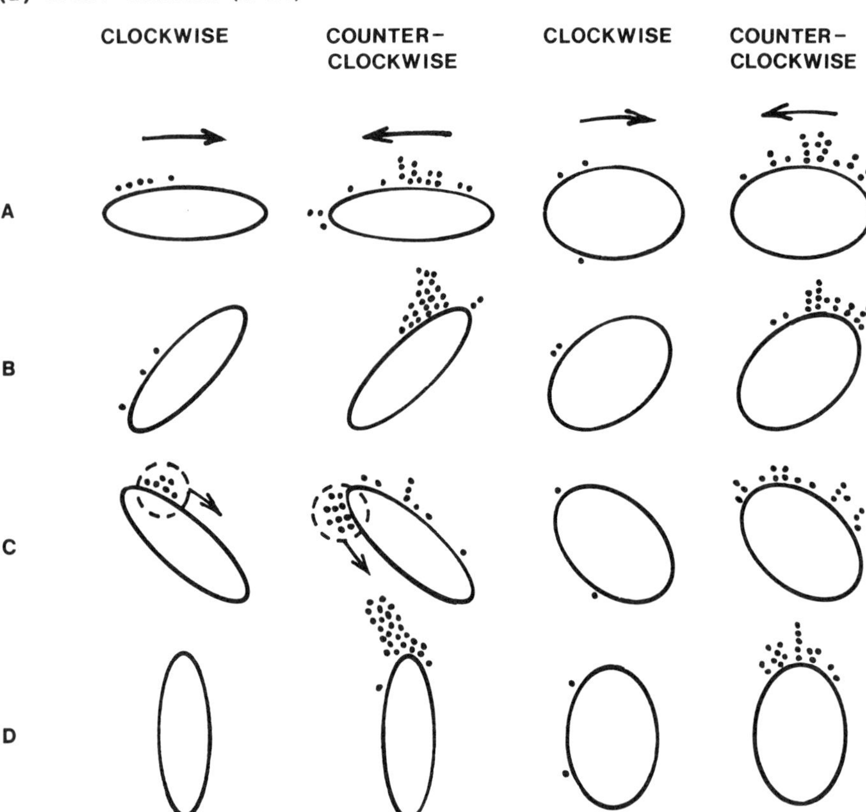

Fig. 4.8. Starting location and direction of rotation in the production of ellipses by 21 right-handed (a) and 14 left-handed adults (b). There were ellipses of two degrees of eccentricity, narrow (left) and broad (right). Each was presented in four orientations, (a) to (d) and (e) to (h). Starting positions for clockwise and counterclockwise rotation are plotted separately side by side. Each point is one subject's starting location.

as Fig. 4.8 shows. Also, as I mentioned earlier, ellipses produce a bigger difference in starting position between right- and left-handers than do circles, perhaps because placement on the page is not so easily defined by the top-center position.

Developmental changes

Before tackling the mechanisms of production, I should like to elaborate on the developmental material, for irrespective of what gives rise to rotation or causes

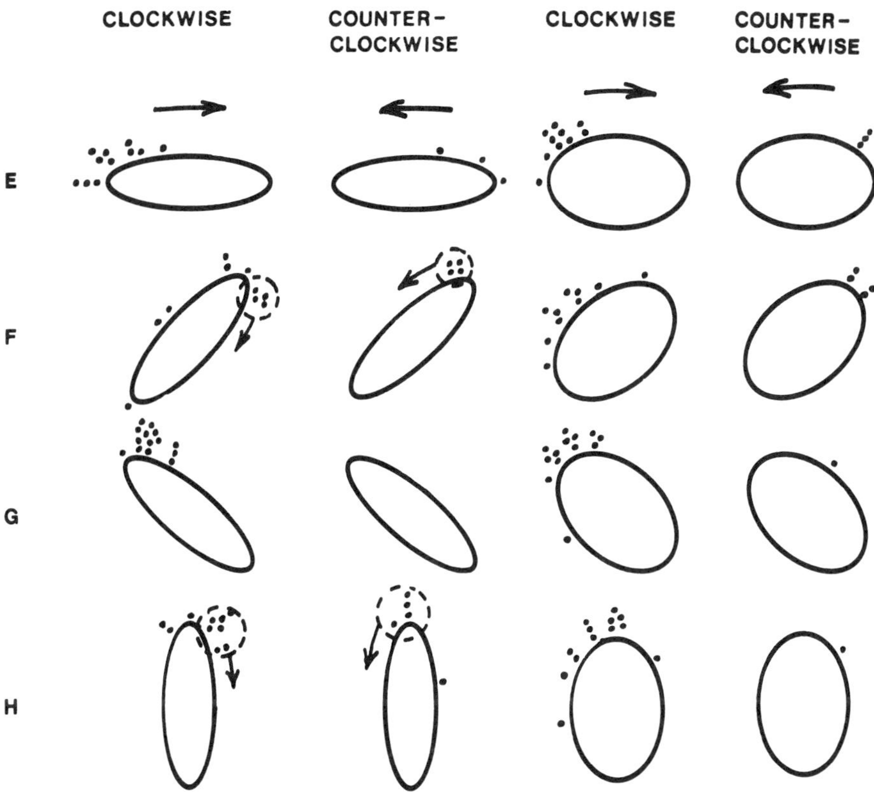

In general, clockwise rotation starts on the left of each figure, counterclockwise on the right. The points enclosed in broken circles in (c), (f), (h) suggest that the start-rotate principle is modulated by a tendency to move along the long side of the more eccentric ellipses.

it to alter, the relationship between starting position and rotation is not just an adult phenomenon; it seems to prevail in childhood and is apparent very early, as we saw in the case of early letter production.

As I stated earlier, there is a change in Australian right-handed children's circle production from clockwise to counterclockwise rotation between 3 and 6 years of age. I had available a wide sample of videotapes from nearly 50 children in this age range, and drew a substantial sample of unanchored circles – features like faces, wheels, and circular decorations. It included only circles that were free-standing, or if they belonged in a context, were drawn first so that starting location was not dependent on other features of the drawing. The drawings from each child were produced over a period of up to five or six months and in a typical case there might be 40 or 50 circles available for analysis from a single child.

The relevant question is, of course, whether or not the rotation change in these children is associated with a change in where the circle starts. At the age of 3 to 4, most circles were drawn clockwise and the most common region for starting was the lower left, so that children were drawing upward to the left, just as adults do from this position. At 4 to 5 years, the situation is mixed not just across children, but within the sample from each child. Two-thirds drew in both clockwise and counterclockwise directions, and commonly did so from two different regions: bottom left (clockwise) and top left (counterclockwise). There were only 11 children in the oldest group (5 to 6 years), but they tended to show the standard adult pattern, counterclockwise from top or top left. In short, both within and across the performances of the children from 3 to 6 years, the global principle of a nexus between starting position and direction of rotation holds.

During the time the children were going through this change in circle production, they were also changing their preferred starting position on other drawing tasks, so that by the age of 5 or 6 they drew sets of lines and traced clusters of dots from a position to the left of that at which they began the circles. The two changes involve a convergence from different origins and by different paths. Dot tracing begins at the bottom right and generally progresses upward and then to the left; the construction of circles begins at the bottom *left* and moves directly upward, so many of the younger subjects display starting positions on one task that are the opposite of the other. The early appearance of the nexus between start and rotation and this lack of coordination between circle and other starting position development makes a straightforward theory of circle production based on conventional starting location difficult.

Mechanisms of circle production

I do not want to dwell too long on the question of mechanism, because although I have pondered it for some time, I do not see the situation clearly and we may well need further studies of motor programming of the hand and arm to solve the problem.

As we saw in this and earlier chapters, right-handers drawing straight lines and arcs adopt starting positions consistent with preferred hand movements, these two forces being roughly encapsulated in the 11-to-5 axis. Since there is a disjunction in left-handers between starting position and stroke preference, we can usually look to the performance of the left-handers to assay whether some phenomenon is tied to one force or the other. Consider what happens when we apply this logic to the present case. We discover that for left-handers, the separation between the two directions of rotation in the upper half of the circle is a mirror image of that of the right-handers, an outcome consistent with stroke preference. By contrast, in the lower half field, the boundary is aligned with the 11-to-5 axis, suggesting a possible link with starting position. The natural inference is that the left-handers' performance is sensitive to both forces.

The principal problem with this resolution is that we hardly wanted a link with stroke preferences, since as I observed earlier the main fact we are trying to explain is that the initial directions of movement in circle production for right-handers are completely the reverse of what straight-line stroke preferences would prescribe. For the left-handers, stroke direction is not completely at variance with circle production, but it is only in the small region at the bottom of the circle that the two are congruent, as Fig. 4.9(a) shows.

There is another mirror-symmetrical process that could be invoked as a partner of starting position in controlling these performances – namely, the "natural" rotational movement of the two hands, the "eggbeating," nonfigurative rotation of the hands that is clockwise for the right and counterclockwise for the left. This scarcely provides a solution for our problem, however, since if it were biasing the left-handers' performance, we might expect it to be expanding the region of counterclockwise rotation toward the left instead of contracting it back toward 1 o'clock, as in Fig. 4.9(b). As with stroke direction, this element is congruent with respect to its distribution but antithetical with respect to direction.

Two starting positions?

The most direct way to implicate starting position is to suggest that when subjects draw from a gap, they have a choice between two end points, which although only a millimeter or two apart, are in fact at different distances from the 11 o'clock position. If they chose whichever end is closer to 11 o'clock, most of the rotation patterns I have reported would prevail. This argument requires that when working from a dot or at their own nominated starting place, the subjects treat that point as having a dual aspect (as the beginning and end of the circumference) and define the segment nearer 11 o'clock as the beginning and move that way. That they do not often use the 11 o'clock location itself as a starting position is explained by the need to locate the circle by beginning at top center, as I suggested earlier. I don't find myself in great sympathy with this view, since it demands that all subjects adopt the interpretation of gaps, dots, and chosen starting locations on a circle as being like an opening, and it makes their respect for 11 o'clock sound a little like a duty. It also causes problems with the developmental data, since we found the start-rotation nexus in young children whose respect for 11 o'clock is not yet established. I should prefer an explanation better rooted in the practical logic of the situation.

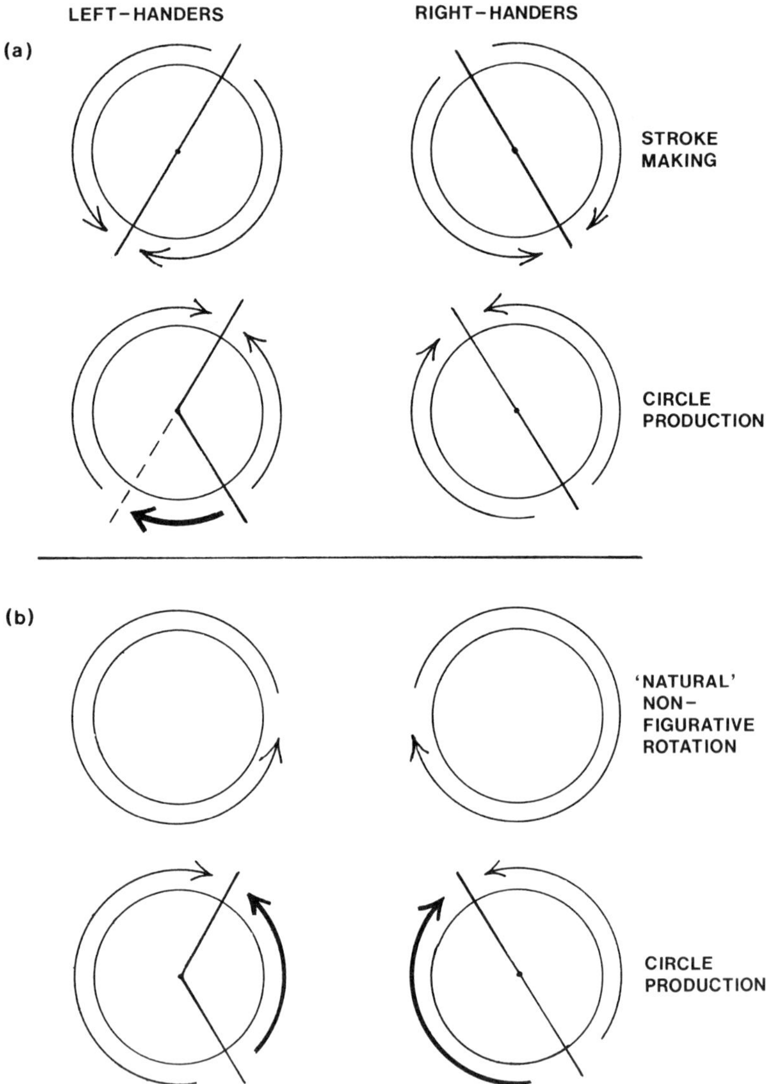

Fig. 4.9.(a): Relations between straight-line production and circle production. Straight lines tangential to the circle are drawn in the direction indicated, whereas the initial movement in constructing circles is almost entirely the reverse. The exception is a small segment around 6 o'clock (dark arrow). (b): Relations between the "natural," "nonfigurative" rotation of the right and left hands in adults according to Thomassen and Teulings (1979). For the left hand, the larger segment of circle production runs in the reverse direction to the "natural" rotation, and for both right and left most circles are drawn in the reverse direction.

Let us return to a reconsideration of starting position itself. I made the suggestion in an earlier chapter that the assumption of an 11 o'clock starting position by right-handers is not an empty convention, but rather represents the point from which all the various favored strokes can most readily be made. *This would suggest that there is a corresponding "natural" starting position for left-handers at 1 o'clock* that is overridden by our writing practices which have evolved for the convenience of the majority, who are right-handed. I also showed that the most severe limitation on the scope or range of movement of the hand and fingers around a natural resting position is in the direction toward which the drawing arm points (11 o'clock for right-handers, 1 o'clock for noninverted left-handers), and this recommends those locations as natural starting points.

This circumstance becomes relevant when we consider some observations made from videotapes of hand position and movement while subjects were drawing circles. The tapes show that when they are required to begin a circle from a low starting position, some subjects automatically and quite unconsciously place their hands on the paper surface at a point higher than they normally would for such a start. In this situation, their fingers are strongly flexed or bunched together. They are, in fact, placing the heels of their hands in just the position they would adopt if they were about to construct the circle from the top. The first movement they then execute is to exploit this "cocking" of the fingers by extending them, producing for right-handers the movement toward 11 o'clock. (Fig. 4.10 shows a tracing from a videotape of this sequence of events.) This phenomenon, if general, would see the paths followed as simply the most direct route to the maximum extension of the fingers (which occurs at 11 o'clock for right-handers and 1 o'clock for left-handers). When I make these movements with my own right hand, I am aware of a feeling of freedom of movement as I rotate clockwise from a position near the bottom of the circle. This view is consonant with the statement of Thomassen and Teulings (1979) that there is a preference in adults for extension first. (Note, however, that one can't apply that principle too generally without falling foul of the whole phenomenon of straight-line production.)

I shall have to leave the account at this point. I am quite unsatisfied with my efforts to make sense of the main effect. I feel, on the one hand, that the key to the matter lies in mechanics and motor programming, and the performance of the left-handers seems to call for an explanation that has more than one component in it. Furthermore, notions of hand preparation of the sort I have illustrated in Fig. 4.10 do not seem to me to be robust and universal enough to carry the weight of such widespread and uniform effects as those we are trying to explain. I myself have seen people following the patterns I have described using movements that are directed from the shoulder, so that a finger-extension theory hardly seems apt. To cap it all, having developed an idea about "natural"

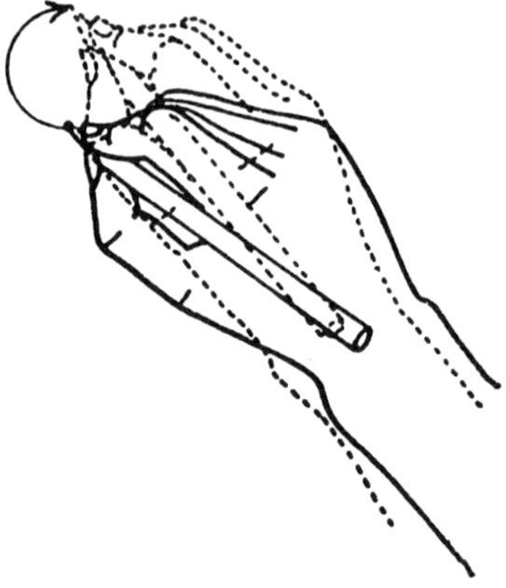

Fig. 4.10. Tracing of a videotape record of a right-handed subject drawing a circle from a dot near its lower extremity. The solid lines show the hand in its initial position, with fingers more strongly flexed than is usual. The dashed lines show that the drawer moved the whole hand and arm upward slightly, but at the same time extended the fingers. This suggests that the drawer is trying to compensate for the more restricted scope of the finger toward the top left by placing the hand a little higher on the page than usual, with fingers flexed, and beginning the circle with an extension of the fingers upward to the left.

starting positions for right- and left-handers at 11 o'clock and 1 o'clock, we are confronted with the fact that when these two groups do show a difference in starting position (for example, in drawing ellipses), the left-handers start near 11 o'clock and the right-handers near 1 o'clock!

But to look on the positive side, what we have laid down is an empirical foundation that suggests (1) a disjunction between certain curvilinear forms and others (arcs versus circles and ellipses); and (2) a strong general principle that direction of movement around circles is contingent on starting position, a principle that applies to right- and left-handers and to children, and even extends to the production of noncircular forms such as triangles, quadrilaterals, and straight lines. (3) As a side effect, the inquiry has thrown up again the possibility that for left-handers there may be two definitions of a preferred starting position, one to the right that is less used but is determined practically by the limitations on scope of the fingers, and one to the left that is often in evidence and arises from our writing practices.

Circle discontinuities and calligraphy

Nothing has been said so far about the actual trajectory of the line in circle or arc production beyond starting points and direction of movement. When I came to analyze the structure of a variety of written scripts (Burmese, Thai, Hebrew, Arabic), I found that few of the "round" characters produced by my informants were in fact properly circular. They tended to progress instead in a number of shallow arcs linked by more sharply curved transitions. A similar phenomenon appears in the production of letters by very young children. Indeed, some children copying such characters as the letter "C" for the first time actually make it with two separate strokes, drawing two flattened arcs that intersect at the left extremity of the letter.

A recent microanalysis of arc production by adults carried out by Abend, Bizzi, and Morasso (1982) shows that although smooth trajectories are occasionally produced by adults, the most common trajectory of the hand in inscribing arcs of 180 degrees is made up of from two to four shallow curved segments, with smooth transitions of a shorter radius of curvature. The arcs were considerably larger than those I have been describing (8 to 16 cm radius) and the hand grip was different, but the effect was very robust. The trajectories were similar whether the subjects followed their own path or conformed to a guide, whether they worked with a fist or with a finger grip. Abend et al. found that at the points of maximum curvature the speed of movement fell momentarily, so that instead of the whole movement gradually accelerating to a maximum and then declining, as is typical of a straight trajectory, they found that in most instances there were discontinuities or multiple peaks in the function relating speed of movement to position along the arc.

This segmentation of a curved or circular path into a number of relatively flatter regions is very pronounced in script production and has a significance that extends far beyond the technical questions of control in a biomechanical system. It is an important element in the esthetics of calligraphy. The beauty of much high-quality script arises from the systematic and sensitive modulation of curvature, from the movement from flattened to accelerated segments. Arabic script provides excellent examples. At the extreme, the original Kufic was often completely transformed from curved to rectilinear forms, so that circles were represented as triangles, squares, and rectangles. But short of this there were many versions in which the pen moved sharply between a succession of shallow curves. The effect of such discontinuity was enhanced by the action of the flattened tip of the pen that produced a ribbonlike line, narrowing and widening. A decorative Arabic script like Thuluth (Thoulthii) owes much of its beauty not just to the rhythm of tight and open curves, but to the asymmetrical sweep of the leading and trailing edges of the pen. (Excellent examples are to be found in Lings and Safadi, 1976, and Massoudy, 1981.) The same conversion of smooth into discontinuous curves is seen everywhere in script, from the earliest Egyptian hieratic script on papyrus (Möller, 1909) to modern italic script (Fairbank, 1968), and even in such areas as musical notation (Bent et al., 1980). The effects produced have their origins in the performance of the calligrapher working with pen or brush, but are preserved for their esthetic impact when the scripts are realized in ceramic tiles, painted in outline on glass, carved in stone, modeled in plaster, or in the case of modern Latin typefaces, designed and re-created by computer (Knuth, 1978).

With this chapter on curvilinear forms, I have completed my treatment of what might be thought of as the "phonological" aspects of drawing performance. I shall now describe some evidence on how meaning combines, complements, and competes with the formal geometric constraints.

5 The impact of meaning on executive strategies

The study I am about to report shows that what a drawing *represents* can affect the strategy of its production; final execution is not by any means monopolized by the formal geometric aspects of making lines on paper. To give a simple example, an arrow pointing to the left is, geometrically, a horizontal line with a pair of shorter oblique lines running diagonally back from its left-hand end. Formal graphic constraints invite the right-handed drawer to make the major stroke from left to right, but its representational significance may promote the reverse, a stroke that moves in the direction the arrow points. This does not mean that geometric constraints become irrelevant. Rather, the drawer's action in any particular instance may result from cooperation or competition between the two forces, geometric and semantic. The context of drawing may modulate this interaction, biasing it in one direction or the other. The more the context emphasizes meaning and the less routinized it is, the more likely it is that semantics will prevail over geometry at the point of action, should they be opposed.

Drawing and speech

Before outlining an analysis and demonstration of this interplay in drawing and copying, I should like to compare the structure of drawing and speech production from this point of view. On the whole, semantics and pragmatics do not intrude on mainstream executive processes in speech. Although linguists explore the mutual interpenetration of pragmatics, semantics, and syntax, they tend to observe a division between them and speech execution, which is assigned to the "phonological component" of language organization. Prosodic features of language such as intonation and stress which carry meaning and intention, represent an important exception, as do certain devices in literary language – poetry in particular. Here substance and intent may directly modulate the acoustic pattern and so codetermine its form. But in ordinary speech there still remains a substantial buffer between meaning and intention on the one hand, and the details of execution on the other. This is because spoken language is heavily codified compared to drawing. By saying that language is codified, I simply mean the fact that one cannot normally decipher what a speaker is expressing in an unknown foreign language by trying to map sound directly onto referent. Even when words are onomatopoeic, they are not like free gestures. They have been "frozen" into the language system and are hardly more variable than the mass of opaque signs with which they are mixed. Drawing, on the other hand, is a strongly mimetic system that usually requires only a little enabling experience to make it transparent to an audience. On the production side, even simple drawings require a degree of instant invention analogous to that involved in descriptive gesture. Drawings are produced by actions in which meaning and pragmatics may be actively involved in determining the form, direction, and sequence of strokes.

Similar drawings with different meanings

The following study was engineered to demonstrate the intrusion of meaning into graphic execution under circumstances in which geometry is "clamped" or rendered invariant to a large degree. This was accomplished by having subjects reproduce standard designs to which different meanings were attributed.

The subjects were two groups of adult subjects, mixed male and female, all right-handed, none with special graphic skill or training. There were 16 subjects in each group, each of whom was tested individually so that the direction and sequence of drawing movements could be documented on videotape. Each subject reproduced the same 37 designs. These were arranged in columns of 8 or 9 down the center of 33 × 21 cm sheets. Each design was 2–3 cm high. Subjects produced their copies down a column to the right, and to the left of each design was a short title or description. These titles differed from one group to the other. For example, a design comprising three vertical lines with horizontal lines running across top and bottom was described as "the Roman numeral III" or "ladder on its side." A line with a triangle above and below was entitled "pyramid and its reflection," or "diamond with a cross-line." Many of the designs and alternative titles are displayed in Fig. 5.1. The study was conducted in the context of other drawing and copying tasks, and the overall instruction was to draw the designs quickly and "in a straightforward way." No specific reference was made to the captions, and no subject specifically inquired about them. It is fair to assume, however, that no subject failed to read them.

Starting position, stroke directions, and ordering of strokes were analyzed for each subject on each design. The aim of the analysis was to separate drawings into two classes corresponding to the two descriptions. Knowledge of membership of the groups was suppressed during the coding. The segregation of different strategies involved little ambiguity in most cases, and the classification is shown in diagrammatic form on the right side of Fig. 5.1. In these diagrams, the convention was adopted of reproducing the initial stroke or strokes as continuous lines and later lines as interrupted. Only in a very few instances were strategies mixed or not able to be assigned unambiguously.

Fig. 5.1 includes 3 typical designs for which there was no semantic effect and 13 for which a significant effect occurred. The examples of nonsignificant outcomes will be mentioned first. They represent cases in which geometric constraints are very strong or in which semantic interpretation prescribes the same procedure for both versions. The formal constraints governing performance on the first two items of Fig. 5.1 are starting position, stroke direction, and anchoring. The third design is affected by asymmetrical conformity and economy in line production. The first design resembles the Greek letter π. It was labeled either "table" or "archway or doorway." Evidently any contrast in priority between table top and legs on the one hand and uprights and lintel on the other were not strong enough to override formal constraints. Virtually all subjects (31 of 32) adopted the same approach: start at top left, left-to-right horizontal, followed by two verticals anchored to the horizontal and drawn in the favored down direction, left before right. A similar strategy dominated by geometry was adopted with the second design, which resembled a rotated "K." The third design, "letter M on a line," or "two witches' hats" was *not* constructed top to bottom by most subjects. A majority of 19 laid down the bottom stroke and added a zigzag above it. This strategy was favored because it avoids having to align the bottom points of the "M" in space, does not require the horizontal to be drawn through three specified points, and has the advantage of producing the horizontal as a single stroke rather than as two separate "hat brims." In other words, the economy of the formal approach dominates the situation regardless of semantics.

When we consider the remaining designs in Fig. 5.1, it is helpful to recognize that the forms are made up entirely of straight lines, circles, arcs, and dots. The only variation that can be expected is in sequencing and direction of strokes; there is no scope for expressing meaning in contour. Designs 3 and 4 were described either as transformed block letters or as folded papers. The analysis of production strategies divides the copying procedure into two stages: the laying down of an enclosed "frame," followed by the addition of detail. The semantic interpretation controlled what was to become frame and what detail. The initial frame for the "folded paper" version was typically a five- or six-sided polygon (the envelope of the figure) into which right-angled elements were inserted. Subjects interpreting the designs as letters laid down the outline of the "L" or "T" and usually added strokes across internal angles. Representation thus governed the basic segmentation. We should note that construction within the sub-

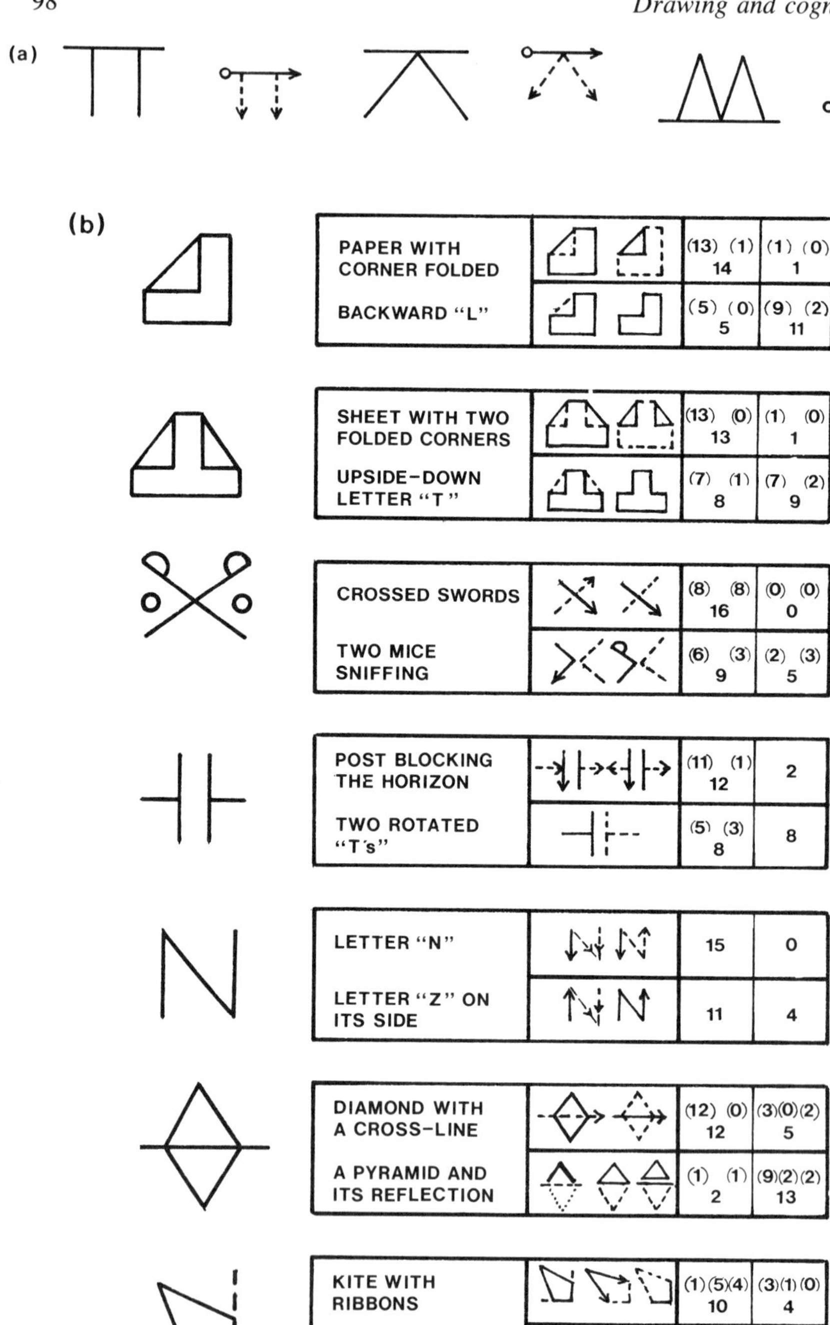
(a)
(b)
PAPER WITH CORNER FOLDED
(13) (1) 14
(1) (0) 1
BACKWARD "L"
(5) (0) 5
(9) (2) 11
SHEET WITH TWO FOLDED CORNERS
(13) (0) 13
(1) (0) 1
UPSIDE-DOWN LETTER "T"
(7) (1) 8
(7) (2) 9
CROSSED SWORDS
(8) (8) 16
(0) (0) 0
TWO MICE SNIFFING
(6) (3) 9
(2) (3) 5
POST BLOCKING THE HORIZON
(11) (1) 12
2
TWO ROTATED "T's"
(5) (3) 8
8
LETTER "N"
15
0
LETTER "Z" ON ITS SIDE
11
4
DIAMOND WITH A CROSS-LINE
(12) (0) 12
(3)(0)(2) 5
A PYRAMID AND ITS REFLECTION
(1) (1) 2
(9)(2)(2) 13
KITE WITH RIBBONS
(1)(5)(4) 10
(3)(1)(0) 4
CORNER OF A SQUARE
(0)(0)(4) 4
(6)(2)(2) 10

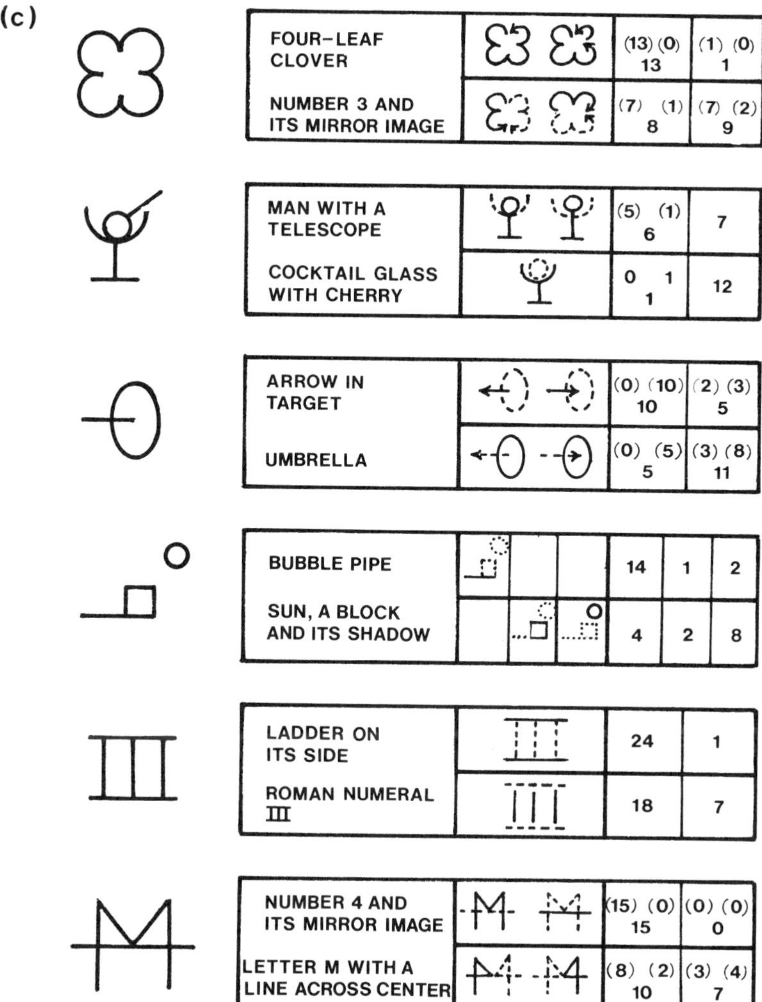

Fig. 5.1. (a) Three designs that were drawn in the same manner irrespective of their identification. (b) Designs, captions, construction strategies, and data for the study of effects of semantics on production. Each of the designs on the left was accompanied by one or other of the two captions in the second column. Production processes were analyzed into two or three broad types reflecting one or other of the meanings of the designs. Solid lines indicate early strokes, interrupted lines later strokes. Values in brackets show the frequency of each construction strategy; values below are their sums. High values in top-left and bottom-right cells indicate a positive relationship between the caption and the corresponding graphic strategy.

components of the figures (that is, within the frame and within the accretions) follows formal executive principles – starting location, paper contact, and so on. This does not mean that all strokes were constructed in an identical manner from one version to another; rather, they are geometrically appropriate when the drawing task is viewed not as the production of the whole design, but as a sequence of two or more subcomponents chosen and ordered on semantic grounds.

The sixth design in Fig. 5.1 (two "crossed swords" or two "mice") shows this same history of perceptual segmentation based on meaning, followed by formal execution. The "sword" version is represented by two lines crossing at right angles, the "mice" by two rotated Vs meeting at their vertices. The execution of the subunits is geometrically orthodox: right downhill diagonal before left, left angle before right, arcs representing "sword handles" and "ears" anchored to the ends of lines, circles drawn counterclockwise from the top.

The final example of the same sort comprises a pair of verticals with horizontal lines meeting them on either side. It is described alternatively as "post blocking the horizon," or "two rotated Ts." The first description produced a segregation of the two center lines from the collinear horizontals; the second produced a segmentation of the left from the right halves of the figure. The segmentation showed itself in two ways, in order and in stroke direction. Order was determined semantically, stroke direction geometrically, and again in that order. The "post" version was commonly produced in the order: left vertical, right vertical, left horizontal, right horizontal. The rotated Ts were produced in this order: left vertical, left horizontal, right vertical, right horizontal. All verticals were drawn top to bottom, but the horizontals varied. When the horizontals represented the horizon behind a post, both were drawn left to right. This conforms to normal stroke direction and contravenes anchoring, but is supported by a need to keep the two collinear strokes aligned. By contrast, in the T versions, the horizontals were usually drawn outward. Collinearity gave way to the anchoring of the left horizontal to the left vertical when the two were drawn successively.

The picture that is emerging consistently in all these cases is that of semantics intruding on execution only to the point that a basic decision is made to start with one representationally defined unit of the design or another. From that point execution is governed only by geometry and formal constraints. Does this mean there will always be an ultimate "articulatory" stage in drawing from which meaning and intent are excluded? I do not accept this view. Rather, I believe that in these cases there just happens to be no strong semantic motivation for varying strategy beyond the basic perceptual segmentation. Partly this is a product of the designs, which systematically exclude one important arena for the exercise of representational forces in stroke production, contour. Furthermore, there are one or two examples within the designs of semantically (or at least symbolically) motivated line production: Item 8 (Fig. 5.1) comprises three zigzag strokes and is described either as the letter "N" or the letter "Z" on its side. All subjects with the figure labeled "N" started at the top left. Four of those drawings it as a "Z" started at the bottom left and drew upward. There is no geometric support for this, nor can it be described as perceptual segmentation followed by meaning-free execution.

Subsequently a more comprehensive study was conducted on the production of rotated capital letters, both in alphabetic order and text. This tendency to preserve the original upright letter as a model for production, rather than simply following the geometry of the new configuration, was not uncommon.

Rotated alphabetical letters

I shall briefly describe the outcome of the study of rotated letters because although it is rather contrived, it illustrates the interaction between the characteristics of subject matter, geometric constraints, and the use of prior experience with the symbols in determining strategy. The first circumstance we need to note is how many majuscule Roman alphabet letters are either right-to-left symmetrical (A, H, I, M, O, T, U, V, W, X, Y) or have a left vertical (B, D, E, F, K, L, P, R). Only four letters invite a start at the right (C, G, J, S). When letters are presented "upside down" (that is, rotated through 180 degrees), some remain unchanged (H, I, N, O, S, Z), some present an accessible top-left start (A, C, G, M, N, X, Z), and many have a downstroke on the *right* with added detail anchored to it on the left (B, D, E, F, K, L, P, R). For this reason, one has to make a careful assessment of the geometry of the rotated letters to establish what invitations they offer the drawer or copier from a formal standpoint. It is against this background that one can assess the degree to which graphic performance is controlled by a memory of the normal configuration of the symbols.

Fig. 5.2 shows the outcome of a study of 20 right-handed university students copying inverted letters or constructing them from memory. Each square of Fig. 5.2 represents a frame on which all letters may be projected. The frame is divided into nine regions, and the values within these regions form a matrix that indicates the percentage of subjects in the group who began the various letters at that location.

The first data matrix shows performance on letters of the normal upright Roman capital alphabet. The second matrix is a rotation of the data of the first and indicates what subjects would do if they were to preserve exactly their memories of symbols in upright positions and use them exclusively as a guide for production. Matrix 3 is theoretically derived. It shows what would be expected if the subjects treated rotated letters simply as new geometric shapes and followed formal constraints as we understand them. The remaining matrices show actual performances under various conditions: copying and drawing from memory the rotated alphabet and the sentence "THE QUICK

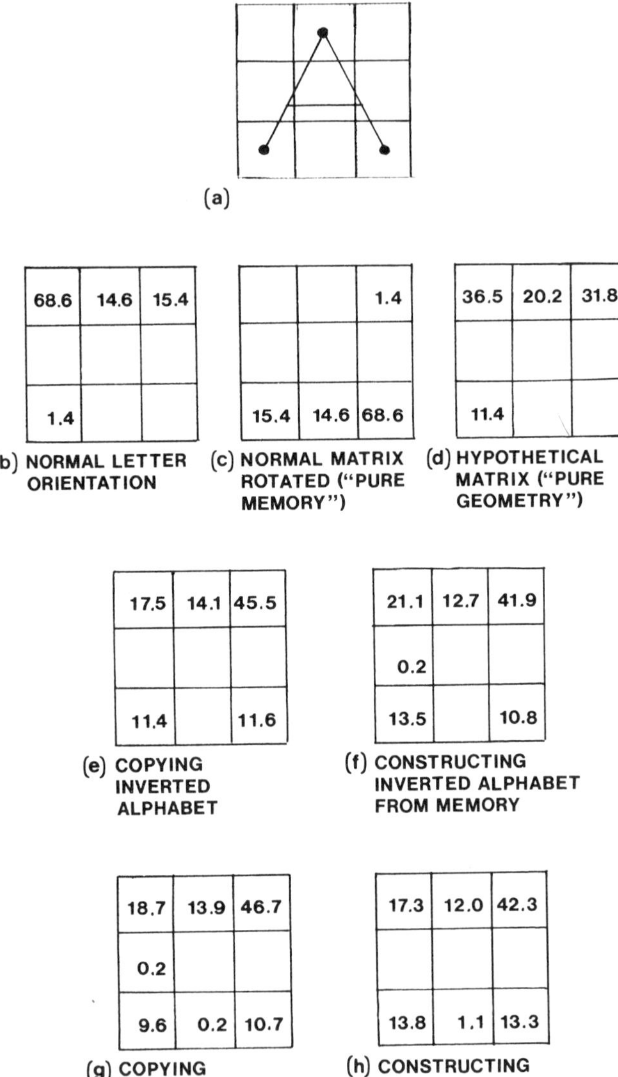

Fig. 5.2. Percentages of subjects starting normal and rotated letters at various locations. (a): Example of the matrix superimposed on the letter A. (b): Starting locations for majuscule Roman alphabet in normal upright position. (c): Matrix (b) inverted to indicate what the distribution of starting positions in reproducing inverted letters would be if only memory of past production governed performance. (d): Hypothetical matrix of starting positions if performance was dominated only by current geometry. (e) to (h): Starting positions in copying and drawing inverted letters in alphabetical order and in text of THE QUICK BROWN FOX JUMPS OVER THE LAZY DOG. Data are from right-handed adults.

BROWN FOX JUMPS OVER THE LAZY DOG.'' The pattern that emerges is much the same under all conditions of copying and drawing. Both the new geometry *and* the trace of what the construction strategy was prior to rotation play a role. (Values in the top left-hand corner are ''pure geometry''; those in the bottom right ''pure semantics,'' if we can use that term to refer to the mental representation of a symbol in its unrotated state.) The generally high values in the top right cell seem to be due to a shift in starting position from left to right associated with the fact that the letters in inverted series progress across the page from right to left. Subjects began at the right not only with letters like B, D, and E, which now have their single vertical on the right, but with many symmetrical letters like A, H, U, and V.

As might be expected, particularly when working without a model, a proportion of subjects made errors in inverting letters. In cases like S, N, and Z, this can be attributed at least in part to a conviction that letters *ought* to be transformed by rotation, when in fact they are not. In other instances (like J, P, and R), the letter is sometimes drawn as a vertical mirror image. Possibly it is the difficulty of orienting the symbol correctly that leads subjects to preserve their old construction strategies. In other words, the task context predisposes them to concentrate on representations previously established rather than on new geometry. This view is supported by a numerical analysis of performance on drawing the inverted alphabet from memory. A certain group of letters (C, G, J, S, and Z) were quite regularly drawn upward from the bottom even when a top starting point was available (43 percent of all cases). It is just this group of letters that has the highest rate of error: 28 percent, compared with 3 percent for all other letters.

In earlier paragraphs I have prevaricated about how best to characterize this intrusion of old strategies into the production of letters in new orientations. Current geometry is not monopolizing production, yet the competing force is not strictly semantic, since it does not reflect the impact of what the symbol *means*. Rather, it shows the impact of the memory of past construction driven by earlier geometry. To sustain an argument that semantics intrudes, we need a different type of example. We therefore turn to a final category of drawing in which semantics can be expected to show itself at the level of final production.

The expression of action in stroke making

I mentioned at the outset the possibility that, in drawing an arrow, subjects may absorb into the act of drawing the direction of flight or projection of the object being represented and in so doing override their formal geometric preferences. This is in fact borne out by the evidence, as the diagrams in Fig. 5.3 show. The same 20 subjects who wrote inverted alphabets were asked to draw arrows,

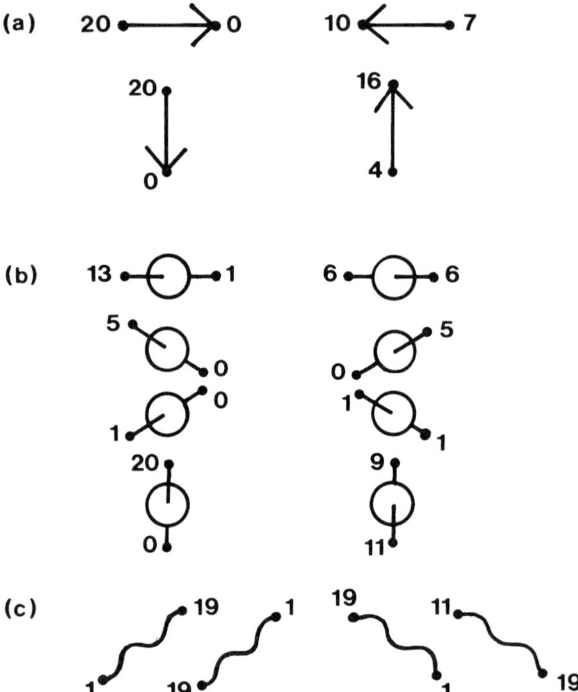

Fig. 5.3. Representational or semantic effects on stroke making. Values indicate the number of subjects starting the figure at the point indicated. Subjects were instructed to draw (a): "An arrow pointing right," "An arrow pointing left," and so on; (b): "A ring with a stick passing through it from the left," and so on; (c): "A snake going up to the top right," and so on. Dots with values beside them indicate the number of right-handed adults beginning at that point. [The diagonal lines in (b) were produced in response to instructions that the stick be drawn passing through from left or right.]

spirals, lines passing through circles from one side to another, and snakes moving in one direction or another.

The aim was to promote the expression of action in execution without using language that was an executive instruction. The circle and line design was specified as ". . . a ring with a stick passing through from the right (left, above, below)." The wavy lines were ". . . a snake going up to the top right (top left, bottom right, bottom left)." The subjects were instructed beforehand how to represent the snake so that geometric language was kept out of the specifications. Another instruction was to draw ". . . an arrow pointing right (left, up, down)." As the values in Fig. 5.3 show, the dynamics of the object descriptions were in fact translated by many subjects into action that competed with geometric constraints.

What these studies have shown is that meaning does not necessarily produce a graphic plan and then pass control over to a purely geometric executive component. Representation may play a role in execution first through the segmentation it imposes on the structure of subject matter, which in turn affects strategy, and in particular the order in which parts of a drawing are laid down. Once such segmentation is accomplished, it may be implemented by stroke making that is geometrically determined. Final stroke making, however, will not always follow current geometry; in the case of rotated letters, we saw the residues of old geometric relations interacting with the new. Finally, examples have been given of motion and orientation of objects being expressed in the direction of strokes used to represent them. Here semantics and geometric constraints interact directly.

There are unlikely to be any fixed rules that specify the relative strengths of representational and formal influences on graphic action. Whatever accentuates meaning in the mind of the drawer may enhance its penetration into the output stages of production, and whenever drawing becomes repetitive, whenever it is transmitted from person to person without reference to meaning, geometric forces will tend to dominate production.

Production history and semantic preoccupation

The tension between meaningful form and geometric routine prompts the following suggestion about the use of details of production history as a way of analyzing artistic performances outside the laboratory. My expectations would be that if any representational drawing is repeated often enough in a standard form (or is reproduced by someone who is not a party to its representational or pragmatic significance), the order of construction will be driven more and more by purely formal principles of the sort described in earlier chapters. A simple example of this is found in drawings of the human figure that use circles for head and body and straight lines for arms and legs. While one keeps the semantic point of paired arms and paired legs in mind, they will be drawn in that fashion – two arms, then two legs. But when children have repeated this many times so that drawing figures has become an almost mindless routine, it is common for the arms and legs to be drawn as four radiating lines in a single counterclockwise sweep around the body.

It would be a valuable exercise to document stroke by stroke the sequence of production of art works in cultures when designs are produced regularly and adapt slowly to try to make a link between the domination of production by geometry and the degree to which the producers of the artifacts have ceased to be preoccupied with signification. In analyzing Sepik River art, for example,

Forge (1971) suggested that the producers of the art continue to be governed by the representational or symbolic significance of what they paint without necessarily acknowledging it. This allegation would certainly gain support if it could be shown that their production sequences still reflect this signification. Indeed I should think that all documentation of graphic and other productions, whether in primitive or in technical societies, should include information on process if this can be achieved nonintrusively. It may even be possible in cases where the production process is relatively robust to go back over the sequence with the artists to secure their reflections on the process. I feel that it is enormously difficult to make complete analytic sense of any graphic work on the basis of products alone.

Drawing from verbal description

I wish now to tackle the question of meaning and production process from a different direction to see how the structure of language can affect the process of production, and how in turn the process of production can affect the choice of how space is represented in drawings.

The most direct explanation of how a drawer proceeds from instruction to finished graphic product is as follows: The linguistic description of what is to be drawn is decoded and results in some perceptual-cognitive representation in the mind of the subject, perhaps in the form of an image or some other quasi-spatial scheme. The subject then simply puts into operation a set of graphic skills and procedures to represent this scheme as a drawing.

The following study shows that this simple sequence of events may not adequately account for what occurs. In the first place, it supposes that once the linguistic form has given rise to some "picture in the mind," it is no longer of any importance in affecting the output process; and second, that the pathway from internal representation to graphic product is a one-way street. This experiment will show first that the linguistic form can affect the output process without necessarily being coded in the spatial representation, and second that the internal spatial representation may be modified in important ways as a result of events occurring during the output process. This is achieved by manipulating the verbal instructions to subjects so that they are biased toward a method of proceeding with drawings that conflicts with their graphic preferences, and under the dual pressure of linguistic and graphic constraints, change their representational strategies.

The study was conducted using 10 right-handed university students. They were given a 10 × 15 cm pad and pencil and asked to portray a number of simple object arrays. These included four types of object: "a small ball," "a large ball," "a rod," and "a square plate." In every case the instruction took

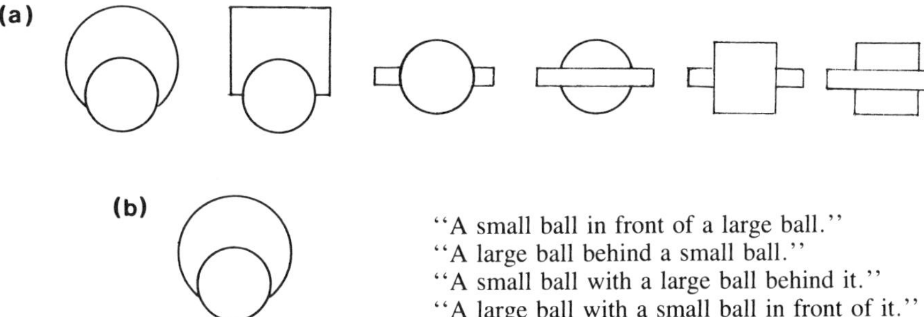

Fig. 5.4. (a): Experimenter's version of the six object arrangements described. (These were not shown to the subjects.) (b): The four descriptions of the first object arrangement. Similar descriptions were generated for all object pairs. The first two descriptions have less focus on the first-mentioned object than the latter two.

the form of a statement about a pair of these objects in front of or behind one another. The investigator's version of the six arrangements of pairs of objects used in the study are shown in Fig. 5.4. These pictures were not, of course, shown to the subjects, who were given instructions like those at the bottom of Fig. 5.4. As usual, all performances were videotaped, and the order in which the objects were drawn and the strokes used in their production were transcribed from tape.

Two different randomly mixed linguistic forms were used. One was the simple form "A in front of B" or "B behind A" ("The square plate in front of the rod"). The second form focused on the reference object. (The reference object in "A in front of B" is B, since the first mentioned object's position is specified in relation to it.) The strongly focused description took the form "B with A in front of it." B in this case is not only the reference object, but it is mentioned first and is referred to a second time by the pronoun "it" at the end of the phrase, whereas A is mentioned in the context of the subordinate preposition "with." All these features contribute to exaggerated focus on the first-mentioned object in the second sentence form.

The results showed two main effects: the proximity of the object (the closer object being drawn first more often than the remote), and the order of mention (with the *first-mentioned* being drawn first). When the linguistic form had weaker focus ("A in front of B"), the order of drawing the objects was most affected by proximity, with the object closer to the observer in the description being drawn first. The order of mention was less important, although nonetheless present (Table 5.1). When the linguistic focus was stronger, with the reference object first, the subordinate "with," and the reference term in pronoun form

Table 5.1. *Number of drawing performances by 10 subjects drawing pairs of objects. The typical weak linguistic form of description indicated at the right.*

	Closer object drawn first	More remote object drawn first	Total
First-mentioned object drawn first	41	23	64 "A in front of B"
Second-mentioned object drawn first	37	18	55 "B behind A"
Total	78	41	

Table 5.2. *Number of drawing performances in response to the more strongly focused description indicated by typical sentences on the right.*

	Closer object drawn first	More remote object drawn first	Total
First-mentioned object drawn first	56	42	98 "A with B behind it"
Second-mentioned object drawn first	18	4	22 "B with A in front of it"
Total	74	46	

again at the end of the phrase, the order of mention effect became dominant (Table 5.2).

We can make the following comment on the outcome: First, why would the closer object be drawn first? This cannot be attributed to linguistic factors, since the closer object appears in all possible linguistic contexts: as subject, as object of preposition, as first and as second mentioned, and with both spatial prepositions. The reasons are almost certainly graphic or perceptual. In order to explain why, it is first necessary to explore the representation of space in a two-dimensional drawing. We will consider the treatment of objects that do not completely occlude one another. If two objects are mentioned in a description, it is a rare subject who draws only the front object, even when it is large relative to the distant object and might in reality fully obscure it. That strategy is ruled out by a type of tacit cooperative principle between drawers and their audiences not to exploit such possibilities except perhaps as a joke. This principle is closely

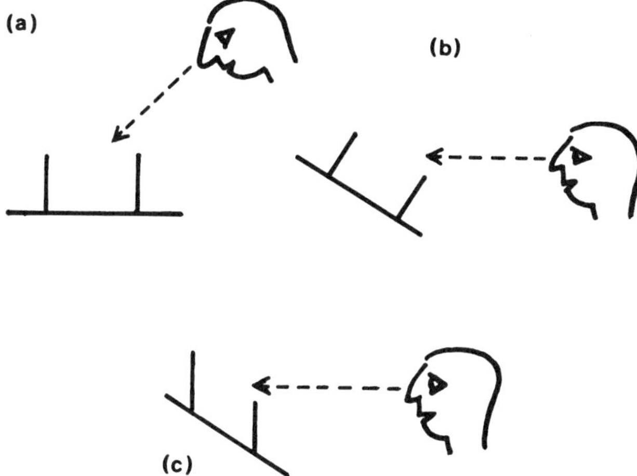

Fig. 5.5. A high viewpoint (a) or a surface tilted toward the observer (b) places objects vertically with the closer near the bottom. Subjects commonly draw such arrangements as if the objects themselves were perpendicular to the line of sight (c).

related to the conversational agreements found in verbal dialogue to provide all expected material.

The next graphic possibility is to make the objects concentric. This involves adopting a line of sight that runs perpendicularly down "through" the page, and is universally used in technical drawing. It is not widely used in vernacular drawing for the following reason: In simple line drawings where only one version is given of the subject matter, concentric outlines are ambiguous. A square in front of a circle, a square lying on a circle, a square inside a circle, a circular disk with a square hole in it all have an identical representation. Mutually overlapping boundaries, another possibility, also have a representational function of their own: They portray transparency or the emptiness of skeletal structures. Mature drawers tend not to use them to represent opaque solid objects partially occluding one another. We are left with two other devices, partial overlap and complete separation. Later we discuss the principles governing the choice between them, but here we must examine the direction in which offset or separation ordinarily occurs.

A very common practice among adults and all but the youngest children is to project horizontal surfaces obliquely up the page as though we were looking down on the tops of objects or as though the surface on which they rest were tilted up into our horizontal regard, as in Fig. 5.5(a) and (b). This descending line of sight or tilted substrate would in the real world cause a foreshortening of the objects and allow us to see their upper surfaces. The vernacular drawer often draws each object as if it were being viewed from in front, but arranges them as though the array was seen from above, as in Fig. 5.5(c).

The next question is this: Why has the vertical been chosen so often as the appropriate dimension along which to separate the objects? The first reason is its relatively uncommitted status in graphic representation. The horizontal is needed to represent lateral displacement, so a horizontal separation used to represent depth might well be misunderstood. The vertical is in theory needed in a similar way to code vertical displacement of objects, but the representation of two unsupported objects located vertically with respect to one another is rarely needed, so the vertical dimension can be more readily exploited. The other very obvious reason why vertical displacement is used to represent depth arises from our regular visual commerce with small objects in the world. The majority of such objects we see and interact with are below our line of sight. If they are substantially above eye level, they have to be near the edge of a support (as on a shelf), on a transparent support, hanging, dropping, or flying. Howard and Templeton (1966) discuss this issue of common perceptual experience and sum up by saying: ". . . there are more things that stick up than hang down." We have to crane, stand, or climb to see objects in depth above our current line of sight, or have the support on which they rest tilted or lowered.

All these circumstances put us into one or the other of the situations portrayed in Fig. 5.5, where the more distant object is above the closer. In this sense, the portrayal of the closer object near the bottom of the page is not arbitrary, but the outcome of several factors:

1. Graphic communicative agreements to include all relevant objects.
2. Pressures to overlap or separate objects in depth rather than to portray them concentrically.
3. The definition of the remote edge of the page as the "top" or "upper," a natural product of swinging our normally horizontally oriented gaze down to inspect the page or other drawing surface (perhaps combined with our experience of such surfaces raised to a vertical position for inspection).
4. The need to use a dimension other than the horizontal, which already codes lateral displacement, and the relatively uncommitted status of the vertical from this point of view.
5. The common visual experience of seeing everyday objects in depth most often lying vertically displaced, with the more distant above the closer.

We can now turn to two matters that relate to the actual laying down of strokes on a page. Formal starting position constraints among this population of English-speaking literate adults prescribe that the unit of a drawing about to be constructed start nearest the 11 o'clock position, other things being equal. The subjects in this experiment follow this principle in the way they construct each form, beginning the rectangles, for example, at the top-left corner. If an elongated form such as a rod is interrupted by another form placed in front of it, the left-hand half of the rod is usually drawn before the right. Circles are drawn starting near the top; and if a rod is represented by a single continuous or dashed line, that is begun on the left.

The drawing of an object low on the page (the "closer" object according to the earlier analysis) before one higher on the page contravenes this starting position principle. Another important graphic principle accounts for this inconsistency: avoidance of anticipated embedding. As we have seen, embedding refers to the interruption of the boundary of one object by that of another. Anticipated embedding means starting with the interrupted boundary, estimating the size and position of the break, and fitting the complete boundary of the "front" object into the gap – a procedure requiring more planning and control of line than simply building the incomplete boundary around the complete. If subjects represent space vertically in their drawings with the remoter object above the closer, if they fail completely to separate the two objects, and if they follow the normal starting position preference for the upper form, anticipated embedding is inevitable.

Before looking at some evidence about this, it should be pointed out that there may be some perceptual-cognitive preference for drawing front to back, working on the foreground forms first, that is independent of graphic difficulties. In painting, for example, the situation from a technical point of view is somewhat the reverse of line drawing. If a complex object is completed in the foreground, background features have to be painted around them. Particularly with opaque media, it is sensible to complete the background material and superimpose the foreground when the background is dry, although it requires discipline to do this. The issue is complicated by questions of speed of work and drying time of media, and it is clear from inspection of the work of many *al primo* painters such as the Impressionists, who on principle worked quickly in oil, that they worked front-to-back, either because of their interest in the salient foreground material or because it was easier to paint foreground objects positively and fit more amorphous matter like cloudscapes or sky around them. The alternative was to delineate the boundaries of foreground objects negatively with the edge of the still-wet background pigment, an elaborate form of anticipated embedding.

In the simple case of drawing geometric forms from verbal description, there is evidence that the graphic constraint on anticipated embedding is very important, overriding any starting position constraints and often affecting the way space is portrayed. To show this, I have extracted all the drawings of the two circular objects ("A small ball in front of a large ball," and so on) and arranged these in a series on the basis of the device used to represent space. The series runs from "concentric" (Table 5.3 top) to "separated" (bottom) and includes all the strategies mentioned earlier, such as transparency and embedding. The

Table 5.3. *Percentages of drawings of two balls adopting various representational devices. Most of the drawings in the right-hand column were produced in response to linguistic descriptions that focused strongly on the more remote object.*

Representational device adopted	Closer object drawn first	More remote object drawn first
Concentric	11	15
Boundaries touch	12	9
Embedded	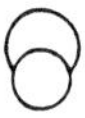 53	8
Transparent	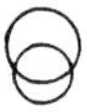 6	32
Separated	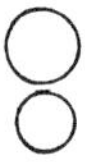 18	35

series generally represents a progressive rising of the point of view of the observer from immediately in front of the objects to obliquely above them. Two of the representational devices in the middle of the series (''embedded'' and ''transparent'') adopt the same viewpoint but differ in that the embedded omits an overlapping boundary that remains in the ''transparent.'' The percentage of drawings using the various strategies are classified according to the order of drawing the two forms. Most of the entries in the first column (closer object drawn first) were produced when the linguistic form was neutral. Most of those in the column headed ''more remote drawn first'' were produced when the linguistic form focused strongly on the first-mentioned object and that object was in the background.

When the closer object is drawn first, most of the subjects build the second object around it to produce an embedding. When under the pressure of linguistic emphasis the subjects begin by drawing the rear object first, they either break one of the well-observed taboos – making opaque objects transparent – or they change the representation of space in the drawing to one with a high viewpoint so that the boundaries do not interrupt one another.

This outcome shows that to understand how a drawing is constructed, both from the point of view of process and product it may be necessary to consider:

van Sommers: Drawing and Cognition

ISBN 0-521-25095-1 hard covers

ERRATUM (1984 printing)

Figure 5.6 on p. 113 omitted the dark arrows referred to in the caption. The correct figure appears below.

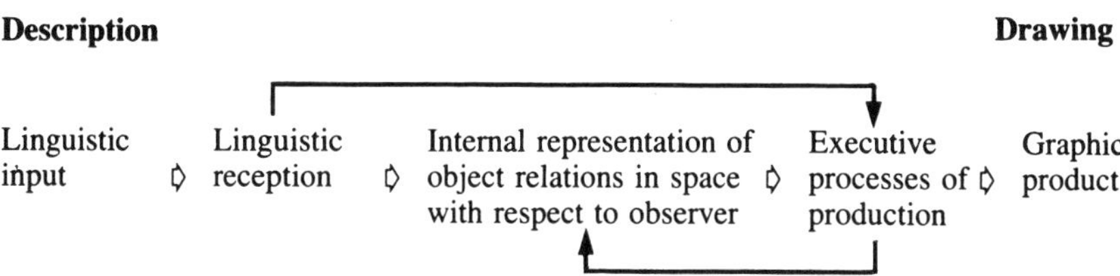

Fig. 5.6. Hypothetical sequence of events from hearing a verbal description to producing a drawing. The dark arrows represent minimal changes in the model required by the study of the effects of the linguistic form on representation of objects in space.

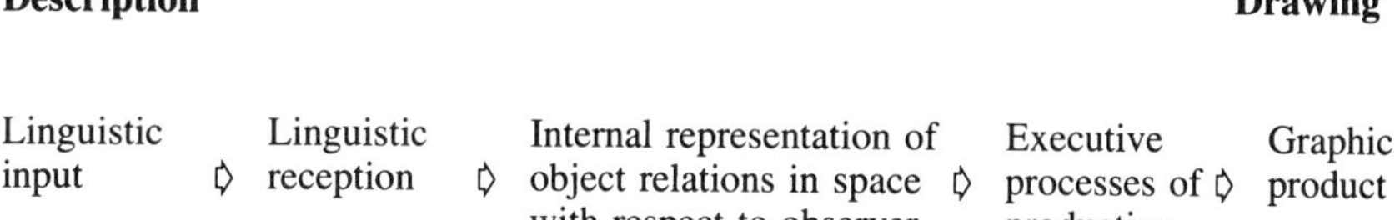

Fig. 5.6. Hypothetical sequence of events from hearing a verbal description to producing a drawing. The dark arrows represent minimal changes in the model required by the study of the effects of the linguistic form on representation of objects in space.

1. The focus of the linguistic form.
2. The tendency for the first mentioned form in the description to be drawn first.
3. The formal graphic constraints, such as starting position and avoidance of preplanned embedding.
4. The relationship between space being portrayed and the frame of the page (nearer objects closer to the drawer at the "bottom" of the page).
5. The possibility that to conform to graphic constraints, such as avoiding anticipated embedding, subjects may alter a representational aspect of their drawings, namely, space itself.

There is a possibility of another ingredient: some tendency to give graphic priority to closer objects, based perhaps on their relative perceptual importance. This was not traceable in this study.

Overall, the study shows that the simple view of the drawing process shown in the linear sequence of Fig. 5.6 must be amended to include the links from linguistic input to execution and from execution back to internal representation (dark arrows). Linguistic inputs are not simply converted into a static visuospatial representation and then dumped; aspects of that input can control graphic execution. Graphic execution in turn can throw up problems that affect the internal representation of space. Although it is not evident in this study, there is little doubt that subjects, having established a vertical overlap or a separation to represent depth, would if it were required of them continue to use that spatial framework for any subsequent graphic work in that frame. In other words, the executive processes could alter the visualization of space beyond the stage at which the conflict between execution and representational intention initially occurred.

We have dealt here with a variety of intrusions of meanings on executive processes. The discussion has been constrained to a certain degree by the need to show the simultaneous application of formal and representational constraints on the processes of drawing compilation, while at the same time allowing us to specify when and how they operate. Because the lines we specify geometrically carry meaning in a relatively direct way, there is no barrier to the interplay between formal and semantic factors. Nor can we assume that both will always be present during execution. Sometimes semantics does stop short of the production stage, especially in frequently repeated performances. Sometimes the geometric factors are so dominant or the semantic so weak or nonspecific that we see no evidence of the latter. When it does reveal its presence, semantics may specify only part of the process, as when it prescribes a particular segmentation of the production process, after which only formal constraints apply. Sometimes the task of keeping track of the form (as in the inverted alphabet study) forces semantics to the fore: Sometimes force or motion in what is represented has echoes in the motion of production.

A reverse process is also possible. Rather than semantics intruding on geometry, the formal graphic constraints may force us to revise our representations, as we saw in the portrayal of space. The upshot is that although they may be segregated, semantics and formal processes are ultimately capable of interpenetration, with semantics in particular intruding intimately into all aspects of production – form, direction, and sequence. At a later stage we will see that such intrusions are not restricted to semantics narrowly defined, but apply also to the broadest interpretation of meaning and intention.

6 Simple representational drawing

In the analysis of spoken language, it is a commonplace to distinguish between the literal meaning of what is said and the intention or the "sense." The first comprises the domain of semantics, the second the domain of pragmatics. If we apply this categorization to drawing, we might say that the analysis of how people represent objects and events they have been asked to portray lies squarely within the semantics of drawing. As we will see, however, one is obliged to conduct any inquiry into semantics with an eye on both the impact of formal executive processes and the social context of the drawing act, matters that are not themselves semantic.

The drawing task and its social setting

The task given to adult subjects in this investigation was simply to draw common objects. The 25 subjects were university undergraduates and junior staff of the psychology department who drew among them 100 common objects. Each subject was given a booklet of A4 paper, each page of which was divided into quadrants with a title typed in each: "ball," "bell," "belt," "bow tie," and so on. Each group drew a little over 50 objects.

Before describing some of the features of their drawings, I should like to comment on the broader context of the task, since the outcome cannot properly be understood simply in terms of the narrow specification of materials and instructions. It seems certain that average educated people in Western society produce more drawings in their first 15 years in response to the demands of educational institutions than during the remainder of their lives. This institutionally directed drawing can be put into three categories: First, there is drawing done as an accessory to other schoolwork – illustrating text, producing maps and diagrams, drawing figures for geometry. Second, there is drawing done in drawing or art class, presumably to cultivate drawing skill and to encourage "artistic self-expression." Third, there is drawing done as "recreation," drawing as a privilege or time filler. Drawing in this last context often joins music and to a lesser extent physical activities as a commodity to be offered and withdrawn as incentive and sanction.

It is only in the first of these three categories that drawing has an instrumental function; that is, that drawings are geared to some task other than production and perhaps display. If a graph or geometric figure is produced in mathematics, it is probable that the student will be using it or is supposed to be using it to identify terms, to illustrate relations, or to help problem solving. For the most part, however, drawing in pedagogical settings is not instrumental, but is treated as an end in itself or a sphere in which execution is a training exercise for later performances of the same sort.

The background of school drawing is relevant to research on drawing. When researching graphics, it is likely that we simply re-create the obligatory, almost motive-free drawing situation so familiar in the school situation: We provide chair and desk, drawing materials, and topic, and subjects move easily into the role. To a degree, the experimental situation re-creates the power relations of the pedagogical situation. It is significant that across all the thousands of occasions on which we have entered into this relation with adults and children, never has any subject asked the question, "What is the drawing for?" We will see in a later chapter that outside the school and the laboratory, drawers often have some specific cognitive or communicative task in hand. They draw to organize their thoughts or to instruct an audience. (This topic of the pragmatics of day-to-day adult drawing will be explored in greater detail in Chapter 11.)

Of course, acting as a "subject" for research psychologists has an independent history of its own. Some participants at least assume that the object of the inquiry is to map individual differences in graphic ability, or some personal characteristic like creativity or imagination. We found in the early stages of research that this led a few subjects to proceed in an idiosyncratic or obsessive fashion, trying, for example, to complete every drawing without raising the pencil from the page, and we therefore routinely established a low-key and practical approach, instructing subjects to proceed in a "straightforward way." The significance of these excursions into the sociology of the experimental drawing situation is that they bear on one of the central issues of drawing: the selection of features to be represented in drawings and the level of detail to be portrayed. When there is a specific task of communication, its nature will dictate the content and comprehensiveness of the performances. The same issues will apply that are enshrined in Grice's (1975) cooperative principles regularizing relations between speakers and audience: quantity, quality, relevance, and so on. By contrast, when a drawing is produced in a pedagogical frame or within the "motiveless" context of the unexplained psychological investigation, there are no local or specific task requirements to point subjects to one level of detail or inclusivity or another. We will therefore be asking what principles determine content under such conditions.

Before tackling this issue, I should like to link this inquiry to the questions raised in earlier chapters about formal executive constraints. If these constraints are held to be at all comprehensive, they should certainly manifest themselves in simple representational drawings; and they do.

Formal constraints in representational drawing

Fig. 6.1 shows starting positions and initial stroke directions for a sample of 16 objects drawn by 21 right-handed adults. This particular subset of objects was selected simply because the form in which they were drawn was consistent enough to permit economical summary, but the same effects are evident everywhere. Fig. 6.2 shows stroke direction from objects whose orientation is not conventionally determined. A pencil or a rake, for example, does not have to be drawn in an upright or horizontal position as does a milk bottle, a door, or a car. Strings on balloons and smoke from cigarettes are anchored to the main object but are free to lie in a variety of orientations. In fact, these lines tend to conform to the diagonal from top right to bottom left.

Do these consistencies in production have any impact on the drawings produced? It is remarkable how many objects, rulers, ladders, bats, chains, brooms, even peapods and worms are drawn reclining obliquely between 1 o'clock and 7. It is difficult to say how much this oblique orientation reflects an intention to show the object leaning or receding in depth and how much it is due to preference in line production. There is some representational (as opposed to geometric) justification for drawing an object in an oblique orientation, although semantics will not necessarily explain *which* oblique position. Although it is not so obvious with a narrow object like a ruler or a broom handle, the oblique position is often a way of displaying an object in three dimensions. This is clearest in the case of a cubic object, where horizontal or vertical orientation displays only one or two sides. Adopting a high viewpoint and turning an object with one edge toward the viewer exposes to view all three facets of the form. At the same time, the high viewpoint is most characteristic of the way we look at the many small to medium-sized objects in daily life. The main flaw in this argument is that quite often objects drawn in the oblique orientation are in fact *not* drawn in three dimensions, but more like a plane tipped up on one corner. Under such circumstances, we are invited to believe that this is simply conformity to preferred line orientation or a simplification of a generally used three-dimensional portrayal.

None of the representational considerations explains why the 1 o'clock to 7 oblique is so much more common than the 11 to 5. This certainly looks like a

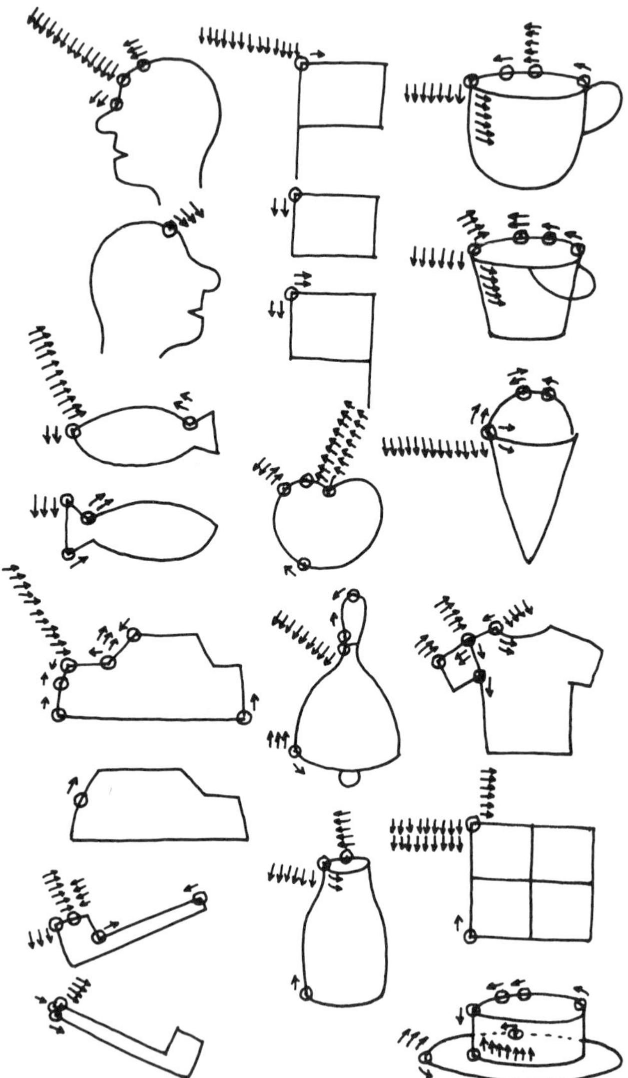

Fig. 6.1. Starting positions and direction of initial stroke in drawing a sample of common objects by right-handed adults. The outlines are in some cases simplified from the originals and in the asymmetrical objects (left, top center), two or three versions are provided since the orientation varied somewhat across the sample. See text for a discussion of the relationship between starting location and the direction in which these asymmetrical objects commonly face. The second to last object is a window.

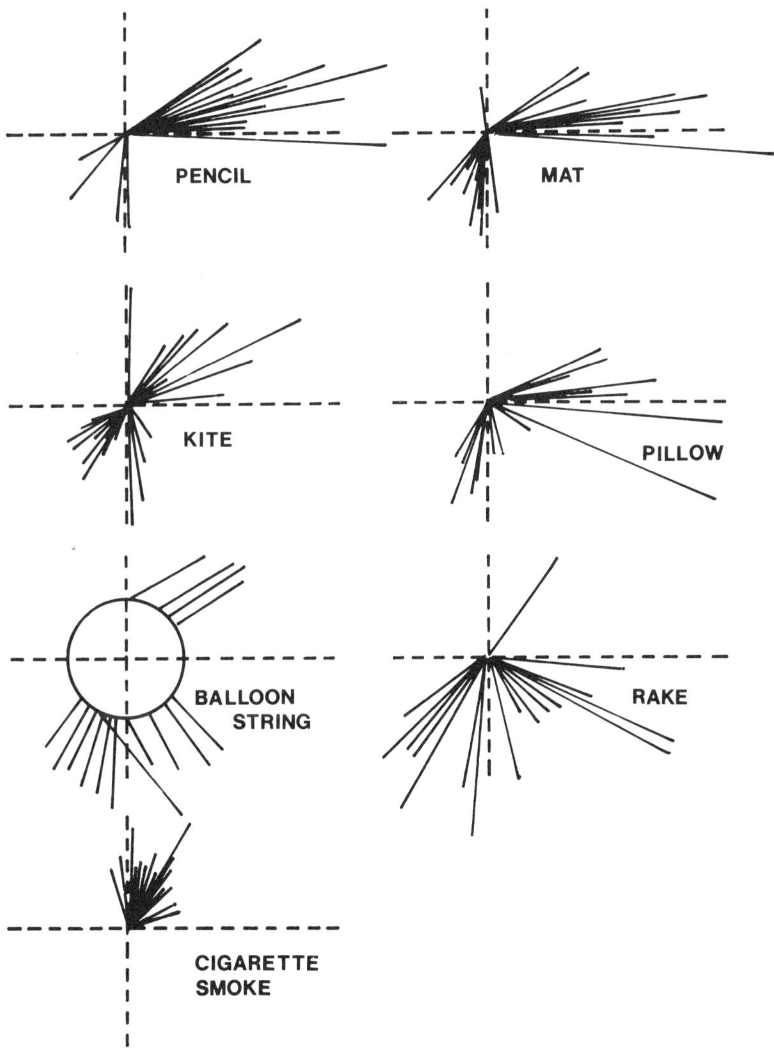

Fig. 6.2. First-stroke direction for seven objects in which the lines are not tightly constrained by semantics. In all cases, the stroke starting point is at the center of the plot.

matter of graphic convenience, and as I mentioned earlier, the tendency to have objects recede to the right is not restricted to untrained drawers.

The facing of objects

There is at least one other important characteristic of drawing of simple objects that can be attributed to formal constraints: the ''facing'' of objects. It can be seen from Fig. 6.1 that most of the profile faces (18 of 21) are turned to the left, as are most of the cars. Glasses have lenses to the left, pencils have points to the left, spoons and pipes have bowls to the left. On the other hand, most flags fly right, and cups and buckets have their handles to the right.

Does this reflect a visual preference independent of execution? One simple way to test this is to ask subjects if they prefer the appearance of objects in one orientation to another. This was done with a separate sample of 22 adult subjects. They were presented with a set of 8 × 15 cm cards on which were sketches of 30 of the objects featured in the drawing study, portrayed at the level of detail similar to or a little above that produced by the subjects. There were two drawings on each card, one an accurate mirror image of the other (Fig. 6.3). The subjects were asked to sort the cards into five piles to indicate visual preference. The criterion for sorting was whether ''one looks more natural or more normal than the other.'' ''Which orientation looks better to you?'' Cards to which they were indifferent were placed in a central pile; strong preferences went to the right and left, weak preference in between. Subjects were told to treat each pair as a separate judgment and not strive to use all categories equally. The relative positions on the cards of right- and left-facing objects were counterbalanced across subjects, and objects like pencils, brushes, and scissors, which do not have a canonical position like buses, cars, and cups were presented twice in different vertical orientations.

The first prediction I set up was that choice would be congruent with the way subjects drew objects. This was *not* upheld across the items as a group. Next I predicted there would be a preference for objects that slanted from top right to bottom left (33 of the 43 cards contained obliquely oriented objects to which this characterization could be applied). This was supported very weakly. (Sign test $z = 2.263$, $p < 0.05$.) Finally, looking at individual items (with confidence levels adjusted for the large group of items), we find that for a certain minority of items subjects did show a reliable preference: They preferred cups and scissors with handles to the right, balloons with strings to the left, flags with poles on the left, buses with motors to the left.

The only objects portrayed on the cards that in real life have an intrinsic right-hand orientation were scissors and TV sets, and subjects showed weak preference for right-handed scissors and a TV with controls on the right.(This latter pref-

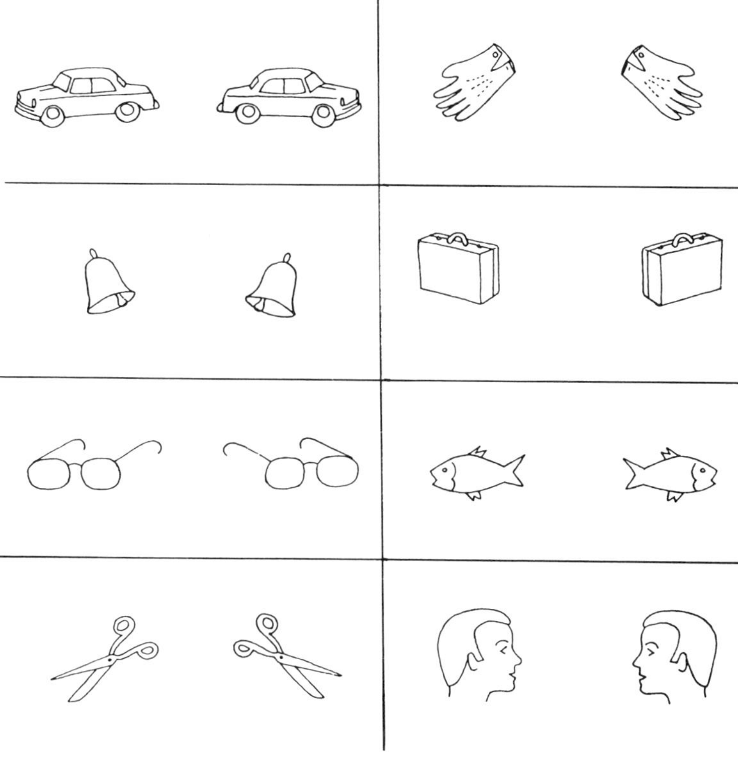

Fig. 6.3. Examples of cards used in tests of preference for visual orientation. Subject sorted cards into five categories indicating no preference or a strong or weak preference for one orientation over the other. Right-left position on cards was counterbalanced across subjects.

erence was shared by a smaller group of left-handers who are apparently not alienated by sets that require them to reach for the controls across the screen!) Next, right-handers prefer cups with handles to the right; left-handers prefer the reverse. (This element of "graspability" applies to the scissors too, confusing the outcome for left-handers.)

Finally there is the right-floating flag. This is perhaps the only item whose preferred orientation is related to graphic representation, and I have little doubt that the causal path begins not with visual preference, but with graphic execution itself. The first component subjects draw is almost invariably the flagstaff, on the left, and the borders of the flag, anchored to it, run out to the right. It is difficult to find a flag in any Western reference book that does not fly right (see for example, Smith, 1975). The practice has clearly become conventionalized, and the constant pictorial bias most likely affects visual preference, which is strong and consistent in both right- and left-handers.

Having established that direction of facing of sketches is not likely to be determined in the majority of cases by a visual preference, we can return to a consideration of the graphic forces, and here the principle used to account for the orientation of the drawn flag can be generalized. That principle has two aspects: (1) At which location on the *page* will a drawing start? (As we have seen, other things being equal, this is top left.) (2) At which location on an *object* will drawing begin? This will vary from object to object. When drawing a head in profile, subjects usually begin with the face, not the back of the skull, so profiles usually face left. A similar salience bias applies to cars, fish, shoes, pipes, glasses, cutlery, the spines of books, the quills of feathers, the blades of tools, the fronts of houses and kennels, the heads of dogs, crocodiles, birds, and so on. Conversely, all the details that are added to the body of an object – the handles of cups, pans, and buckets, the strings on balloons, the tails of cats and kites, wings on spectacles, feathers and flowers on hats – all tend to be anchored at their left ends and like the flag, extend to the right.

I should now like to leave these orientational aspects of the drawings and turn to three issues concerning their content: (1) How do the social context and expectations affect the outcome? (This has already been discussed in general terms, but will be examined in a little more detail.) (2) How are representational problems solved, in particular the issue of ''contrastive identity'' – that is, the need to key a simple drawing to the object it is meant to represent and no other? (3) How is the problem of gradation of detail handled? To answer this question, I shall have recourse to the idea of a ''profile of detail,'' a way of characterizing objects that shows why performances may differ quantally rather than continuously in level of detail portrayed.

Drawing in the laboratory

''Demand characteristics'' are familiar enough in psychology, and they apply to drawing as much as to any other performance. If in another context I ask subjects to indicate their tolerance of sensory isolation, it makes a difference to the outcome if they are civilians expecting to spend the afternoon in a laboratory and be home for dinner, or army personnel released from duty for a month to test their ability to withstand the stress of prolonged incarceration. Likewise, if I recruit subjects to serve as volunteers for an hour and present them with a booklet 12 pages thick each with spaces for four small drawings, they are unlikely to fill the first compartment with detail comparable to a Dürer engraving even if they had the skill to do so. The situation and our instructions place a firm upper limit on graphic obsessiveness.

It is mutually understood that the "audience" (the experimenter) is familiar with the objects being portrayed and will not be misled by simplifications. Hence in drawing a bicycle, the frame and the wheel spokes could be drawn as lines of the same thickness without undue concern. It is in this sense at least that the drawings are to some degree codified versions of the objects they represent, or at least depend on recognition of shared experiences.

Next, there seems to be an implicit "leveling" of the degree of detail from drawing to drawing. To take an example, one list of objects in this study included a bicycle and a baby carriage ("pram"); the other a car, a bus, and a wheel. When one counts the features portrayed or the number of strokes devoted to the one item common to all these objects – the wheel – we find that it varies over the range of 9 to 1. On cars and buses, wheels are shown simply as circles. On the pram and bicycle, the modal representation includes a rim and spokes; the wheel drawn alone typically includes rim, tire, hub, and spokes. Or again, a flower pot alone is rendered on the average with 6.3 strokes; when it is incorporated into a representation of a Christmas tree, the number of strokes is halved (3.1), with a corresponding fall in the number of features represented.

This does not imply that each drawer devotes the same quantum of graphic effort to each subject, but rather that the drawer effects a compromise: Complex objects require more complex drawings, but not in direct proportion to their complexity. This compromise may not in actuality represent a mechanical trade-off between complexity and the principle of least effort, but rather be due to a shift from internal to external contextual support for the interpretation of each component of a drawing as one moves from simple to complex subject matter. This idea should become clearer when we have explored the question of representational adequacy and in particular representational contrast.

Representational contrast

When a window is drawn on the front wall of a house, it can safely be portrayed simply as an unadorned rectangle. Proportions, size, number, and lack of contact with the boundaries of the wall define it as a window. If it were smaller and one of many rectangles, it might be a brick; if it were vertically elongated and anchored to the lower edge of the building, it would be a door. If it is very elongated and makes contact at top and bottom, it is a downpipe or a chimney. When, on the other hand, a window is drawn as a single object, not in the context of a wall (which itself is defined by the presence of a roof and even the window), it must be distinguished internally from similar rectangular forms representing mats, stamps, envelopes, table tops, football fields, and so on. Likewise, the wheel can be represented as an unadorned circle on a bus, but when portrayed alone needs the support of internal circumstantial detail: tire, hub, spokes. The minimal isolated clock face is not an empty circle as it might be on a clock tower or a wrist, but a circle or ring of dots enclosing an angled pair of hands. Without the hands, the circle could be a ball, a porthole, a ring, and so on. This suggests that given that the overall level of detail implicitly or explicitly set by the situation and provided by the drawer is low, the minimum elements are constrained on the one hand by support available from other parts of the drawing, and on the other by the need to distinguish the object represented from other candidates.

How is the contrast set of candidates determined by the drawer? The particular list encountered on a particular occasion is obviously important, as is the history of its unfolding. But with the very first object, the drawer must set a standard. The first object in one of our booklets was a "ball." Most subjects drew a circle with arcs within it representing pattern or perhaps reflecting the spherical shape. The first cylindrical object in the same booklet was a barrel. Most drew this with curved sides, and many drew staves or bands. Neither of these representations would absolutely distinguish the objects from a terrestrial globe on the one hand and a bongo drum on the other, but the items themselves set a level of familiarity that would ordinarily exclude these more exotic items.

The language of specification is an important source of orientation. "A clock" calls for a different level of specification from "an ormolu clock" or "Big Ben," and again this is not just a matter of the particular item, but of the context of all items as they unfold. Without having conducted the study, I would guess that "book" might elicit a different level of detail in the context "Grandfather clock, bowling ball, Union Jack, briefcase," compared with "clock, ball, flag, case." Nor is it simply a question of the specificity of objects as objects; the representational similarity in the context of the medium is important. In the current study, for example, "a box" follows "a block." Two subjects of a group of 12 drew both as unadorned cubes, but the remaining 10 added detail to identify the box: lids, internal lines, and so on. This situation repeats itself throughout the data, each object having its minimal hallmarks. A small circle set at one side of center turns a rectangle into a door, an arc above or to one side makes a vessel a bucket or a cup, a flame makes an elongated rectangle a candle, a double arc joined to the top of a horizontal rectangle identifies it as a suitcase.

Subjects working under such circumstances are not profligate with these identifying features. They portrayed a rectangular mat as a square with fringes, or with texture, or as a parallelogram (to suggest that it is a member of the smaller subset of rectangular objects that is flat and lies below eye level on a horizontal surface). Few drawers provided more than one clue at a time. A donut was always represented as two concentric circles or ellipses with added detail. It sometimes had an irregular outline, was dusted with spots (sugar?), or was shadowed or crosshatched to indicate contour, but rarely was more than one of these hallmarks present.

There is nothing compelling about this level of economy. It is traceable, as we have seen, to a particular combination of pragmatic circumstances that include the language and the scope of the specification of items and the range of their varieties, the expressed or implied attitude of the investigator, the type of materials supplied, and the announced duration of the experimental session. The pragmatic forces also extend outward to include the power relations between subjects and investigators in the university subculture and even perhaps to the society and to the cultural period more generally, which prescribes a certain restraint in obsequiousness. Subjects permit themselves to display skill gratuitously, but not effort.

At this same level of the "presentation of self in the drawing context" is another compromise: that between the demands of representational adequacy and consistency. A sudden change in the level of detail by a subject represents an admission of earlier misjudgment and raises the possibility of revision. In fact, no subject backtracked to amend a drawing that was rendered ambiguous by the nature of succeeding items or conspicuously upgraded the level of detail. Because the situation relieves subjects of any final responsibility for accurate recognizability (since, as I said earlier, the task is not crucially communicative), it is probably more important to press on without substantially altering style. In so doing, the subjects are implicitly throwing the responsibility back onto the investigator and giving themselves a vote of confidence in their initial judgments about the level of detail.

Prototypicality and aspect

So far my emphasis has been on discriminability within a hypothetical contrast set. This is not all that is involved in choice of level of detail. There is also a sense of "prototypicality." A passenger car without wheels is unlikely to be confused with a Christmas tree or even with a delivery van, but drawers do not omit wheels. Wheels are so important to the prototypical car that their omission can be construed only as a significant communicative or expressive act (or a joke). I do not wish to explore the details of prototypicality too far because I do not regard these details as central to drawing itself. That most land vehicles have wheels is a fact of technology, not a facet of the science of drawing. If one wants to explore why drawings of clocks have hands, those of windows have multiple panes, and those of aircraft have propellors, one is rapidly drawn out of the realm of graphics into the order of the world. In another generation clocks will have digits and windows single panes and aircraft will be jets. The explanation is not to be found in graphics or in the psychology of "prototypes," but in the technology of products.

There is perhaps one exception to this. James (1982) made the observation that simple representational drawings often have an old-fashioned touch to them, and this is to a certain extent my experience. Whether it is simply a transmission from older illustrated books I am not sure, but people do tend to portray trains as steam locomotives, and baby carriages are rather Victorian. I suspect there may be a number of reasons for this. First, the retreat from the modern is also a retreat from the particular. If I choose to draw a modern chair, I might be led into drawing my own furniture and find myself engaged in a memory search and an inappropriate level of realistic detail. In addition, many objects of an earlier period wore their function more transparently in their aspect. A steam locomotive did not conceal its crew, its fuel, and its combustive processes in the way a modern diesel does. The engines of buses have disappeared into a rectangular exterior, microwave ovens resemble television sets, and so on. So drawers may simply feel that the best and quickest way to provide a recognizable version is to call up an era when function was more evident from form.

Another aspect of prototypicality is the choice of *aspect*. Subjects so regularly dispose their objects in a recognizable orientation that we almost forget cups could have their handles toward us or be viewed from above, and so on. There is a great deal of agreement between subjects on the "standard aspect," the main differences being related to inclusivity (whether to include a holder with a candle), stylization (whether to draw a fish as a circle and triangle and a cat as three circles or to attempt a "naturalistic" version), depth (whether to draw a dog kennel front-on or in perspective, a ring in profile or rotated toward the viewer), and finally real-world variability, especially of objects like umbrellas and books, which can be portrayed open and in use or closed.

Profiles of detail

We have been exploring so far what might be called "the dynamics of the minimal." What happens when for one reason or another a drawer moves in the direction of including more detail?

I asked several adults to produce two sketches of each of 30 objects, the first more detailed than the second. The group of features omitted from the simple versions fell into a relatively small number of classes. First, there were what might be regarded as physical components of objects in the sense of concrete items: hubs on wheels, curtains on windows, holes in belts. These by no means monopolized the situation, however; and I shall mention five other categories of change: contour, texture, decoration or symbol, solidity, and numerousness of repeated elements. By *contour* is meant the delineation of the external shape or envelope by controlled, curved, or hatched lines rather than straight lines or smooth arcs. (In their simpler versions, objects were often built up from primitive regions: a car from a lower elongated rectangle with a smaller one joined on above it, a fish as a circle with a triangle for a tail.) *Texture* refers to marks that indicate the nature of surfaces: smooth arcs drawn within the boundary of a balloon, parallel ridges around a carrot, flecks on a basket to represent cane. *Decoration and symbol* include patterns and borders on clothes, designs on flags, and so on. They seem often to have been added to complex versions in order to be deleted from the simple. *Solidity* includes all efforts to represent surfaces and depth: using pairs of lines to delineate slender objects as regions and adding further lines to suggest depth. Sometimes the regions in the "complex" version were made opaque to contrast one surface with another. The "complex" objects also included more instances of a repeated motif: more teeth in combs, strings in racquets, spokes in wheels, pages in a book. Finally, subjects seemed to feel that a carelessly drawn version was "simpler," and many pairs of drawings differed only in this respect.

This particular technique of exploring the hierarchies of detail within subjects is not without its problems. What is remarkable about the transition from "complex" to "simple" is how minimal it often was, and how often the basic strategy of production was preserved from one to the other. Subjects complained about this task as they complained about no other. They seemed to find it a great effort to "push apart" the two versions of objects. As we will see in later chapters, drawers in general seem to have difficulty producing a really divergent version of an object they have already drawn. So with the exception of the changes associated with primitives – delineating contour *versus* rhythmical strokes and standard regions – many of the changes are rather cosmetic. For this reason an alternative technique, that of looking across a series of productions by different subjects, may be a more useful way for us to understand the range of possibilities in the selection of graphic detail.

Fig. 6.4 shows a sample of the variation in the portrayal of clock faces, clock hands, and windows across a group of subjects. The source of simplicity or complexity of representation here is somewhat ambiguous, since the economy may lie in the drawers' productions or in the reality of the object they draw. (Some clocks have nothing on their faces but four marks or four numbers; some windows comprise little besides a simple glazed opening.) But assuming we are working with a standard object of some complexity, it is possible to have more and more detailed versions of it. If we explore this range, we are likely to find the progression to be quantal rather than continuous, to rise in irregular steps. These steps are determined by an interaction between the profile of detail of the real object, the perceived effort required to negotiate this profile, and the incompatibilities among different devices for representing detail.

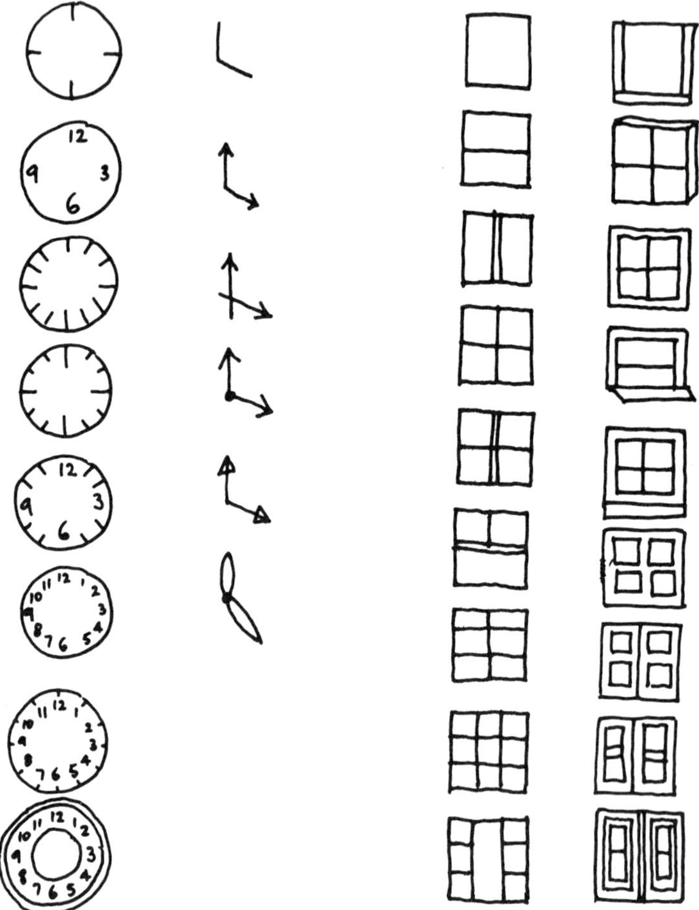

Fig. 6.4. Samples of clock faces and hands and windows from drawings of common objects by adults.

By a profile of detail, I refer to a hypothetical plot of the number or fineness of details from the grossest and most salient to the most intricate. In Fig. 6.5 there are four representations of a pocket calculator, each including more detail. If a decision is made to upgrade detail from one level to another, drawers commit themselves to a certain increment in observation, care, and sheer graphic work. For example, as one moves from (1) to (2), the portrayal of the lower keys of the calculator involves first their segregation as a separate group, and then the delineation of a pair of concentric boundaries. To move up to putting numbers and symbols on the keys or around them, or even more, to represent each key

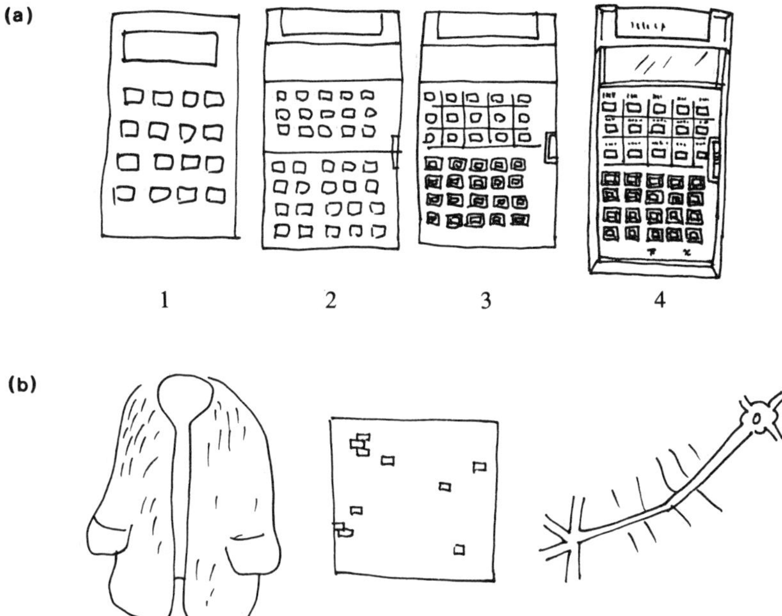

Fig. 6.5. (a): Four versions of a pocket calculator showing different levels of detail. (b): Detail can be shown economically by providing samples, often on an exaggerated scale (fur coat, brick wall, map with indication of multiple cross streets).

in depth, involves more work than was involved in representing the whole calculator at the simplest level. Of course, there are devices for achieving economies. It is common to move to a new level of detail by providing a sample of new features – a scattering of bricks across a wall, a few lines representing hairs on a fur coat, three or four lines running across a main road on a sketch map to indicate an unspecified number of cross streets. These economies are often signaled by a deliberate looseness of style (lower drawings, Fig. 6.5).

The graphic devices used to represent features at one level are often incompatible with a higher level of detail and have to be scrapped. So the continuous line expressing the boundary of a fur coat is out of place when all the individual filaments are to be drawn. Sometimes subjects add three-dimensionality to an object simply by duplicating the boundaries along two sides. In other cases, this change requires a fundamental revision of the strategy of representation. Moving to new levels of detail may require the whole scale of the drawing to be altered.

These various considerations – the physical reality of the graduated structure of the object, the priorities applied to each in terms of contrastivity and prototypicality, the amount of observational and graphic effort involved in representing each increment of detail, the availability of summary devices, and the occasional need for new scales and revised strategies of representation – all combine to provide what I call the ''profile of detail.'' It is along this complex profile, in some respects unique to each individual, that the selection process moves under the pressure of pragmatics.

7 Difficult graphic tasks: A failure in perceptual analysis?

It is never easy to prove in any graphic context that a failure in performance is due directly to a failure in perceptual analysis. There will always be a storage stage, however brief, between attending and acting during which information may be lost or distorted. Even when people are copying, they are continually switching backward and forward from inspecting the model to monitoring their own performance, and when the model is removed before drawing, as it is in many of these studies, storage must necessarily intervene.

Building a case for defective perceptual analysis in drawing is not made any easier by the ability of subjects to recognize relatively accurately designs that they cannot draw. Even when working from memory, they can usually select the design they are attempting to produce from a set of distractors in an "identity parade," even when the distractors are more like the model than their own completed versions. Subjects may fail to copy a design when given generous time to inspect it, yet it is inconceivable that they would fail to recognize differences between the model and even quite subtle variants of it under such inspection conditions.

Why then raise the issue of defective perceptual analysis as a serious issue? The first reason is that there seems to be evidence from the nature of errors in drawing and copying that something associated with perception is often involved. Second, the argument from recognition tests that has just been outlined is not as clear-cut as it may first appear. I will tackle the latter problem first and then turn to the data.

Recognition and analysis

The key to the "recognition" problem is structural redundancy. A design such as the "trinacria" or three-armed swastika [shown as (d) in Fig. 7.3] is susceptible to a number of different perceptual analyses: It can be seen as the letter "Y" with three arms added, as a set of three-angled components rotating around a center, or even as a cube with three sides omitted. Any one of these would

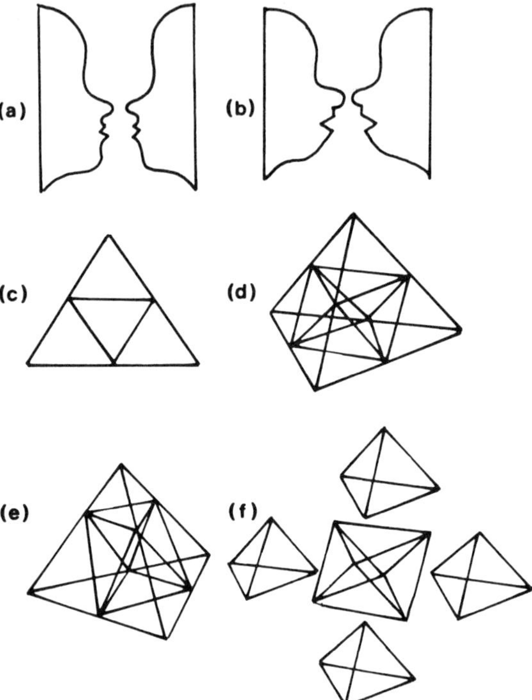

Fig. 7.1. The array (a) could be distinguished from (b) without the goblet shape between the two faces being perceived. Four frames shaped like (c) could be assembled into the tetrahedron (d), which in turn could be recognized as different from (e) without the internal structures shown in (f) being extracted perceptually. These examples illustrate that a perceptual analysis that permits successful recognition may not detect all the internal relationships within a model. Some of these relationships may be more useful than others in compiling drawings.

be adequate for recognition, but as we will see not all are equally suitable as a basis for drawing.

Put another way, there are many internal geometric relationships within complex figures, and any one subset of these may uniquely specify the design for recognition purposes. Fig. 7.1(a) shows one of the many multistable figure-and-ground illustrations found in psychology texts. A subject who fails to discern the "vase" or "goblet" in this picture may nonetheless easily distinguish the whole design from a variant such as (b). Fig. 7.1(c) shows a large triangle with a smaller triangle upside down within it. If four such units made of thin rods were assembled together into a tetrahedron (d), one could easily distinguish it from a variant (e) without noticing that it has an octahedron in its interior, or that the whole interior space of the object can be divided into an octahedron and four small tetrahedrons. The external characterization uniquely specifies the object. The internal structures, being in this sense redundant, are not necessary for recognition.

If we have subjects draw this construction, they could not put together the four sides correctly without incidentally portraying the internal structures. In the unlikely event that we could get a subject to see the figure only as a collection of subcomponents (f), drawing would be exceedingly difficult. The first perceptual analysis makes the production feasible, if not easy, and automatically ensures that the unnoticed internal relationships are intact. The second is complex, lacks cohesion, and would provide a precarious route to portraying either the internal or the external geometry.

This example suggests a way to define easy topics and competent drawers. A complex object may be easy to draw if it readily presents its most graphically useful face to the observer. The other side of the coin is that the graphically competent eye *may* be the one that routinely extracts from objects that internal structure which leads most surely and economically to a faithful reproduction. Such a skill could be based on specific graphic experience, as when sophisticated drawers use a perspective frame to organize rectangular or quasi-rectangular objects in space. They do not necessarily gaze at each chair, desk, or stairway trying to flatten it into a two-dimensional plane, but rather set their perceptual apparatus to organizing the object in three coordinates and their internal generating equipment into the corresponding routines calibrated to the needs of the case. When competent drawers lack appropriate learned strategies, they may exercise a type of graphic intelligence to solve new problems of perceptual analysis posed by complex subject matter.

Although such ideas about easy subject matter and competent drawers may seem plausible, even banal, I am not putting them forward as matters of fact. They are propositions that ought to be tested against reality, and indeed part of the present investigation addresses the question of whether competence can be traced to consistently felicitous perceptual analysis.

Returning for a moment to the structure of objects: The example of the polyhedron deals with a form for which there is one best interpretation that simplifies graphic reproduction. This may not always be the case, of course; much complex subject matter is less cohesive. To take a less geometric example, consider the drawing of a hand shown in Fig. 7.2(a). This object incorporates a set of internal relationships that are incapable of concise summary. They nonetheless have to be unpacked perceptually and resynthesized graphically. The details of Fig. 7.2(b) indicate some of the features of curvature and dimensionality that are essential for an adequate representation of a finger: The "print" surface of each joint has a changing radius of curvature that repeats itself to a degree with each segment. Each joint is of a certain length and at an angle to its neighbor. All

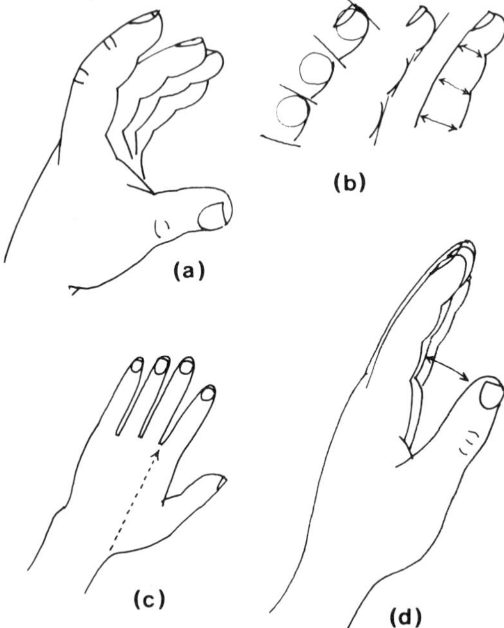

Fig. 7.2. Even a subject as familiar as the hand (a) incorporates internal geometric relations that normally pass unnoticed. To draw a finger adequately, one must simultaneously take into account regularities in curvature, length, slope, and breadth (b). When viewed from the back, a line projected upward from the wrist will commonly pass between the index and second finger (c), and when the "flat" hand is viewed from the side, the thumb is often held well forward of the palm (d). Such features usually remain unattended to by the owners of hands unless they have to inspect them for purposes of graphic reproduction.

must maintain a certain distance from the line that delineates the back of the finger, and so on. There is no geometric algorithm that solves these problems economically; the drawer must detect each feature and handle the heterogeneous collection simultaneously.

I do not believe that normal perceptual commerce with objects is adequate to this task. Nothing is more familiar to us than the backs of our own hands, yet most of us have a very inadequate graphic knowledge of them. Few of us notice that the line of our wrists on the thumb side usually passes between the index and second fingers of our hands, Fig. 7.2(c), unless perhaps we set ourselves to draw it; nor are we ordinarily aware that when we rotate our open relaxed hand to regard it from one side, the thumb may stand well clear of the palm, Fig. 7.2(d).

So far I have sought to establish that in spite of our success at recognition, perception may ill prepare us for representation. I now wish to illustrate the way that perception or decisions based on perception may penetrate into drawing and copying processes.

A study of imagery and drawing competence

The present inquiry began in the context of an imagery study. The question was this: Are "good" visual imagers better than "poor" in drawing from memory? The imagery test used was adapted from that of Slee (1976). It is entitled the "Visual Elaboration Scale" (VES). Subjects are asked to imagine an object (such as a cup on a table) and are then interrogated about the visual details of their images. The test has proved useful in predicting recall of appearances. In her original study, Slee showed significant correlations with visual memory tasks involving subtle variations in appearance of familiar nameable objects and in short-term memory for meaningless visual configurations. The VES was adapted slightly to group administration and given to 200 first-year university students. The 22 best and 24 worst performers on the test were given the drawing and copying tasks.

The VES scale turned out to be a very poor predictor of performance in either drawing from memory or copying complex designs. Good and bad drawers were almost exactly split between good and poor imagers, as measured by the scale.* The performance of subjects on the drawing tasks themselves, however, repaid the analysis, because they reveal perceptual and executive processes rather different from "imagery copying," and I will describe some of the individual strategies in a little detail.

The materials used in the study comprised an assortment of designs drawn in black ink on plain 12 × 8 cm cards which subjects had first to draw from memory and later copy. Several designs, such as a simple overhand knot, a figure-of-eight loop, a swastika, a three-link chain, and an unfolded cube, we can assume were quite familiar to the adult subjects. Some slightly less common designs were gleaned from anthologies of symbols (Dreyfus, 1972; Helfman, 1967; Hornung, 1946) and from commercial logos published in the press.

The designs may be sorted into two main classes. The first had a simple planar geometry. Three examples are shown in Fig. 7.3(a), (b), and (c). These items

* It is perhaps worth noting that Slee tested her subjects on the task devised by Brooks (1968) of naming corners of a printed "F." She found the *poor* imagers on her scale performed better than the middle or top group when they had to imagine the "F" and mark letters on a code sheet. Middle-level imagers were most disadvantaged. The top group showed intermediate levels of interference. As we will see later, there is some indication that competition between generating images and inspecting the already completed components of drawings may be involved in certain drawing tasks, so that at least on these items strong imagery may not be a particular advantage.

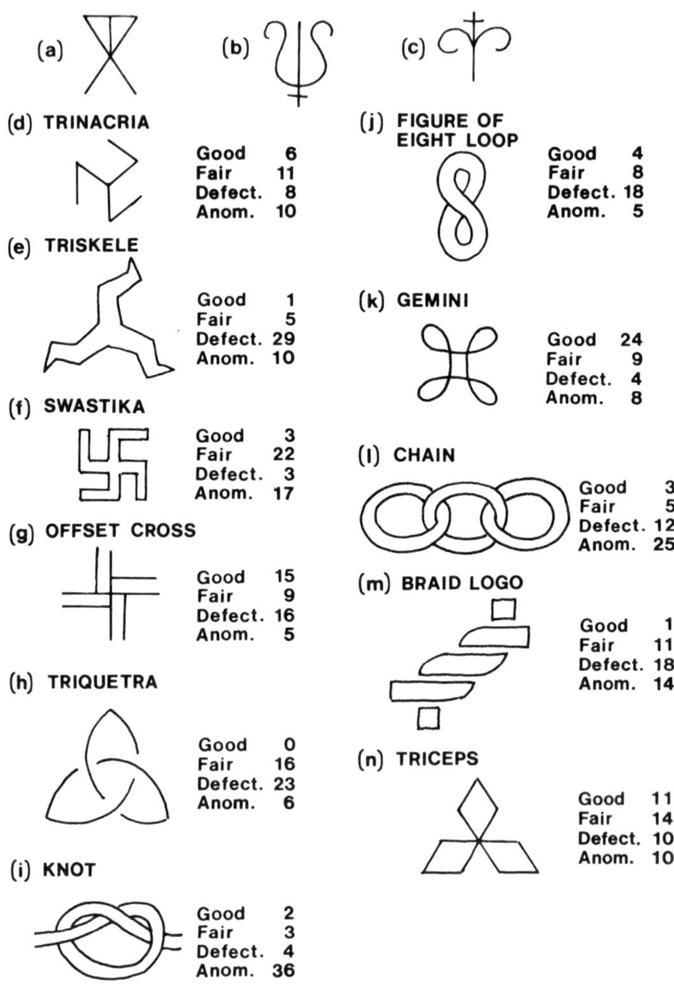

Fig. 7.3. (a) to (c): Designs of this type produce success rates of about 90 percent under 5-second inspection conditions. (d) to (n): "Difficult" items. These items were presented singly on cards to be drawn after a 5-second inspection. Later they were copied while the design was in full view. The numbers of subjects from the sample of 45 making a correct version ("good"), a version with misalignments or errors in important dimensions ("fair"), drawings with clear structural defects ("defect"), or a distinctly anomalous structure ("anom.") are shown. These values refer to drawing from memory. No consideration is given to how economical or "elegant" the production process was.

presented few problems to subjects either in copying or in drawing from memory (five-seconds inspection time immediately prior to drawing). They serve to establish that all the subjects had at least minimally adequate perceptual, memory, and graphic competence, and these items will not be discussed further.

A careful scrutiny of the geometry of the "difficult" items reveals certain recurring features that are usefully listed and described before we tackle the drawings made from them:

1. *Rotation of elements*. Most items are radially symmetrical, comprising a basic unit that is rotated and repeated three or four times. The swastika and three-legged triskele are familiar examples. There are five others among the set: (d), (g), (h), (k), (n). Note that "rotation" is an ambiguous term. It can mean a geometric property of a design or a process in a drawer's mind. We may find it convenient to describe a design as involving rotation, yet some subjects may not carry out rotation if they have a substitute structural interpretation to guide their actions.
2. *Serial anchoring*. Items such as (g) and (h) contain lines that successively intersect with their neighbors as they rotate. In (i) (a simple knot) and (j) (a figure-of-eight loop), this mutual or serial intersection appears without symmetrical rotation.
3. *Breadth*. The knots, the swastika, and other items contain double boundaries. When such boundaries are curved, subjects have to analyze the fate of the two edges by a type of mental rotation that tracks each line of the pair to its destination.
4. *Continuity and occlusion*. The Gemini symbol (k) is continuous without overlap. The triquetra (h) comprises a line that is continuous, but where it forms an intersection with itself, a gap is left in one component to indicate *overlap* or *occlusion*. In the knot, loop, and chain (l), the overlap is signaled by intersection of pairs of lines. In (m), which is a logo based on a two-strand braid, the designer has left gaps at the points of overlap to produce a stylized horizontal structure. This design therefore has two distinct levels of structure: the two-dimensional, which comprises an oblique stack of components, and the three-dimensional, which comprises two twisted and interlocking strands.
5. *Collinearity and parallelism*. The Mitsubishi logo [triceps, (n)] comprises three parallelograms meeting at a point. Their sides are collinear with those of other parallelograms at both the center and the perimeter. In the trinacria or three-armed swastika, the external arms are parallel to the central strokes.

This review by no means exhausts the properties of the designs, and other features will be mentioned later where necessary. Note that some properties like serial intersection or overlap are more fundamental to the structure of figures than those like parallelism, which may be neglected without doing topological violence to the design.

Attempts by subjects to draw these figures will now be reviewed. The first comment to be made is that the subjects, 45 right-handed university students, had great difficulty with many of these items. In the extreme case, only 2 of 45 subjects could reproduce a simple knot from memory even after inspecting a clear drawing of it for 5 seconds. Only 3 made a correct version of a three-linked chain or a swastika, and none could reproduce the triquetra properly. Even under copy conditions, several of the items were beyond the capacity of many. Of the sample, 18 of the 45 made substantial errors copying the triquetra. Half the sample made errors copying the knot, and many who achieved a reasonable facsimile did so by leaving gaps to be filled in with short makeshift strokes.

Five seconds is a short inspection time, but subjects treated it as if it were time enough to acquaint themselves with new designs or to remind them of those with which they were already familiar. The scoring procedure was not unreasonably strict. Items did not have to be elegantly drawn or even accurately proportioned. A "good" version simply meant that there were no topological anomalies, serious misalignments, or transparencies.

Although the values I have quoted testify to the overall difficulty of the items for this sample, they reveal nothing about the structure of the performances. That requires a closer examination of each item. The object of this analysis is not primarily psychometric; that is to say, I am not attempting merely to establish a system of scoring to improve the reliability of numerical values, or even to place them on more analytically valid footing. Rather, I have attempted throughout to throw light on the drawing process itself and the way perception and production are implicated within it. There is no standard technique of drawing analysis that will do this. Each design and each subject's version of that design must be examined stroke by stroke as they were compiled to bring out the sometimes unique logic of the performance. The whole philosophy behind the analysis is essentially *rationalist*. It does not conceive of subjects as simply more or less haphazard copyists, but as intelligent individuals working out the best solutions to graphic problems.

One of the daunting aspects of a project such as this is the realization that in studying attempts to reproduce a dozen or so forms, one seems to be trying to assay a forest by examining a fistful of plants. I do not believe that the proper response to this problem of scope is to back off into a more cursory study of a larger corpus, but rather the reverse, to push the analytic process to the limit and to leave it to time to show how general the products of analysis are. As we progress from design to design, principles of some generality do in fact emerge.

The spectrum of performances

I begin the analysis with an item of moderate difficulty, the three-armed swastika (trinacria). Fig. 7.4 shows a full range of attempts at drawing this form from memory. They are classified vertically into four groups: good, fair (adequate topology but failure to observe parallelism), defective (correct central intersection but inner or outer strokes incorrectly oriented), and anomalous (drawings in-

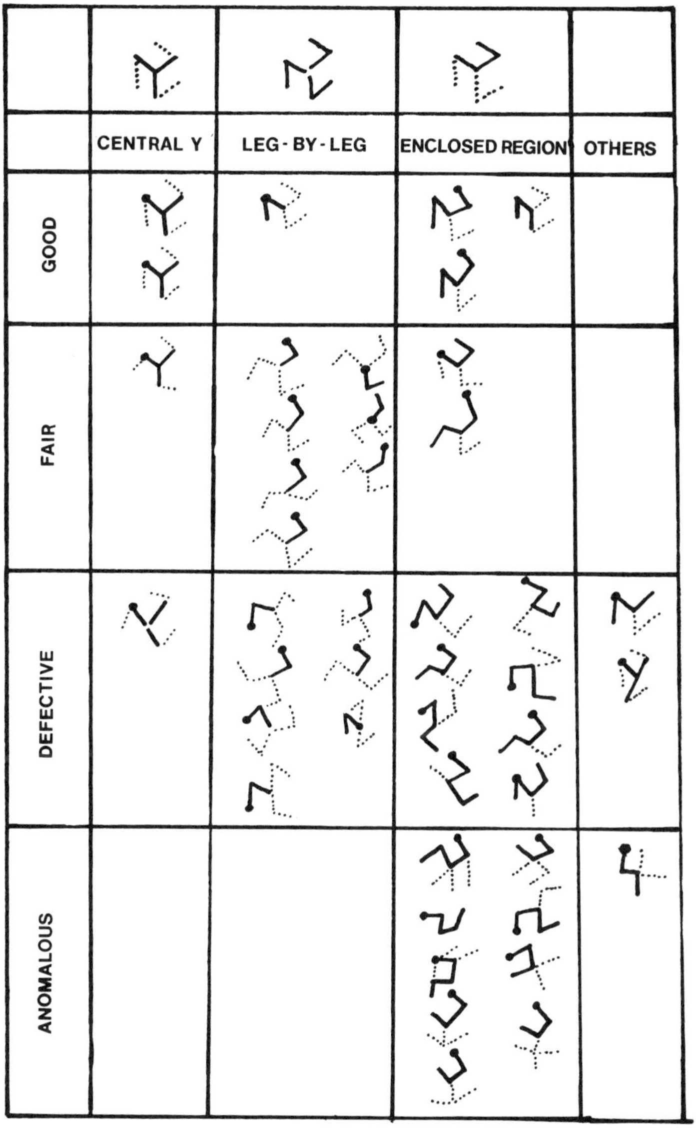

	CENTRAL Y	LEG-BY-LEG	ENCLOSED REGION	OTHERS
GOOD				
FAIR				
DEFECTIVE				
ANOMALOUS				

Fig. 7.4. Trinacria. Three principal methods of segmenting the figure are shown across the top. The horizontal divisions segregate the attempts to reproduce the figure from immediate memory into four grades. Dark lines indicate early strokes in subjects' performances. Circles show starting points.

corporating multiple intersections or no intersection at all). Fig. 7.4 is also organized into columns that indicate the structural approach, established by tracing the progress stroke by stroke. The three alternative perceptual segmentations are: (1) central Y, (2) successive arms, and (3) three sides of a quadrilateral region.

If one compares the production routines within each grade of success in drawing the figure from memory, it will be clear that the Y configuration is relatively more heavily represented in the "good" and "fair" categories. The strategy of constructing successive arms (drawn either out from the center or in from the periphery) is heavily represented in the "fair" category, in which parallelism of the outside strokes is not observed. The approach that begins with the building of a three-sided quadrilateral (with or without a side arm) is most common in the defective and grossly defective categories.

Rotation of elements

Why do particular strategies lead so often to substantial defects or complete confusion? First, consider the "arm-by-arm" strategy. Many defective drawings are produced when subjects recognize that there are three identical arms but fail to have them all rotate properly about the center, reversing the second or third arm. This is also a common problem with one of the most difficult items, the three-legged Isle-of-Man symbol, or triskele. Here too, subjects may construct a pair of legs in proper coordination, but fail to rotate successfully forward or backward to the final leg. Perhaps because the three-legged symbol has the configuration of a conventional human figure at its base, more than a third of the subjects began by drawing these two lower legs and tried to add a third above them. Six succeeded, eleven failed (Fig. 7.5). It is possible that some of the latter were seduced by a desire to have the upper part of the figure point to the right with the lower pair of legs. But the task of rotating the image of any angled element through 120 degrees while inspecting the sections of the drawing already completed is extremely difficult. (This is the Brooks effect, to which I referred earlier.) Some subjects appear to simplify the task for themselves by extracting only the feet from the rotation pattern, and there are instances of correctly oriented feet on wrongly oriented legs. The problem of mental rotation we have encountered in these two designs will reappear in other contexts, and we will encounter it in figures that are not radially symmetrical.

I might add that one strategy was even more prone to error than starting with the lower pair of legs, namely, that which begins by conforming to normal starting position at the top of the figure. Nobody succeeded in making an even passable design using this method, and all but one of the worst nine attempts adopted this approach. (There is, of course, a problem of direction of causation

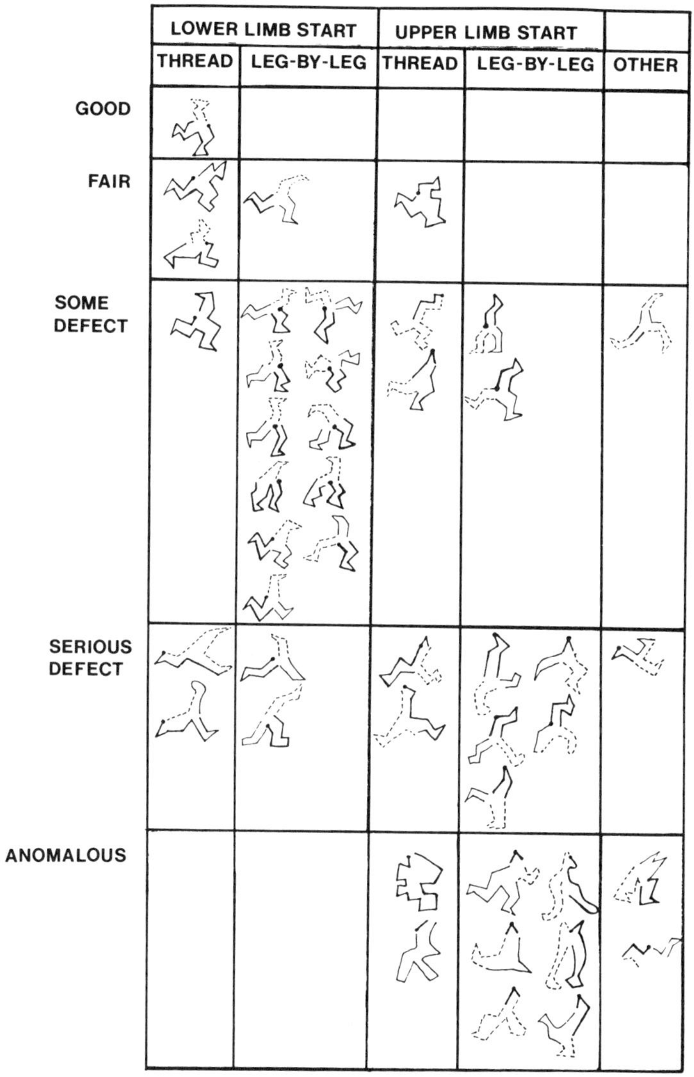

	LOWER LIMB START		UPPER LIMB START		
	THREAD	LEG-BY-LEG	THREAD	LEG-BY-LEG	OTHER
GOOD					
FAIR					
SOME DEFECT					
SERIOUS DEFECT					
ANOMALOUS					

Fig. 7.5. Triskele (Isle-of-Man symbol). The vertical divisions separate two strategies associated with starting location. Those in the left two columns start their constructions with the lower limbs of the figure, those in the middle columns commence with the upper. (Minor strategies are in the far right column.) The vertical subdivisions distinguish between those who thread a path beyond a single leg and those who build up the figure one leg at a time. Darker lines indicate early structures laid down. The circle shows starting location. The horizontal divisions mark the quality. In this case, the "defective" category has been subdivided into two. (In scoring, errors in orienting the foot are regarded as less serious than omitting the lower leg or rotating it in the wrong direction.)

here. Perhaps it is not the high starting position that causes difficulty, but rather that subjects who have not established a systematic approach have no reason to do anything but commence at the top.)

Remote consequences of early faults

I should like now to return to the first design, the three-armed swastika, to describe another strategy strongly associated with error, in this case the ''open box'' configuration shown in Fig. 7.6(a). The difficulty here resides in a subtle aspect of the design, the shape and orientation of the first region drawn. It is worth pursuing because it illustrates a common situation encountered throughout drawing and copying and is relevant to drawing tasks commonly used in studying brain damage and perception.

Fig. 7.6(a) shows the correct shape and orientation of the upper three strokes of the trinacria design. The area embraced by the strokes is a rhombus with an open side facing toward 10 o'clock. The only two strokes that can legitimately be built from it are the two verticals shown. The left vertical is the one most commonly chosen for the fourth stroke. If the three initial strokes have produced a region that is too square or faces upward, a vertical stroke, which is the next line needed, will form an acute angle, Fig. 7.6(b) and (c), that is unacceptable to the drawer on two grounds: First, no such acute angle appeared in the original; and second, the effect contravenes the equality of the three regions of the figure. Subjects therefore typically add a line at right angles, in Fig. 7.6(d). Once a rectangular ''dipperlike'' form of this sort has been produced, the situation is almost unrecoverable.

Many of the defective versions involved the addition of the final arm in line with one or other of those already produced, as in Fig. 7.6(e) or (f). This is not necessarily due to a misperception or distortion of the figure in memory. Rather, it appears to represent another attempt to conserve certain geometric properties of the design, in this case equivalence of shape among areas enclosed by the arms. The difficulty, of course, is that the rectilinearity of the first part of the drawing has left the drawer with 245 degrees to partition and a choice between three equally unsatisfactory alternatives: to align left, to align right (having in both cases three similar arms but a large open area), or to drop down vertically and sacrifice identity between the enclosed areas.

This speculative but very probable history of successive acts and decisions has been spelled out to illustrate the cumulative process common to much drawing by both adults and children. Certain figures and certain approaches make the initial orientation of lines disproportionately critical. An error at the beginning of the process of execution produces consequences that are geographically and temporally remote from the site of the original miscalculation. This becomes

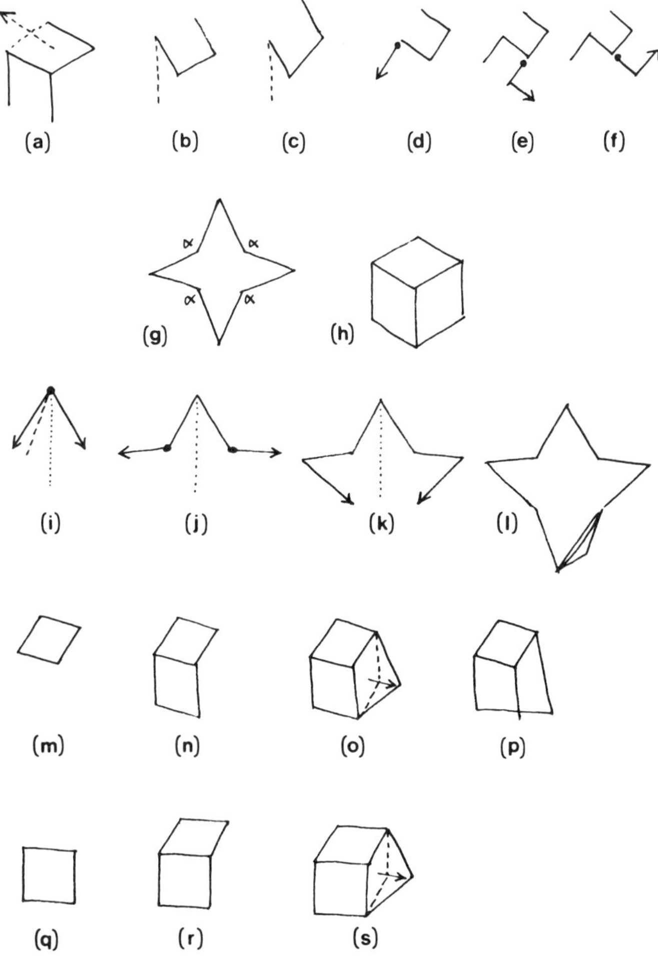

Fig. 7.6. Row 1: problems arising from drawing the trinacria from three sides of a quadrilateral (a). If the quadrilateral is misaligned (b) or distorted (c), it invites an oblique rather than a vertical attachment (d). Once this has been added, incorrect versions (e) and (f) are very probable. Similar cumulative effects occur in constructing the star (g) and cube (h). (See text for details.)

especially important when the location of conspicuous error is used as a diagnostic pointer in studies of brain pathology. Consider the two designs in the second row of Fig. 7.6, the four-pointed star and the cube. The star has relatively broad points. As a consequence, the four angles marked α are close to 180 degrees. In this situation, the orientation of the very first stroke the subject lays down will be critical. The initial stroke is almost always the left side of the upper point, followed by its right-hand neighbor. The two are usually drawn symmetrically about an imaginary midline, so that an initial stroke that is too far from the vertical, Fig. 7.6(i), is likely to be followed by a matching stroke to the right. Two strokes follow to the sides, drawn almost horizontally, Fig. 7.6(j), to achieve an appropriate angle α. The next two strokes drop down to make the width of the side arms of the star match the upper. Prospects for a clean finish have now vanished. Curved lines, gaps, and overdrawing supervene, and typically show up in the bottom right quadrant, where the drawing ends.

In the case of the cube, minor deviations in shape and orientation of the first-drawn face (usually the upper or the left face) show up in the last-drawn face at the bottom right. Subjects, having been shown a cube with three similar faces, draw the second face to match the first in shape and area. The result, shown in Fig. 7.6(n), is a pair of faces aligned at a very open angle, far from the ideal 120 degrees. The boundaries of the third face will be pulled out to the right, Fig. 7.6(o), or given a horizontal base, Fig. 7.6(p), in an effort to increase the area. This flat-bottomed effect, usually seen simply as a sign of "poor perspective," is found widely in the drawing of solids and is sometimes in reality a testimony to the drawer's faithfulness to one aspect of the design (equality of areas of faces) when confronted with a graphic dilemma that is ultimately traceable to an apparently minor misalignment at the commencement of construction. Perhaps the most common source of this problem is a tendency to start a cube or rectangular prism with a square or rectangular face (bottom line, Fig. 7.6).

Since the distortions of a conventional cube are usually found at its base, we tend to interpret them as a contamination of a perspective view with a side elevation view. This is not necessarily the correct explanation. As the facsimiles of Fig. 7.7 indicate, this expansion of the face of a solid can occur in many contexts, and may even be found in a face earlier in the sequence than I have specified as in Fig. 7.7(b). (The solid lines in these diagrams show actual lines drawn in a sequence from top to bottom. The broken lines show where strokes should have been made at each stage to preserve normal conventions of perspective. Arrows show departures from these norms.) It can be seen that distortions occur whenever earlier strokes set the stage for too narrow or too broad representations of faces. Historically, the striving after an appropriate balance in area among the sides of a solid at the expense of parallelism of its edges (or linear perspective) contributes to the phenomenon of reversed perspective. Reversed perspective, found in pre-Renaissance European art and in the art of many other cultures, involves the divergence of receding edges rather than the convergence with which we are familiar (Edgerton, 1976). In some cases, the artist wished to enclose an object (a panel, an opening, or even a reclining figure) on or in the receding surfaces, so the need for greater area was also a practical

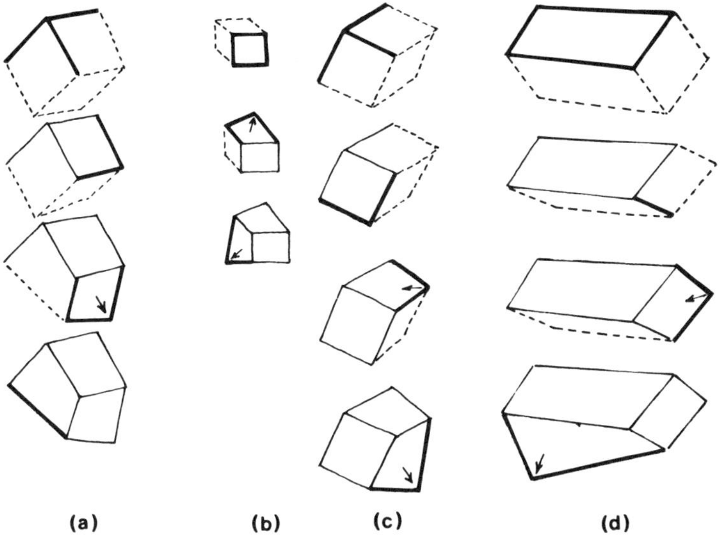

Fig. 7.7. Distortions of the boundaries of solids that arise from a need to preserve equality between areas of faces are not restricted to the lower edge of prisms. These examples are taken from adult subjects' drawings of prisms in various orientations. The dotted lines indicate the form the prisms would take if subjects kept edges parallel. Arrows show how edges are misaligned to control area. (Construction sequences are read from top to bottom.)

necessity. In the present context, it is a device forced on the drawers by early miscalculation.

This phenomenon of the "roosting of graphic chickens" is familiar to all who monitor production processes in children's drawings. Much of the charm of young children's draftsmanship arises from the compromises forced on them by the unanticipated consequences of earlier actions and from the pragmatic and unself-conscious manner in which they tackle the graphic problems so produced.

I will now proceed to the closer analysis of five further designs, each of which exemplifies a facet of the complex relation existing between perceptual analysis and production. I will then approach the question of individual differences, asking whether we are dealing simply with different perceptual analyses made haphazardly, or with a type of systematic perceptual selectivity by subjects.

Complex relations between analysis and error

The analysis of drawings of the Mitsubishi logo built from three parallelograms meeting at a point reveals a paradoxical linkage of strategy with success or error. Three major approaches emerged (Fig. 7.8). The approach of rotating around the three parallelograms produced more errors than successes. But the errors, when they occurred, were not gross anomalies, but misalignments of the components. The second common approach combined an upper diamond, a horizontal line, and the balance of the lower parallelograms. It was strongly associated with successful drawing, but also with a cluster of serious anomalies. The third approach was in a sense more analytic. It was based on the extraction of one or more radial lines crossing at the center. When all radials are used performance is usually good, but with one or two extracted there are many anomalies, presumably because the intermediate construction does not provide appropriate guideposts to action. This case indicates that it is not necessarily useful to classify a strategy simply as reliable or unreliable, because an approach that works in a majority of cases may in a minority lead to serious error. Should we embark on programs for improving this type of graphic ability by tutoring people in more subtle perceptual analysis, we might expect a certain unevenness in the outcome just because some drawers will extract structural frames they are incapable of exploiting and will occasionally end up with versions that are less satisfactory than a loose impressionistic attempt.

The triquetra (Fig. 7.9) resembles the two earlier designs in that it is radially symmetrical, but it has a three-dimensional quality. An otherwise continuous line passes over and under itself, producing a set of serially intersecting "lobes." It is a very difficult thing to draw and is susceptible to a wide variety of analyses by subjects. Six versions are shown in Fig. 7.9. No performances captured all the features of the model. When the continuous line was used or subjects constructed the figure from three arcs, they tended to omit the interlocking feature of the design. The continuous line also tended to sacrifice the pointed tips and occasionally led to the complete omission of the central region. The construction based on asymmetrical "lobes" rotated around, Fig. 7.9, produced the rare reasonably acceptable version. Other subjects using this technique made each lobe too narrow, and moving only a quarter of a full rotation at each step, produced either a four-lobed version or a form with an open side that the subject felt obliged to fill with a supernumerary tip. All the designs built from symmetrical V shapes, almond shapes, or a mixture of the two tended to lose the mutual interlocking of the design. The majority of anomalous versions, many of them scarcely recognizable, were pieced together in this fashion.

In the analysis of other designs in the series we have seen how the choice of a particular perceptual organization may predispose drawers to certain sorts of errors. In this instance, the choice of certain structures almost necessarily involves omission of features. Drawing three complete arcs or commencing with a com-

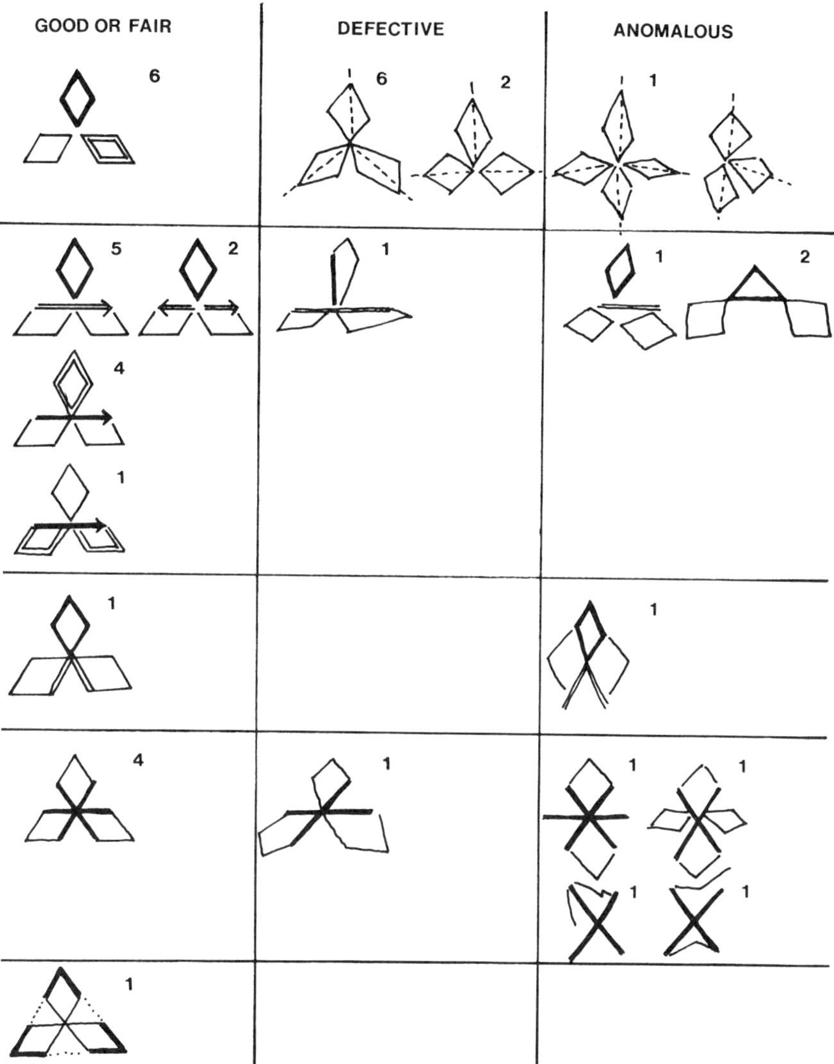

Fig. 7.8. Triceps (Mitsubishi logo). In this figure the four basic strategies and a variant are arranged down the page. Since all the "good" and "fair" versions were similar, they have not been individually reproduced. The values in the left column indicate how many "good" and "fair" versions were produced using each strategy. Likewise, in the two columns demonstrating defective and anomalous versions, numbers indicate how many instances of a type occurred among the 45 drawings in the sample. Dark lines indicate initial strokes, double lines intermediate, thin lines last.

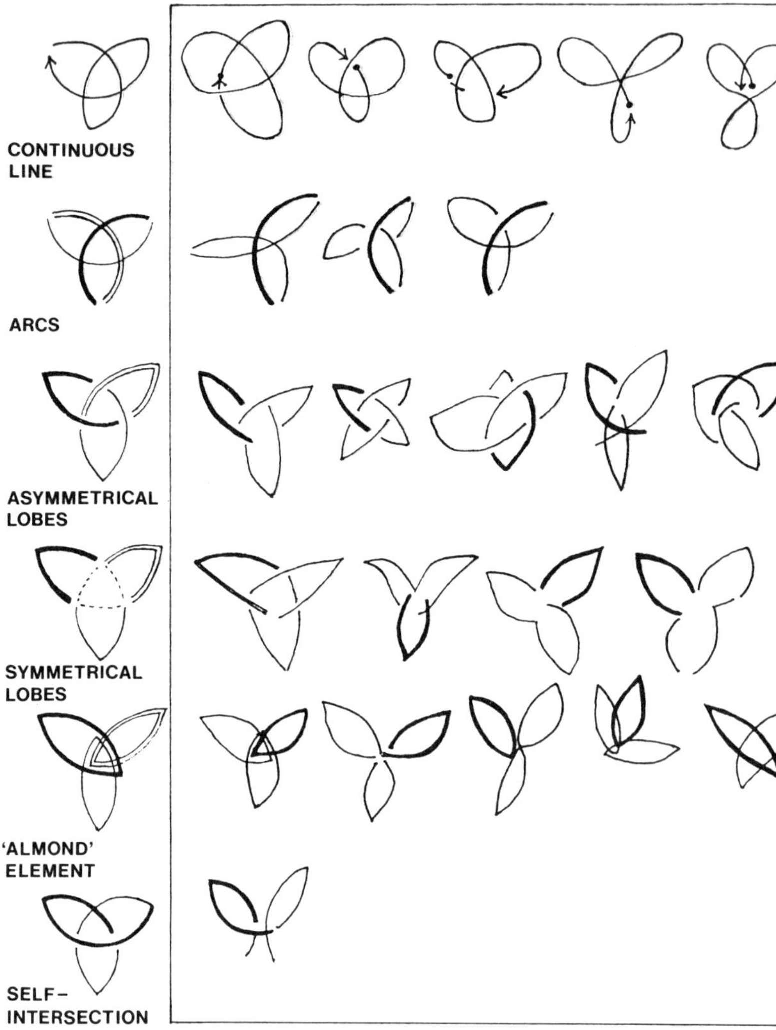

Fig. 7.9. Triquetra. No subject produced a faithful version of this design. The six major strategies used are shown in abstract form down the left side of the figure. Examples of these strategies in operation are shown. Dark, double, and light lines indicate early, middle, and late strokes in compiling the design. (The best version produced was that next to the model in the third row.)

plete petal shape renders incorporation of serial anchoring impossible. In this sense, the tactic produces errors directly and immediately.

Figures translated into a linear skeleton

Many subjects drawing the Mitsubishi logo constructed it by drawing a succession of three narrow diamond shapes and in the process lost much of the alignment of sides of the parallelograms that characterize the design. It is as though they had simply extracted the orientation of the long axis of each parallelogram and retained in memory the fact that each was a diamond shape. The synthesis based on this analysis produced a figure like an upside-down Y with narrow diamonds for arms.

This extraction of the center or axis of a solid figure as a skeleton for reproduction produces its own peculiar difficulties. It can be seen most clearly in the reproduction of the solid swastika. The swastika, probably the most familiar graphic design, yielded a surprising range of defective drawings, 20 of the 45 failing to preserve the distinctive geometry of the figure and only 6 representing the form without shortened arms, offset central intersection, or transparency. One group of subjects proceeded to thread their way around the complete outline, or tried to construct it arm by arm in a rotary journey around the design. The other significant strategy was the familiar one of building the swastika from two zigzag components at right angles, or laying down one zigzag to which extra arms are added. (Only two subjects began by laying down a central cross and adding arms to it.)

The two principal strategies were prone to different types of error. In the case of threading or working arm by arm, subjects utilized a subroutine that had to be rotated through successive 90-degree angles. Some subjects simply failed to keep the routine intact even on the rotation to the second arm, or failed to segregate the new arm from the strokes of that preceding it. Others fell victim to the perceptual difficulty mentioned above of interpreting regions as lines or axes. The four regions enclosed by the arms of a swastika composed of single lines are squares. When the lines are broadened into regions, these areas must become rectangular (Fig. 7.10, top). Therefore if one moves around the figure enclosing squares, as several did, a discrepancy in alignment inevitably develops so that opposite arms do not coincide at the center. If the error is small, the subject may manage to close off the figure without losing the perceptual integrity of the whole. But if the arms are broad and the interior regions made square, by the third arm the alignment is likely to be so distorted that the subject loses the overall pattern and has to resort to ad hoc accretions.

Ironically, it is the subject who is most scrupulous about the length of external arms who is most likely to make this error. This is a classic case of how the

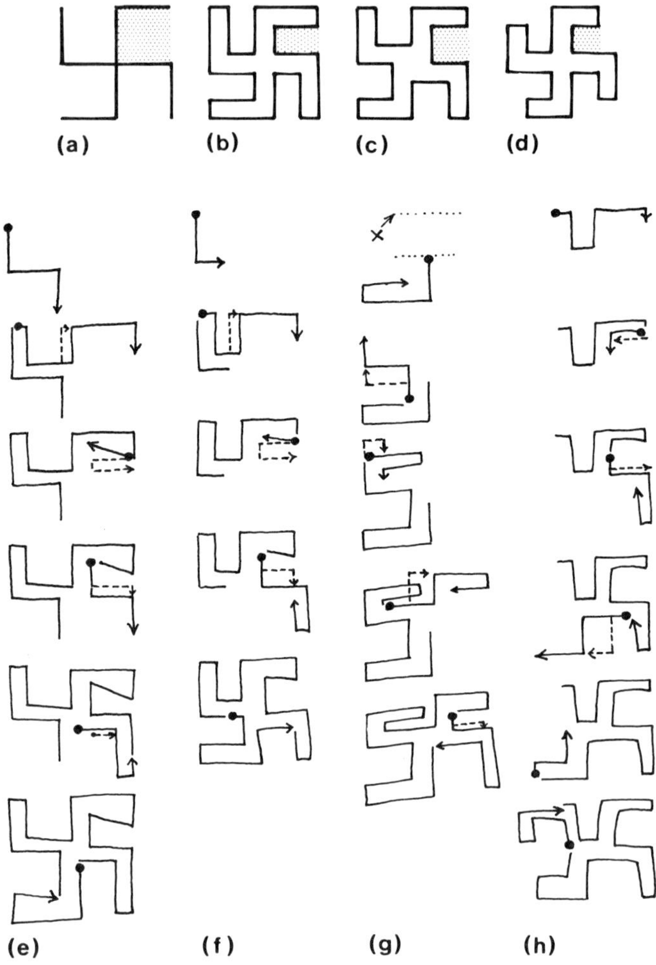

Fig. 7.10. Swastika. *Top:* The areas enclosed within the arms of a swastika composed of single lines (a) are squares; the corresponding regions in a broad swastika are elongated (b). Any attempt to enclose squares in the arms of a broad swastika is likely to result in misalignment of the central cross (c). The problem is not encountered if the outer arms are abnormally short (d) or if the figure is built from a cross or zigzag. *Bottom:* Flowcharts (to be read from top to bottom) showing the step-by-step development of misalignment. In two cases, this led to anomalous figures. Broken lines show hypothetical moves that could have preserved some alignment at each stage. Lines actually laid down usually have some logic to them, given that the aim is to enclose squares within arms. Subject (g) appears to have set an upper boundary (x) to the figure, affecting the third stage of the drawing.

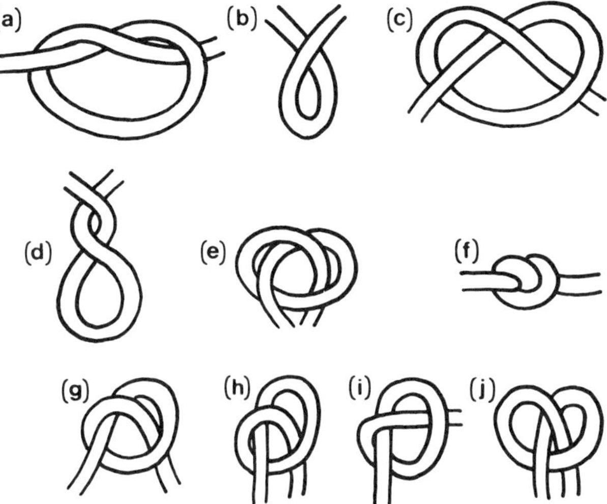

Fig. 7.11. Single overhand knot. (a): Knot to be copied or drawn from memory. (b) Loop with single crossing. (c) Knot in "pretzel" position, with three crossings clearly displayed. (d) Double loop. (e) to (j): The same knot in six alternative configurations.

failure to isolate a redundant internal relationship during perceptual analysis becomes critical when one rather than another graphic strategy is adopted. Subjects can protect themselves against this by monitoring the central alignments, but many appear to assume that threading or rotation around the figure using a standard subroutine is safe and will ensure a proper outcome.

Finally, a few words about the strategy based on one or two zigzags. First, the initial component may or may not be correctly formed. Some subjects, in trying to recall the figure, felt that the components must be more complex than simply three strokes and added a fourth or fifth. Others used two similar and correct components, but crossed them at the wrong point. A large group tackled the problem by laying down one zigzag and adding two angled components to it. The lack of geometric cohesiveness between these added pieces made this a risky maneuver for the less accomplished subjects.

The knot, a problem of enactive knowledge

The next item, the single overhand knot (Fig. 7.11), represents a new departure first because it is not radially symmetrical, and also because it represents an object that each of us has seen and constructed thousands of times. This means that along with visual perception, we must take into account a type of *enactive* knowledge.

The most common product in drawing the knot from memory was in fact far removed from the model; it comprised a simple loop with two free ends. Such loops were themselves drawn in a variety of ways, but they all appear to represent a stage in the production process from which the subjects could see no adequate way forward, and in fact what the subjects had constructed was simply topologically incompatible with an adequate portrayal of a knot. The loop they produced is weakly related to a knot: It incorporates a rounded section and one intersection. A knot, on the other hand, incorporates three crossings in an alternating series.

It is here that we encounter a question of belief based on action rather than on visual observation. After reviewing some of the drawings, I conducted the following inquiry with 10 intelligent adult subjects. I showed them a knot in a cord, then a simple loop, Fig. 7.11(b), pointing out that the loop had a single crossing. I then asked for a snap decision about how many crossings there are in the knot (which I had in the meantime untied or concealed). Nine of 10 subjects unhesitatingly said, "two." Some needed considerable convincing that there are in fact three. The most eloquent way to achieve this was to bring the free ends of the knot down toward the classic "pretzel" shape, Fig. 7.11(c). Even then some wanted to argue that I had surreptitiously tied a different knot! Subjects seemed to agree in retrospect that their belief arose from *tying* a knot, which they said involves making one strand pass "over and under the other." (The most salient of the three crossings, that in the middle, is not immediately connected to the loop below it. Instead, the loop surrounds this intersection and connects to its upper arms, passing over or under the free ends in the process.)

So when subjects approach the task, they are in a curious situation. They are capable of recognizing a knot and distinguishing it from a loop, Fig. 7.11(b), and a double loop, Fig. 7.11(d). They extract certain features, including the crossing, the loop, and the free ends. They probably have a perceptual impression of some reversed curvature and of a level of complexity involving more than one crossing. They also have a belief based largely on action that there are not as many as three crossings. In Fig. 7.12 I have ordered the subjects' actual attempts to reproduce the knot in a series from simple to complex. Using these versions, one can piece together how these ingredients of perception and belief interact with executive processes and mental manipulation to produce the various outcomes.

Tracking pairs of curved lines

Two subjects using a pair of parallel lines to portray a knot allowed them to cross (line 2 of Fig. 7.12). This is an elementary example of a common per-

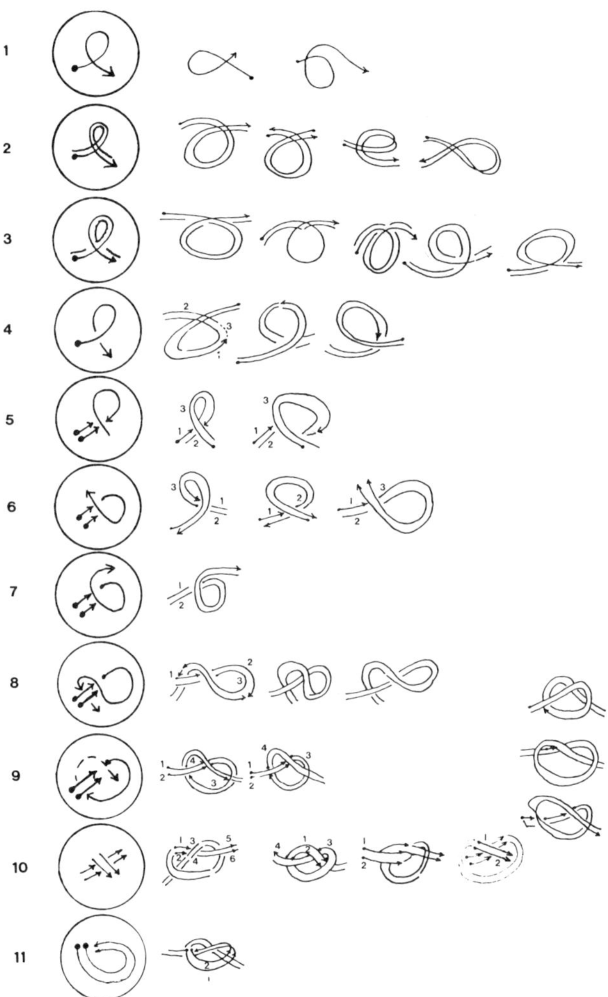

Fig. 7.12. Single overhand knots. Facsimiles of attempts to reproduce the knot from memory. They are arranged from the top: (1) single loops, (2) double loops, (3) single loop with interrupted line, (4) line doubling back upon itself, (5) end of strand with line crossing, (6) gap with line doubling back on itself, (7) strand going to right after traversing gap, (8) strand going left after traversing gap, forming double twisted loop, (9) strand passing below gap, returning through it, (10) to (12) various successful or near successful strategies. Dot and arrowhead indicate first stroke, numbers indicate order. Circles enclose summary of basic strategy.

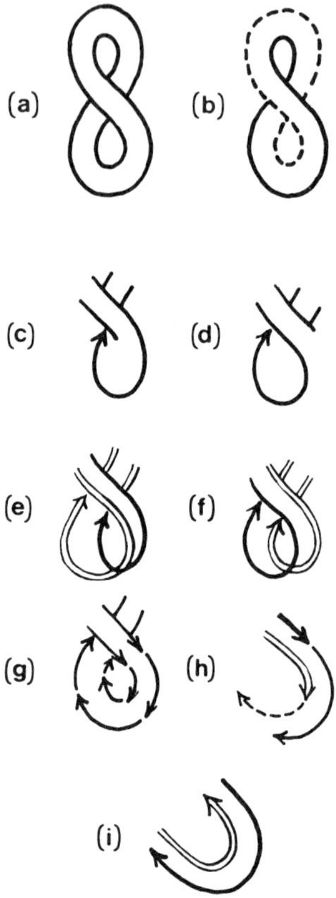

Fig. 7.13. Figure-of-eight band. The symmetrical band (a) is composed of two asymmetrical lines (b). Moderate curvature either brings the outer stroke into alignment with the inner (c) or the inner with the outer (d). In either case, the next stroke must cross (e) and (f). Three strategies to minimize this are small strokes advancing in pairs (g), ''pathfinding'' with one stroke or the other (h), and ''backtracking'' (i).

ceptual-motor problem, that of tracking a pair of parallel lines curving through 360 degrees to their destinations. It represents a variation on the mental rotation process mentioned earlier. I should like to digress for a moment to pursue this question of rotation, using another simpler figure, the ''figure-of-eight'' band (Fig. 7.13). Almost two-thirds of the subjects attempting this design from memory failed to produce a fair version, and in all cases the problem arose from a difficulty in identifying the fate of a pair of lines curving back upon themselves.

First note that the figure-of-eight design, although symmetrical above and below the midline, comprises two interlocking lines each having a larger radius of curvature on one side of the crossing than the other, Fig. 7.13(b). Next note that in order to render these lines correctly, the inner must rotate tightly back on itself while the outer must follow a more generous curve onto its partner, Fig. 7.13(d). When an intermediate degree of curvature is adopted, the rotation leads in either case to an incorrect destination, Fig. 7.13(c), (d), and the situation shown in Fig. 7.13(e) and (f) results. If the two lines could be made to wheel around together, the probability of error would be minimized. The cautious performers will in fact advance the pair of lines in small steps. Two other common tactics are widely used in such cases. One may be dubbed "pathfinding" in which the lines take turns in progressing into unknown territory, Fig. 7.13(h). The other I have termed "backtracking," where one line is taken to a goal and its partner is drawn backward from that goal, Fig. 7.13(i).

Returning now to the knots of Fig. 7.12: The real action begins in row 6 with the appearance of gaps *through which the curving lines return*, a maneuver that involved the tracking of curved double lines described above, with each line having to make contact with an appropriate side of the gap. Ironically, once this return has been negotiated successfully, the situation is at an impasse. There is no way to proceed to produce a successful version of the knot. One subject (number 9) curved tentatively to the right, producing an eccentric loop. The three in line 8 reversed curvature to the left, passed "under" their first strokes, and so produced a representation of a double twist.

The key to the problem is that anyone who utilizes gaps must make two, judiciously placed, *or must resist the temptation to return immediately and directly through the gap recently made*. One promising strategy is to leave a gap, then pass under the strand *below* the gap and return through it from above (row 9). This course of action is demanded by the circumstance mentioned earlier that the central crossover in the knot lies *within* the loop and not above it, and so has to be approached from its upper side. Not only is this action rather complex in itself, but it arises at a point in the process of execution when subjects are most immersed in the task of rotating the two lines of the loop appropriately.

All these difficulties serve to illustrate an important and obstinate problem of memory for designs. Unless drawers have extracted the essential features from a design, they seem incapable of reconstructing it. We and they tend grossly to overestimate the capacity of the imagery process. Drawers tend to launch themselves into a production routine hoping that it can be relied on to achieve the desired effects of partial or complete graphic goals. If it does not do so, they seem incapable of retrieving the original design, unless it is very simple. Even after analyzing in detail dozens of versions of drawings of the knot and drawing it myself many times, it is extraordinarily difficult to visualize it. The information I use myself to reproduce a knot is largely procedural, backed up by some quasi-visual representations of features, themselves linked together by conceptual knowledge. The "window" of visual imagery is extremely narrow and seems not to widen even after long experience.

The remaining seven drawings of the knot, which include the two essentially correct versions (albeit one is left-right reversed!), provide us with a further surprise because they were produced largely by unorthodox means and are not natural extensions of the process I have been describing. Four of them, including the two best, did not commence with a free end of the knot at all, but with the loop or an interior strand within the crossover complex.

At the risk of trespassing on what is to come, we might ask: Who are the nine producers of these successful or near-successful performances? They certainly are not people who have learned a standard trick for producing a knot facsimile. No two follow the same strategy. Nor, it appears, are they a random assortment of people of varying ability who by chance have stumbled on the fact that starting points *within* the knot are safe bets for successful performance. Five of them are among the top eight performers across all tasks. They are either cunning drawers who know best where to begin, or virtuoso performers who can succeed no matter how they start!

Mathematical analysis

Before leaving the task of drawing the knot, I should like to ask whether or not the difficulty of this task can be accounted for in purely topological terms. I do not believe that the problem it presents is simply topological, because the triquetra (Fig. 7.9), the pretzel-like cousin of the simple knot, has an almost identical topological structure (it is simply a knot with the loose ends joined), but it is graphically easier to handle because the three crossover points are equally salient and are thus unlikely to be misread by the viewer.

It is imaginable that a general theory could be generated to deal with the drawing of all knots (trivial and otherwise), braids, and loops as an extension of knot and braid theory. This may be so, but as I have intimated, the theory could not rest simply on mathematical definitions at the level of knot theory. All the knots in the lower part of Fig. 7.11 are topologically equivalent, but they represent quite different *perceptual* arrays. Consequently, they are approached differently by drawers and represent a wide range of difficulty.

To review the situation so far, we have seen that drawing performances appear to follow one or another perceptual organization of a design. This is made possible by the fact that the designs themselves contain not only a cluster of features, but a variety of alternative internal structures, more than one of which can form the basis for a drawing strategy. Certain structural analyses can hardly be used at all without producing errors (for example, using complete arcs to portray the triquetra). Others predispose drawers less inevitably to errors, and these errors may be basic or trivial.

Sources of error arise not just from the perceptual analysis alone, but from an interaction between that analysis and the processes involved in compiling the drawing. The problems associated with mental rotation show this clearly. The first step in a drawer's program is to interpret a design in terms of rotated elements; the second is to develop a suitable subroutine for generating an element; and then that routine has to be repeated in varying orientations and integrated with the strokes already laid down. A faulty subroutine can subvert the drawing process profoundly (as happened for many subjects trying to produce the swastika).

In many cases, perceptual analysis is manifestly deficient. Subjects frequently overlook important relationships, such as the vertical asymmetry of the lines making up the figure-of-eight loop, the alignment of sides of the Mitsubishi logo, and the three-dimensional aspect of the twisted braid symbol. They may not be able to identify the correct shape of subcomponents to which they have reduced a design, or they fail to discover how they are coordinated. It may be, as occurred in the case of the knot, that they bring to the situation an almost unshakable but mistaken belief about the object based on everyday experience of manipulating it.

Another important principle that emerges is the fact that early steps in compiling a drawing may lead to trouble at a later stage and in a different location. This showed up clearly in the examples of drawing cubes, the four-pointed star, the swastika, and the three-armed trinacria, where a slight misalignment of a component can lead to substantial changes in strategy, and in turn to anomalous graphic products. In all the cases we have examined, the history of degeneration or collapse of drawing arose to some degree from attempts by the drawer to honor some relationships recognized in the original model, such as the segmentation of space or the identity of certain elements.

When a subject incorporates a feature in a drawing, we can make a minimal estimate of what perceptual analyses must have preceded the drawing. When subjects *fail* to incorporate features or restrict themselves to one type of structural analysis, it is not easy to specify how impoverished the original perceptual analysis was. To state the matter conservatively, I have simply been arranging drawings into taxonomies reflecting one structural analysis or another. When available information is not utilized by subjects, can we specify why with any assurance? Were the alternative analyses ever made? Were they made but rejected as unsuitable? Might subjects extract features and structures but fail to recall them? Could they be distracted from using them, or find it impossible to integrate them into their strategies by virtue of the particular executive path they have chosen to follow?

The role of perceptual analysis

One approach to these problems is to consider whether there is some regularity to the manner in which a particular individual utilizes perceptual analyses across a spectrum of problems. I should now like to address this issue. The question may be expressed in the following way: Given that success or failure in drawing may depend on the particular perceptual organization used, and given that two or three different perceptual readings of a design may be equally possible, does this imply that success depends largely on the accidents of perceptual analysis?

A contrary (but not necessarily correct) view I expressed earlier was that the sophisticated drawer might perhaps be the one who knows which of a number of perceptual organizations to prefer and follows the analysis that is graphically most promising. If that were the case, we would have to assume that the better performers do in fact extract more than one structure and make a choice between analyzed alternatives.

Good and bad drawers

The problem needs to be approached in two stages: First, to ask whether it is safe to assume at the outset that there are in fact "good" and "bad" drawers. In a sample of 45 subjects randomly performing, some are bound by chance to achieve higher total scores than others. So an analysis to establish whether some do in fact perform consistently better or worse than chance must precede any inquiry about the sources of possible "talent" or "disability." If consistency is proved, the next question is this: Have the good drawers consistently followed more promising perceptual analyses, or do they simply make the best of the analyses they happen to select?

Before embarking on these two analyses, let me briefly review one or two technicalities: First, all scoring in the study was done "blind." Personal details (age, sex) as well as scores on the imagery test were filed until scoring was complete. The only information on protocols was a code number. Each design was analyzed independently from the others to avoid halo effects, and so on. Although the four categories – good, fair, defective, and anomalous – were used for all designs and given similar numerical values, no attempt was made to equalize the proportions of scores in each category across designs. These were based initially on judgments of how serious the discrepancies from the models were in each case.

A standard approach to the question of whether there are indeed consistently good and consistently poor subjects is simply to inspect the range of scores. There were clearly some outstanding performers at both ends of the scale on this criterion. Within a range of scores from 8 (all anomalous) to 32 (all good), seven subjects were within 5 points of a perfect performance, and five subjects were equally close to a minimum score. Another criterion is to ask whether the item scores are highly intercorrelated across subjects, since this would indicate that we are tapping a relatively unified skill with real and systematic variation across subjects. The intercorrelations between items were, in fact, consistently high. We can therefore proceed to an examination of "good" and "poor" groups, and it is probably safe to consider the top and bottom 10 subjects as distinctly different in competence.

Can we now give an answer to the question, are good drawers those who select graphically more appropriate strategies? Unfortunately, we cannot proceed to a quantitative answer to this question because we are locked in a tautology. We define good drawers as those who succeed and good strategies as those characteristic of good drawers! We cannot even solve this problem by independently defining good drawers by evaluating them on separate drawing tasks, because their performances on those other tasks are so highly related to the tasks under scrutiny.

The poor performers

It is possible, however, to gather some circumstantial evidence on the question, simply by looking at the pattern of results that emerged from the study. First, we will briefly consider the 10 poorest performers. They certainly are characterized by a tendency to launch into disastrous strategies. In drawing the three-armed swastika (trinacria), for example, 7 of the 10 began with the hazardous step of building it from a three-sided square and produced many gross anomalies. Another figure they drew from memory was a cross with offset sides, Fig. 7.3(g). One relatively safe approach to the figure is to begin with a simple cross. It is not an especially unusual approach; 17 of the 45 subjects adopted it, but not one of the worst 10 performers began this way. Instead, they attempted to produce the figure from various smaller units. In trying to draw the triquetra, none seems to have isolated the asymmetrical lobes from which it is built; 8 of the 10 used symmetrical elements accreted one to the other.

Finally, I should mention their approach to the swastika. Here we have a rather different situation, for all but 1 of the 10 worst performers adopted an approach that, in theory at least, might be expected to pay off: They analyzed the swastika into crossed components, rather than trying to thread their way around it. But they either misconstrued the shape of the components or failed to have them intersect at the appropriate points. So although they have made one potentially useful perceptual segmentation, they have failed to extend it to a full grasp of the figure's geometry.

The good performers

What characterizes the 10 best performers? Most important is that although inevitably they use more successful strategies, they also seem to have a capacity to use strategies that lead many other subjects into trouble. Consider, for example, the offset cross figure mentioned earlier. Four of the best subjects did not build it from a simple cross, but used exactly that piecemeal approach which in the hands of the poor drawers led to disaster. In producing the three-armed swastika, three of the best subjects produced good versions beginning from the open square so fatal to the poor drawers. In drawing the conventional swastika, many threaded their way around the figure quite unerringly. It is difficult to believe that the poorer drawers could have succeeded by that method, and it is a fair guess that in so doing the more competent performers are utilizing knowledge of important internal relationships that do not show up directly in the structure of their production sequence.

Overall, this informal analysis suggests a rather asymmetrical situation; namely, that poor drawers seem to owe their poor performances to some extent to their incomplete perceptual analysis or their choice of an analysis that is inherently unreliable. The good performers may choose felicitous strategies, but they not infrequently succeed with an approach that gives them little tactical assistance. Put another way, graphically helpful perceptual segmentations of difficult designs may be sufficient to produce good performances, but in the case of competent drawers, they are not necessary.

At this point I wish to desert the analysis of adult drawing performances for a time to consider some processes within children's drawings. This will occupy three chapters; in Chapter 11 I return to adult performances to discuss the pragmatics of drawing in natural settings.

8 Stability and evolution in children's drawings

In drawing, as in spoken language, children's "reception strategies" or understanding of graphics outrun their productive capacities by a substantial margin. Although one might hesitate to characterize children's drawings on the whole as deficient or impoverished, it is reasonable to ask why they do not move more rapidly toward a diverse interpretation of reality in line with their growing sophistication in perceiving and understanding the world.

The possible role of stereotypes

One possible explanation is that graphic inventiveness is restricted by the ubiquity of those public stereotypes that children spontaneously adopt or have forced upon them. Certainly stereotypes and other influences from external models are found in children's drawings, but they are not as pervasive as casual inspection might suggest. Even when children are in close and continuous contact with one another's drawings, there is considerable variety in their representation of even the most common objects. The drawings in Fig. 8.1 are the products of a single class of Australian public school children aged 5.6 to 7 years, drawn on the same day. The variety of forms is striking, and this is typical of much of their drawing. Even when such children do adopt stereotyped formulas, they not infrequently include their own personal versions side by side with the "public" versions, indicating that when stereotypes have been incorporated into a child's repertoire, they do not necessarily monopolize production.

Although personal versions of objects may vary considerably from child to child, the drawings of one child over a period of time may be very repetitious in the treatment of individual motifs. This might be ascribed simply to lack of graphic skills or to the dependence of drawing on certain slowly developing cognitive capacities. Even were such explanations acceptable for the majority of cases, they cannot serve for instances such as that illustrated in Fig. 8.2. Both of these drawings were executed on the same day by the same 7-year-old boy. Drawing A was characteristic of his normal figure drawing at this time and for

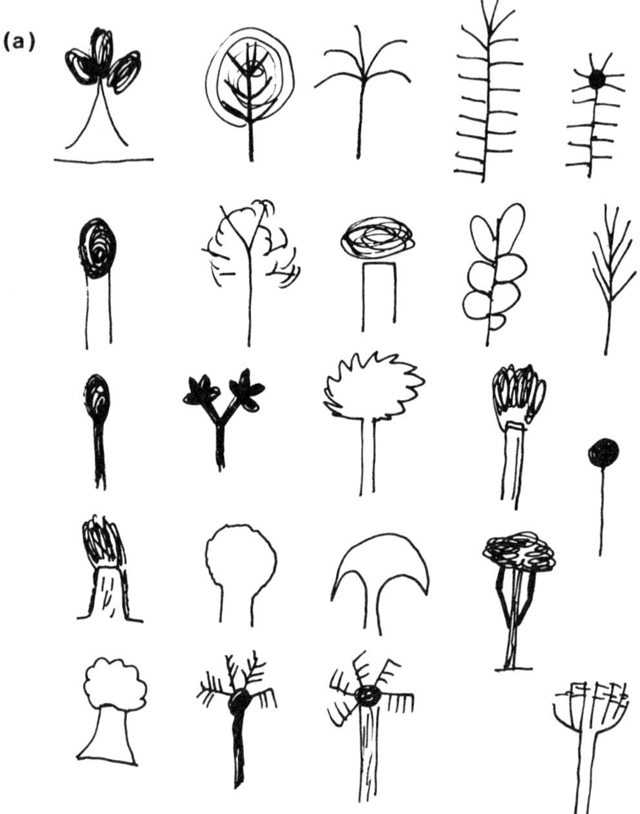

Fig. 8.1. Drawings of trees (a) and noses (b) extracted from drawings produced in a single classroom of an Australian primary school (age 5.6 to 7.0 years).

a considerable period afterward. Drawing B was produced when he was invited to look very carefully not so much at his own drawing, but at the detail of a model before him. The point of the comparison is not to analyze how drawing B was achieved, but why drawings such as A, which is more characteristic of children's productions at this age, come to dominate their normal output.

The objective of the present study is to point up one of the forces operating within the developing graphic competence of children that tends to restrict their productions to certain slowly evolving lines and renders radical innovation and reorientation to the problems of graphic representation less common than cognitive abilities and graphic skills would allow. The study was conducted some time ago under the author's supervision by Sharyn Jones, then an Honours undergraduate at the University of New South Wales (Jones, 1972). The study

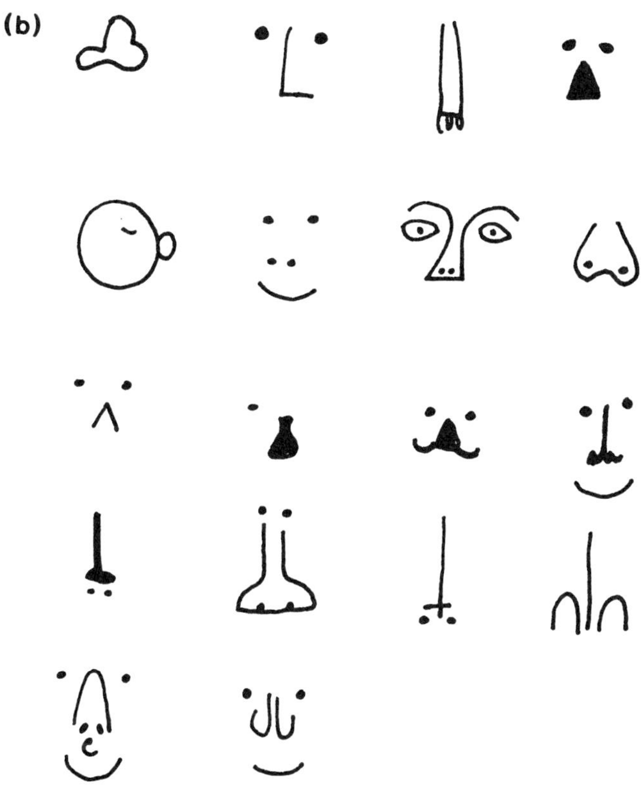

explores to what degree the very act of *producing* a drawing restricts innovation in subsequent drawings. This can occur even when new knowledge has been acquired in the interim and when the children are quite capable, under other circumstances, of utilizing that knowledge. In this sense, the study points to forces within the drawing process itself that tend to restrict graphic development to a slowly incrementing evolutionary process.

Surface and structural aspects of objects

After some preliminary exploration among various small toys and household items, Jones settled on a selection of objects cut from thick paper that could be regarded in two different ways: as a surface pattern, or as a construction. For example, the children were shown an open fan cut from light-colored paper and mounted on a dark card, Fig. 8.3(a). In this form it presented the appearance of a continuous quarter circle, within which the edges of the individual blades

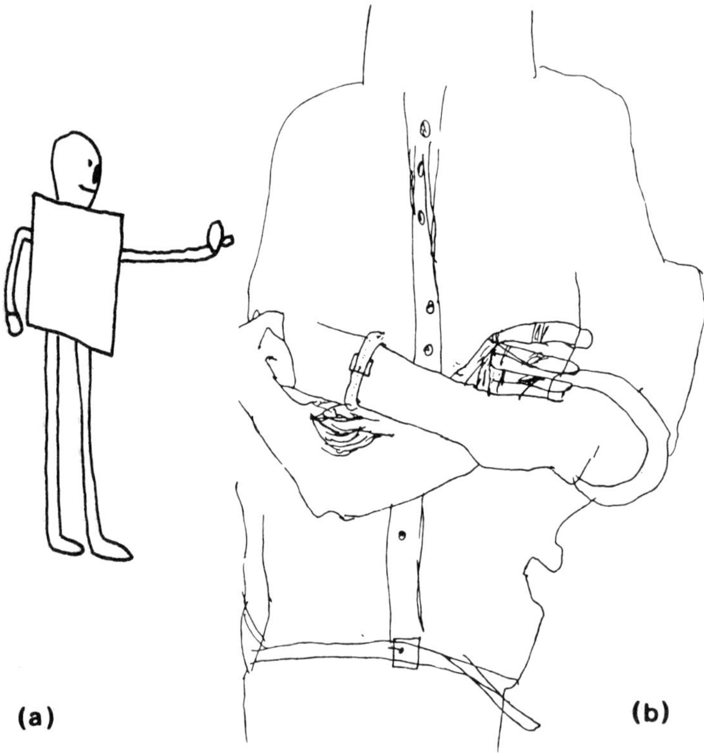

Fig. 8.2. Two drawings of a man produced on the same day by a 7-year-old boy. Drawing (a) was his routine style of drawing. He could be induced to produce drawings like (b) when urged to pay close attention to the model.

could be seen. The fan was also displayed as a series of elongated rectangular blades arranged in an overlapping sequence, and held in place by a small round brass fastener, Fig. 8.3(b). The latter version was a structural rather than a surface version, since it displayed how the fan had been assembled from a number of units. More detail is given below concerning the other items, but they all shared this property of having both an intact and structural form.

The study was conducted twice, the first experiment being used to refine the items for the second. The design of both experiments was as follows. The children were tested in one of two groups, each selected at random from kindergarten and infant school classes. The first group made one drawing of each object after it had been shown to them in its intact form and in the form that revealed its structure. The children in this group were given no opportunity to draw the objects until they had been exposed to both surface and structural aspects. No

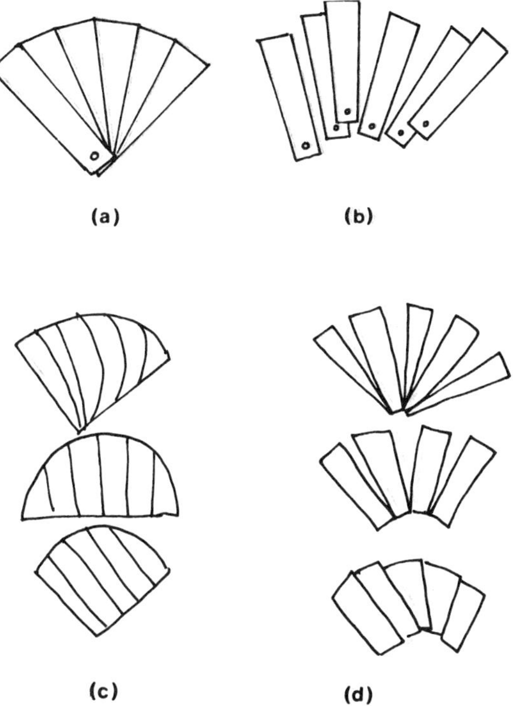

Fig. 8.3. (a): ''Surface'' presentation of a fan, constructed from thick paper. (b): Fan broken into its components to demonstrate its structure. (c): Typical ''structurally naive'' drawing. (d): Typical ''structurally sophisticated'' drawing showing structure not merely as added detail, but in basic graphic strategy.

mention was made about drawing,and no materials distributed, until after all the objects had been displayed, so that they did not even plan drawings until they had all the available information. It was expected that the drawings these children made would reflect structure and not just appearance, and would reveal the cognitive capacity and graphic competence of children of this age to generate drawings that reveal more than surface form.

The second group made *two* drawings of the objects. The first was made when they had first viewed the intact objects. Immediately afterward they were shown the structure of the objects, using exactly the same instructions and procedure as those used for the first group. In this way the two groups of children were given the same contact with the objects overall, the difference between them being that the second group made a drawing after seeing the surface appearance of the object and before being shown its structure. It is the impact of this drawing process on the final drawing that is of interest.

	GROUP 1 One Drawing	GROUP 2 Two Drawings
(a)	Intact Object Shown	Intact Object Shown Drawing 1
	Structural Description Drawing 1	Structural Description Drawing 2
(b)	Maximize structurally sophisticated drawings in drawing 1.	Minimize structurally sophisticated drawings in drawing 1.

Fig. 8.4. (a): Basic design of study investigating the effect of drawing an object before being given structural information about it. In the preliminary study, the aim was to select items that would meet the boundary conditions specified at (b).

In a study of this sort it is not enough simply to select a random set of objects with divergent surface and structural characteristics. The objects and the descriptions that accompany them must be chosen so that there will be a substantial difference between the drawings made after seeing the intact object and those made when the structure has been exposed. In other words, it is necessary to get as many structurally sophisticated drawings as possible from the first (one drawing group) and as few as possible from the second group doing their first drawing (Fig. 8.4). The contrast was necessary since (1) no effect was to be *expected* if none of the group 1 single drawings was sophisticated, and (2) no effects could be *detected* if the group 2 first drawings were already largely sophisticated. The prediction was that if drawing one version exerted a conservative influence on subsequent drawings, the second drawings by group 2 children would remain predominantly naive with respect to structure, rather than approach the level of sophistication of the one-drawing group. If the second drawing does remain relatively naive with respect to structure, the first drawing may be said to be exerting a conservative influence, "immunizing" the child, so to speak, against making use of a new structural approach.

Another requirement of the design was that the drawings should fall naturally into at least two clearly distinguishable classes that reflected the impact of structural understanding. It was not satisfactory if a change could be produced simply by adding detail to the basic form. A "good" item from the point of view of this study was one in which there were two distinctly different approaches to the representation of an object. The fan provides an example: The rectangular components could be (and were) represented in two ways, by the addition of internal details such as radiating or parallel lines within an intact outline, as in Fig. 8.3(c), or building up the fan shape from a series of components, as in Fig. 8.3(d).

The initial group of items contained a number of solid objects – model house, staircase, Chinese doll, book, and lipstick. The variety of approaches to their representation by the 6- and 7-year-old primary school children tested was too wide to permit appropriate comparisons. These objects were dropped or converted to a two-dimensional form, and new items added.

Fig. 8.5 shows all the items used in the final study. On the left is the name and brief description of the item, at the center is an illustration, and on the right is the structural description given. In all cases, the explanation was accompanied by a demonstration of structure using a model resembling the intact object, but with the components freed from the backing so they could be manipulated by the investigator during the structural description. This was, of course, identical for both groups. When the explanation using these loose components was complete, the glued-down version was held up as the model to be drawn.

The subjects of the main experiment were boys and girls aged 5.5 to 7 years (mean age approximately 6 years) from kindergarten and lower primary school classes in Wollongong, a city in Eastern Australia. Items 1 and 7 were administered to 70 children, items 2 through 6 to 140. Boys and girls were assigned in equal numbers to the two groups. The testing was done in groups of approximately 15 children.

The design required that all the children's drawings be classified into two groups: the "naive," which reflected surface appearance, and the "sophisticated," which revealed structure. The preliminary study provided the broad guidelines for this classification, but further decisions had to be made on the drawings in the experiment proper. To avoid contaminating the data by developing the scoring system and scoring on the critical material, two groups of drawings were analyzed first: those of the single-drawing group and the first drawing of the two-drawing group. The categorization was thus established before the critical set of drawings was inspected, these being the second drawings of the latter group. This reduced any unconscious bias in the scoring of these drawings in favor of the hypotheses under examination.

Two statistical tests were applied to the data. One asked: Was there a significant difference between the single drawing done by the group that was given all the information about drawing and the second drawing of group 2, who had all the

(1) "Fan"
Six cardboard rectangles joined at the bottom

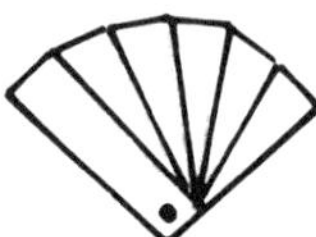

"Can you see this fan is made up of different pieces. You watch and I'll show you how it is made. We start with a lot of strips with a hole in the bottom. Now if we gather them all together and hold them at the bottom near the hole we can join them together by putting a paper fastener through them all. Then when I spread out the strips it gives us a fan. Now I'd like you to draw this fan."

(2) "Stairs"
Four rectangles of card on a dark background

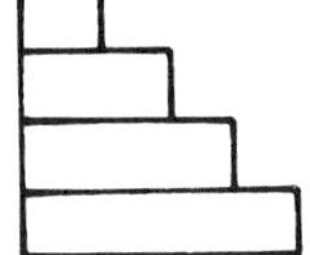

"See this staircase is made up of four rectangles. The biggest one is on the bottom, then the next biggest, then a smaller one sits on it and the smallest one sits on top. They all make up the staircase. Now, I would like you to draw this for me."

(3) "Diamond"
Two triangles of card, the lower slightly wider than the upper.

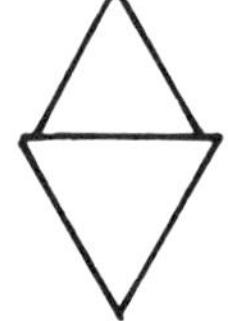

"Can you all see this diamond? Did you notice that when I made it I did not make the two triangles exactly the same size. See the top triangle is a little smaller than the bottom triangle. This makes little ears on the side. Do you think you could draw this diamond for me?

(4) "Flower"
Three card "propeller" – shapes crossing at the center.

"You all know what this shape looks like but notice how it was made. There are three of these propeller shapes and they all cross over and join in the middle and we end up with a flower. I want you to draw this for me."

(5) "Egg"
Two half ellipses, the lower slightly larger in diameter.

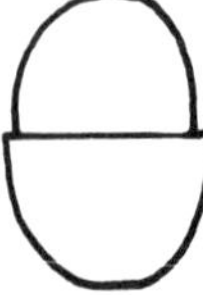

"Did you know that this shape was made from two semi-circles? But notice that the top one is a little smaller than the bottom one so that there are little ears sticking out the side. Now I want you to draw this for me."

(6)"Heart and triangle"
Two figures superimposed.

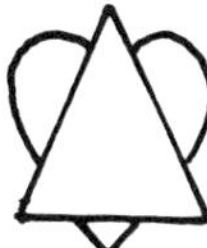

"Did you know that this unusual shape is just made up with a heart and a triangle. I put the heart down first and simply placed the triangle over the top so that when they are together they make this funny shape. Now I'd like you to draw this shape for me."

(7)"Wheel"
Three crossing members, a ring and a disc.

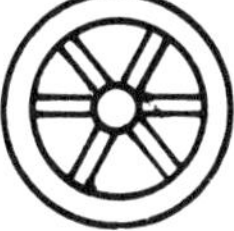

"Did you know that this wheel is made up of three strips which all cross each other in the middle. Next this big spot has been put over where all the strips cross. Then the big rim is put around the outside."

Fig. 8.5. Final set of items used. All were constructed of thick paper of a pale color mounted on a dark background card, or vice versa. The cards were approximately 25 × 20 cm, and the forms occupied most of the card. On the left are names and brief descriptions. On the right are the structural descriptions given to the children.

same information but had produced a prior drawing of the same object? The second test asked: Did the subjects in group 2 change significantly from their first to their second drawing? Some random changing might be expected, so McNemar's test was used, comparing the number of those who changed from "naive" to "sophisticated" with the number who changed in the reverse direction. The expectation was that in spite of the new material given between drawings, the first drawing would stabilize the children's approach and there would be no significant net shift. McNemar's test is relatively powerful statistically, and with a sample of reasonable size should detect substantial systematic shifts.

Both expectations of the study were confirmed. For all but one item, there were a significantly greater number of structurally sophisticated drawings in group 1 than in the second drawing of group 2. For no item was there a significantly greater change from naive to sophisticated than in the reverse direction across the two drawings of group 2.

The first question to be asked is this: Did any feature of the procedure favor the outcome other than some mechanism inherent to the drawing process? Was there, for example, any expectation fostered that the second drawing should be like the first? It seems that the expectations were more likely to be in the other direction. The children in group 2 were given new information and asked immediately to draw again. Many of them added detail to their drawings at this point. What they failed to do was to reevaluate the basic strategy of production to produce structurally sophisticated products like those of their classmates in group 1. Stanton (1973), commenting on this study, pointed out that it bears some resemblance to the phenomenon in thinking of "functional fixedness" (Duncker, 1945) and the "blocking" tendency found by Trabasso and Bower (1968) in classification tasks.

It would be too much to claim that such a tendency to retain a basic strategy and elaborate it rather than change it cannot be overcome. In 1971 McWhinnie reported that provided the instructions were pointed enough, the child's approach to drawing an object can be changed, particularly if the child is shown new drawing strategies. (McWhinnie had subjects draw a tree, and then showed them a variety of drawings and paintings of trees. He reported that 90 percent of the drawings changed substantially.) What the present study shows is that when new information is presented relating to an object itself rather than to the method of representing it, young children tend to lock onto already established strategies. They adapt by elaborating detail rather than altering basic strategies. It may well be this rather than conformity to public stereotypes that gives a stylized quality to their productions.

Jones's investigation of conservatism in children's drawings suggests first that it is an individual process, not an interpersonal exchange. Second, it shows stability not after frequent repetition, but after a single drawing of material that is generally unfamiliar to the children. One item used in Jones's preliminary work was an exception to this rule in that it involved one of the most regularly occurring motifs in Western children's drawings: a conventional square house viewed from the front with a chimney protruding from the sloping roof, Fig. 8.6(a).

Since the house and chimney had to be represented in a structural and non-structural way for the purposes of the experiment, it was cut from thick paper and mounted on a card. To reveal the structure, the front of the house was hinged to open like a book, revealing the continuation of the chimney extending straight down to a fireplace, Fig. 8.6(b). Children in the group that produced two drawings were required first to draw the house with the front closed. Almost half (32 of 68 children) drew the chimney in this drawing at an oblique angle, perpendicular to the roof, Fig. 8.6(c). The house was shown a second time with the front now open to show the straight chimney running up from the floor. The majority of the children who drew the chimney obliquely continued to do so (18 of 32), producing the various versions in Fig. 8.6(d), (e), and (f), with curved, sharply angled, or broken connections between interior and exterior sections of the chimney. This is not because children of this age are inevitably locked onto the oblique representation of the chimney; of the 82 children who saw the opened

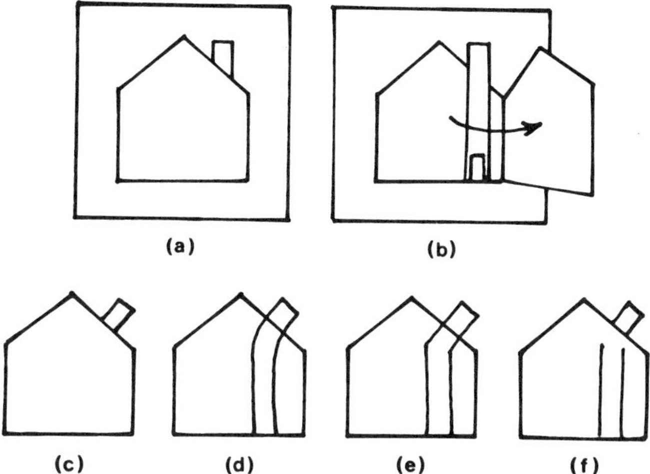

Fig. 8.6. House used in Jones's (1972) study of children's graphic conservatism. (a): "Surface" appearance of model. (b): House front opened to show chimney running down to fireplace. (c): Angled chimney drawn by many children after viewing (a). The adaptations of the oblique chimney to reconcile it with the vertical interior include curves (d), angles (e), and discontinuities (f).

house *initially*, only 7 produced slanted chimneys. The effect seems to be due to the recent experience of actually drawing a slanted version.

Conservatism after a time lapse

Robert Stanton, an honors undergraduate from Macquarie University working on children's graphics, asked whether the effect shown by Jones could be demonstrated with a longer time lapse between drawings. He therefore replicated Jones's study, using the same items and descriptions but adding two extra groups. Both the new groups made two drawings, but between the first showing and first drawing of objects and the structural explanation and second drawing there was a lapse of time, 24 hours in one case and 7 days in the other. This procedure represents a relatively challenging test to the conservatism idea, since the structural explanation is given immediately prior to the second drawing and remote in time from the first.

The results of the study showed a significant difference in the proportion of sophisticated versions of the objects between the drawings of the single-drawing group and all three other groups, including those that received their rebriefing and did their second drawings immediately and those who received it 24 hours and 7 days later. There were no significant differences among these last three groups.

Conservatism and functional knowledge

The next question Stanton set out to resolve was whether the phenomenon was restricted to structural redescription. He selected a new set of items, mainly kitchen implements and tools. The objects were sufficiently exotic in the experience of first-grade primary school children that descriptions of how they were used constituted new information. The effects were not as dramatic as those found with the structural redescriptions, but the overall effect was the same: Prior drawing reduced the number of functionally sophisticated productions.

Conservatism and graphic planning

Stanton added a further procedure at this point. So far there had been no indication of whether it is the drawing process as a physical act that tends to "fix" a strategy in a child's repertoire. Stanton went some way toward resolving this by asking whether the effect required the children actually to put pencil to paper. In the original study and in Stanton's replication, the fact that drawing was involved was concealed from the children of the single-drawing group until all structural explanations were complete. No mention was made of drawing, and drawing materials were kept out of sight. The object of this tactic was to ensure that children did not carry out any graphic planning which might itself exert a conservative effect on their subsequent drawings.

This precaution turned out to have been justified, for Stanton succeeded in demonstrating a conservative effect with a group of 50 first-grade children who did no drawing on the first occasion, but were simply instructed to *think* about drawing. On first presentation of each of the kitchen implements, the investigator said: "I want you to think how you might draw this object." He then handed out paper and pencils, redescribed each object from a functional point of view, and had the children draw each one. Although there were significant differences between planning and actually drawing, both planning and drawing procedures produced a significant lowering of the number of functionally sophisticated drawings. This outcome indicates that the conservative effect is not entirely due to the development of a motor routine, although actually laying down the strokes does strengthen the phenomenon.

Finally, one negative effect found by Stanton is worth reporting. He followed the basic procedure with a new set of objects selected for use with first-year university students. The implements included surgical and specialized drafting instruments, and the explanations included statements about how the devices moved and for what purpose they were used. Although the sample sizes were smaller, varying from 16 to 21 in each group, the conservatism effect seen in the young children was not evident even as a trend. Among the university students, a functional redescription of objects was followed by a modest increase in sophisticated drawings in spite of prior drawing or planning to draw.

It is very likely that the university students picked up the implicit demand to reconstruct their drawings and had the graphic versatility to do so. Whether it is possible to design drawing tasks sufficiently challenging to make such sophisticated subjects retain their original solutions when the situation so clearly invites a show of innovation remains to be demonstrated. It is much more likely that a conservative effect will be demonstrated in older subjects when they are drawing less self-consciously.

Conservatism or evolution

The context of this exploration of the reappearance of certain strategies of portrayal has been the retarding influence it may have on the flexible development of representational skill in children. It is important to recognize that the coin has another side. The development of skill in portraying particular items or classes of items depends also on developing by evolution appropriate methods of attack. When a graphic problem has been solved, it is to be hoped that the useful features of that solution will be incorporated in subsequent drawings. Conservatism could then be seen as simply a derogatory term for developing competence. Perhaps what makes us see the fixity of strategies as a predominantly retarding rather than a constructive force is that in the context in which they emerged, they seemed too invariant. It was not the case that when children had to produce a new drawing they considered a range of strategies and repeated the old one because of its superiority, but rather the old strategy seemed to preempt the invention of a range of new approaches. It remains to be seen whether by sensitizing drawers to what they are doing, one could increase the range of alternative solutions generated and decrease the tyranny of the established graphic solution.

9 Innovations, primitives, contour, and space in children's drawings

The studies of Jones and Stanton on repetitive drawings demonstrated that once children have developed a strategy of representation, they tend to retain it in subsequent drawings even after they have been provided with additional data about the objects they are depicting, data that would normally affect their mode of attack quite fundamentally had not graphic strategy already been developed in their minds or put into action. These experiments provide a model for the emergence of relatively stable individual graphic versions of objects by children and at the same time help to explain why children's drawings are often not as sophisticated as their knowledge. The logic is that children tend to lose their flexibility in portraying things in the very act of generating early versions of them. That is not to say that children's drawings never change, but rather that their drawings often evolve by the modulation or amendment of existing devices, rather than through a revolutionary rethinking of the basic representational strategy.

Where do innovations occur in drawings?

One prediction we can make from this is that when innovations *do* appear in children's drawings, they will tend to occur not in the initial strokes of the drawings, but late in the sequence. To establish empirically whether this was in fact a fair inference, I undertook to collect a substantial corpus of repeated drawings from a group of primary school children.

There were 20 children in the group. Each child drew 12 different objects, half from imagination and half from life. From each child we collected 10 or more versions of each object, the versions being produced at intervals of two to four weeks. This exercise produced a prodigious body of graphic material – in excess of 2400 drawings in all, each drawing accompanied by a video record of the production strategy that in turn could be transcribed and analyzed.

From this body of information it was possible to make analyses that went well beyond the original research question of where graphic innovation occurs. Of the various empirical outcomes one in particular stands out, and it will be discussed and illustrated in some detail. This revolves around the following issue: Given that we believe each child stabilizes to a certain degree on a particular graphic strategy for the representation of an object, at what level does this stabilization occur? The whole tenor of this monograph, concentrating as it has on regularities or consistencies in production acts and sequences, might predispose one to believe that if children repeat themselves, they will do so at the level of physical execution, simply following again and again the stroke orders and forms with which they began.

This is not correct. The salient fact, which can be illustrated at every level of detail, with every child and every topic, is that they do *not* achieve stability of product by rigidly ordered production routines. Their consistency arises from the production in a great variety of ways of what might be called *graphic schema*, or visually equivalent forms.

It would be misleading to say that there are no limits to the variability of attack; as we will see, the performances do on average conform to the executive constraints set out in earlier chapters, and the structure of objects itself gives priority to certain elements. But within limitations of this sort, variability in sequence is the outstanding characteristic of the children's performances, indicating that the conservatism we have discussed operates at a more abstract level than final motor sequence. We will return to this issue more comprehensively in the next chapter. First I wish to outline the procedure in more detail, report the outcome of the inquiry about where innovations typically occur, and raise some issues related to graphic "primitives" and universals of production.

Collecting repeated drawings

The children, 11 boys and 9 girls, aged 5.3 to 6.4 years at the commencement of the study, were attending a primary school in a middle-class Sydney suburb. They were tested individually at one- to two-week intervals, and at each session they drew 6 of the 12 objects that were to become their standard repertoire. At each session they drew 3 drawings from life (shoe, tape dispenser, and so on) and 3 from memory. There were no time limits placed on their drawings. The structure of this timetable meant that the interval between successive drawings of a particular object was always in the range of two to four weeks.

The 6 objects they drew from life were a pair of scissors, a plastic tape dispenser, a single (rather worn) canvas tennis shoe, a clear electric light bulb, a hair brush with a wooden handle, and a punch for cutting a pair of holes in paper (Fig. 9.1). The objects to be drawn from memory or imagination were a bicycle, a telephone, a television set, a crocodile, a baby in a pram, and a man rowing a boat. Children usually drew with felt pens, working on A4 paper in a standard vertical orientation while seated at a low table.

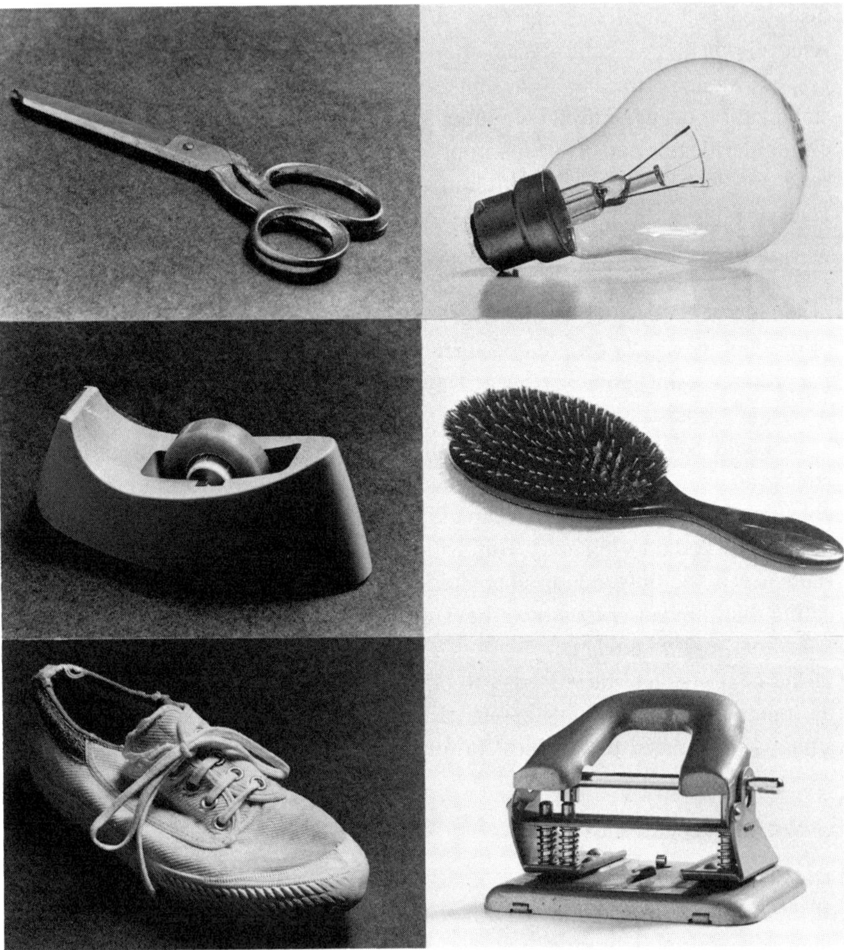

Fig. 9.1. Photographs of the six objects drawn by children from life. From top left: scissors, tape dispenser, tennis shoe, light bulb, hair brush, and hole punch.

On each occasion, the children were urged to produce as good a drawing as possible and to make their drawings "better than the last time." The alternation of the set of 6 objects to be drawn (including on each occasion 3 real and 3 imagined objects) helped to delay the onset of boredom, but the task was necessarily repetitive, and some children understandably required patient encouragement toward the end of the series.

The first method used to track the introduction of new elements in drawings was quite direct: All the individual strokes within all drawings had been numbered according to the order in which they were laid down. Three objects were then chosen for detailed analysis: the bicycle, the telephone, and the tape dispenser. A list was compiled of all the features of each of these three objects that appeared anywhere in the corpus of drawings. These features included for the bicycle such items as handlebar support, left handlebar, left handgrip, bell, lamp, and basket. For the telephone: outer dial ring, inner dial ring, finger hole one, finger hole two to n, cord, plug.

It might be useful before proceeding further to clarify the units of analysis so far mentioned, strokes and features. *Strokes* are units based on drawing actions and are "meaning-free." A stroke begins when the pencil touches the paper and ends when it is removed. A *feature*, on the other hand, is a representational (semantic) unit defined by what it portrays. Some features, like a wheel rim or the filament of a lamp, are almost invariably made with a single stroke, whereas a set of wheel spokes or a basket on a bicycle may include several strokes, as Fig. 9.2 shows. This figure also introduces some other terms that will become relevant shortly, in particular the *subsystem*, which is simply a larger semantic unit than the feature, so that a number of features (rim, spokes, hub) might together make up the wheel subsystem. There is no great theoretical weight behind any of these terms; they just turn out to be convenient for exposition and analysis. But it is important sometimes to recognize when we are talking semantically and when we are speaking of concrete products of action.

The total number of features found in all drawings ranged from 20 for the tape dispenser and 27 for the telephone to 37 for the bicycle, although of course by no means all features appeared in each drawing. The next step in the analysis was to construct a matrix for each child and for each of the objects. The rows were the successive drawings from 1 to 10, and each column represented a feature with entries in each cell indicating whether the feature was present, and if so at what point in the construction of the whole object it appeared.

An innovation was defined in the first instance simply as a feature appearing in a row with all empty cells above it. The question then reduced itself to asking when in the order of construction innovations were introduced and to determining whether they were on the whole early or late. Because there were different numbers of features in each drawing, absolute order numbers were not unambiguous indicators of early or late appearance of innovations, since fifth would be early in a complex drawing with 15 elements and late in a drawing with 6 elements. For this reason, it is helpful for visualizing what is happening to use a display like that in Fig. 9.3. The sequence of production within a drawing where an innovation occurred is set out horizontally, one feature to a cell, and each succeeding drawing in which an innovation appeared for each child in the group is shown set out beneath its predecessor. To help distinguish "early"

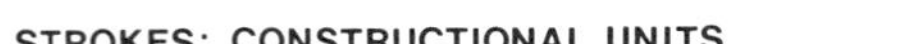

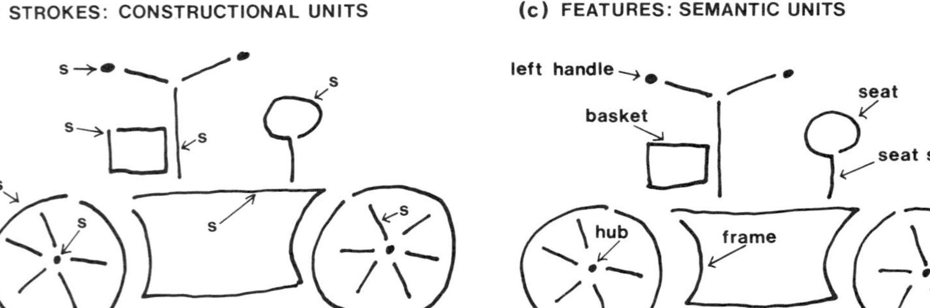

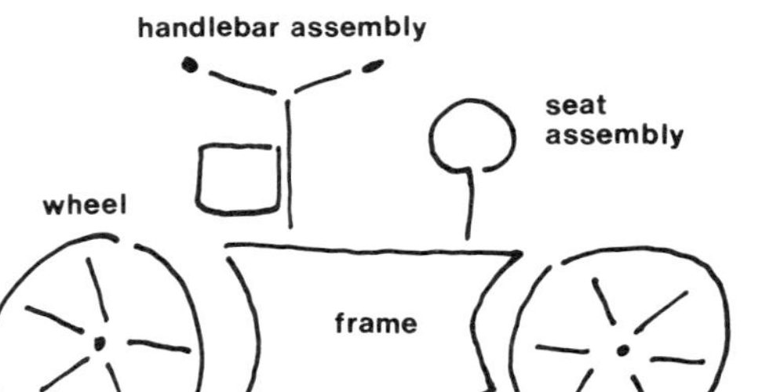

Fig. 9.2. Some terminology: The same (synthetic) version of a bicycle is labeled in four ways. The first two deal with production categories, the last two with representational categories. (a): The drawing is decomposed into the individual *strokes* defined by pencil contact with the paper. (b): The strokes are described according to their control characteristics or similar criteria. (c): The object is broken down into elementary semantic *features:* wheel rim, spokes, and so on. These are used to establish order of production. (d): Larger semantic units (subsystems) usually made up of a number of features used in some analyses of change in drawing across time.

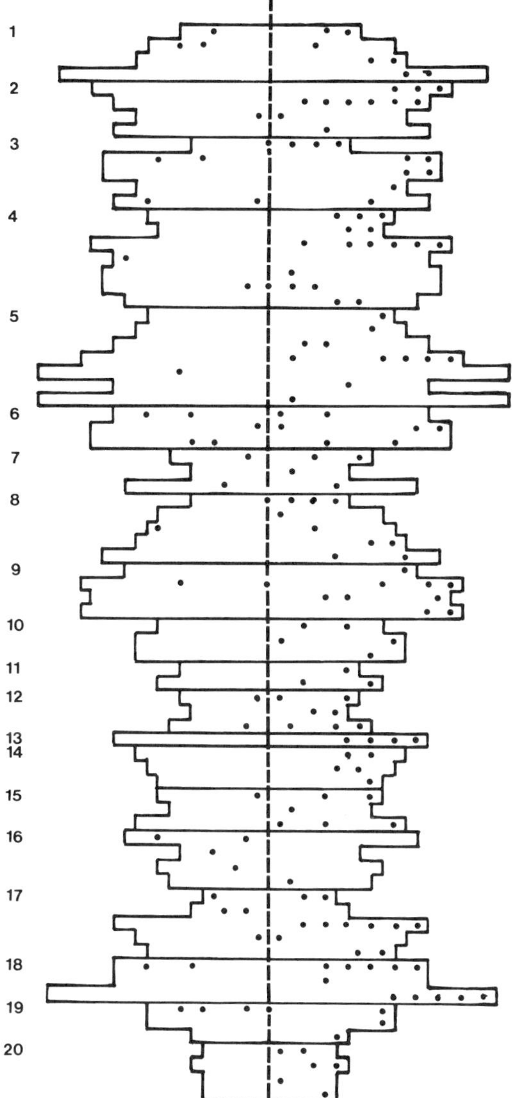

Fig. 9.3. The location of innovation by addition of new features. Each row represents one drawing of a bicycle by one child with features in order of construction. Only drawings in which an innovation appeared are included. Subject numbers are on the left. The length of each segment corresponds to the total number of features included in the drawing, and the segments have been centered so that innovations (black dots) can occur early (left) or late (right).

from "late" in the drawing sequence, each horizontal set is centered about its midpoint. Innovations in the form of additions are marked as filled circles. It can be seen immediately from this display that innovations are concentrated heavily to the right of the midline. That is, they are appearing late in the sequence, as the earlier studies would lead one to predict.

It is my intention to take this analysis of innovation one step further to consider not only the addition of new features, but changes in the way old features are represented. It is also necessary to distinguish the time scale we are dealing with, because of course there are two senses in which innovations of any sort can be said to be "early" or "late": early or late within a drawing, and early or late across a series of drawings. We might think of this as micro- and macro-time, seconds versus weeks. When I said in the previous paragraph that new features are added late in the drawing process, I meant at the microlevel, within the individual drawing sequence. When we ask the same questions about a series of drawings (macrolevel), the reverse is the case. *Fewer* innovations occur as we progress from the first to the tenth drawing. Table 9.1 shows the number of new features added as a function of the passage of the weeks for the three objects we have been analyzing (bicycle, telephone, and dispenser), and the decline in additive innovations over time is consistent. We can therefore sum up by saying that the greatest number of new items are added in the early drawings of a series, but late in the process of drawing them.

Innovation through substitution

The analysis I have been describing does not paint the full picture in that it restricts itself to innovations in the form of additions of features to drawings, and does not document another equally important class of change: modifications in the way features are represented. Such an analysis is rather more exacting. Recognizing new features is easy, but specifying whether features are portrayed by the same or a different graphic device involves multiple comparisons and qualitative judgments. Each individual version of the feature under analysis has to be compared with all the versions of that feature in the earlier drawings of a sequence. For 10 drawings, this demands 45 comparisons per feature per child. In practice this task, although reasonably formidable, is not quite as heroic as it sounds, provided one chooses features that vary distinctly and quantally.

Five subsystems were chosen for analysis: the filament of the lamp, the wheels and the handlebar assemblies on bicycles, the tape reel on the dispenser, and the device used to portray the spatial relation of the reel to the tape dispenser body. In all but one case (the lamp filament), it was possible to identify a range of relatively mutually exclusive versions emerging from the drawings of the 20 children. There were 17 devices used to represent the tape reel, 20 to portray

Table 9.1. *Innovations by additions of new features. The data are from 10 drawings done at approximately 2-week intervals by 20 children aged 5 to 6 years. Three objects are analyzed. The bicycle and telephone were drawn from memory, the tape dispenser while the object was present.*

	Drawing number								
Object	2	3	4	5	6	7	8	9	10
A: Bicycle	52	30	33	21	6	22	12	6	6
B: Telephone	38	21	17	11	6	13	5	4	4
C: Tape dispenser	35	15	17	9	11	12	3	3	3
Mean number of additions	41.6	33.0	22.3	13.6	7.7	15.6	6.7	4.3	4.3

bicycle wheels, and 16 showing the tape reel in relation to the dispenser. In the next chapter, when I spend a little time teasing apart how certain graphic components combine and recombine in a kind of mosaic in the work of an individual child, it will emerge that some of these subsystems, particularly the lamp filament, are not entirely suited to an "either-new-or-old" categorization. Rather, each version shares a greater or lesser number of themes or properties. In the current context, this meant that although one could reasonably dichotomize most versions as innovative or not, for the lamp filament a relative judgment on a 4-point scale was easier to use.

Fig. 9.4 shows one of the matrices generated in this analysis. It is annotated with filled circles that indicate where a new version appears. Some children regularly produce more new versions and backtrack to earlier forms than others, but when the data are pooled across children, we find that innovations of substitution, like innovations of addition, flourish in the early weeks of the drawing series and tend to decline in frequency as drawings are repeated. This is a constant finding across all the items analyzed, including the complex filament structure and the rather more abstract mechanisms by which tape reel and dispenser are integrated.

One might simply think that the children lose interest in making new versions or are satisfied with existing forms, except that only one or two children really stabilized their drawings; most changed continually, even if only to revert to earlier versions. It seems more like a process of imaginative exhaustion; children move about within a limited repertoire. No child comes anywhere near producing all the versions produced by the group. As far as innovative substitution goes, the most that one child achieves is about one-third of the range utilized by the group.

So far I have documented the occurrence of new features and of new versions of standard features over the long term. Both tend to decline with repetition. I have also shown that new features tend to be added late in the sequence of productive acts. Is it possible to round out the picture by indicating whether there is any relation between introducing a new *version* of a feature and where in the individual production sequence that feature falls? In other words, do children have any tendency to stick to an old formula with items they draw first or early?

We could tackle this problem by taking a pair of elements – say, the wheel and the handlebar assembly of the bicycle – and, given that wheels are normally earlier in the production sequence than handles, ask which shows more changes in form. Unfortunately, this is unlikely to be a fair comparison, since there are basic differences between the potential for change from one subsystem to another, and a massive amount of work would be needed to examine enough features to wash out such intrinsic differences. A more economical attack on the problem

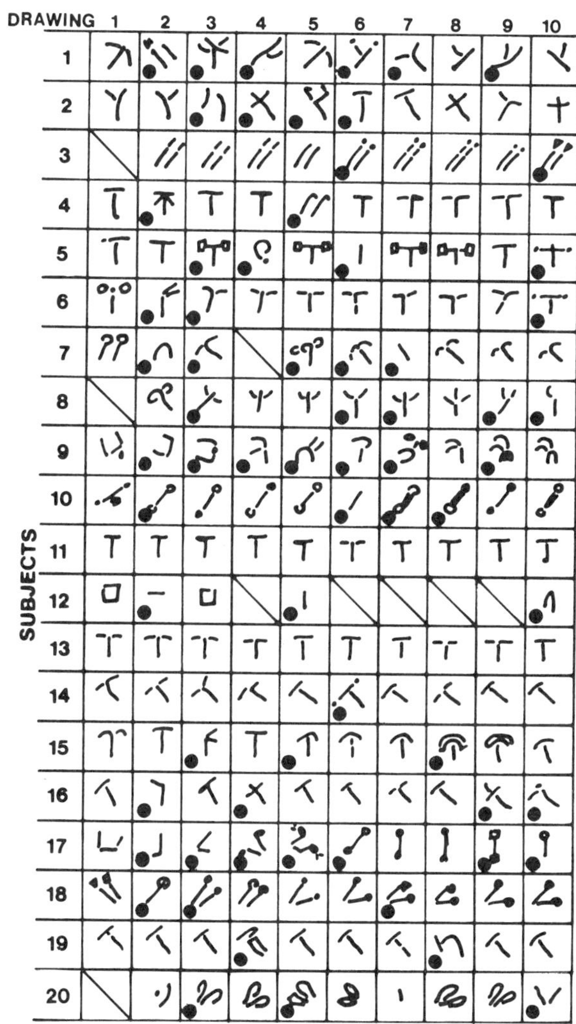

Fig. 9.4. Analysis of innovation in the bicycle handlebar assembly. These are innovations of substitution. The 20 subjects are arranged down the matrix, and the 10 drawings produced by each are shown horizontally. Within each cell is a schematic version of the handlebar structure (stem, handles, and so on). A filled circle in a cell indicates that a new approach has been taken to portraying the assembly. A diagonal line across a cell indicates that the assembly did not appear in the drawing. Judgments were made on the basis of the overall topography of each succeeding drawing of the assembly. I have left gaps between strokes in each diagram that give some feel for the variety of constructional techniques used, but method of construction was *not* considered in classifying a version as new. There is a general though modest decline in the number of substitution innovations across the 10 consecutive drawings. Matrices of this sort were generated for five subsystems.

is to see whether within a given subsystem there is any relation between (1) whether a new or old version of it is used and (2) when (earlier or later) it appears in a production sequence. The object of the whole exercise is to see whether the general model is correct: Drawings tending to stabilize with repetition and doing so through early "conservatism" and late "embroidery."

For each subsystem comprised of one or more features (Fig. 9.2), data were available on file specifying where in the order of construction each feature appeared. There were roughly 200 occurrences of each subsystem, each with one or more features. It was simply a matter of collecting these values together and dividing each by the total number of features in the drawing in which it appeared. This yields for each a value between 0 and 1 that expresses the relative position of the feature within the drawing compilation. For example, features making up the handlebar assembly ordinarily occur about two-thirds of the way through the drawing sequence. This is expressed numerically as 0.67. (There is no conventional name for such values; I simply call them "proportional ranks.") So it becomes a question of asking whether the proportional ranks of new versions are or are not higher than those of old versions.

The outcome of this analysis was contrary to expectations in that innovations of substitution did *not* behave like innovations of addition. Sometimes substitute versions were produced early in the executive sequence and sometimes late, so that when we compare the average proportional ranks for repeat versions, new versions, or versions that represent a reversion to an earlier form, the values are all much the same. What this might suggest is that children are building up their drawings in a particular order, and when they come to portray a wheel, a handlebar assembly, or the reel of tape in a dispenser, they then choose how to represent it. They neither postpone an item because they are going to change it nor promote it to an earlier position in the series.

To sum up, we have a situation in which innovations of both types, additions and substitutions of new versions, tend to be more common in the first drawings of an extended series. In terms of microhistory, however, there is disjunction. Innovations of substitution can be made at any time when the feature or subsystem is being delineated, but new features tend to be included as additions or embellishments late in the compilation of a particular drawing.

The question of graphic "primitives"

I wish to turn away from the problem of innovation for the present and revert to an issue closer to the actual production of marks on the page. And that issue is whether it is fair to describe the drawings of these 5- and 6-year-old children as predominantly an aggregation of standard graphic elements: straight lines, arcs, circles, dots, and so on. Certainly this can be said: From a raw quantitative point of view, the overwhelming majority of strokes can unambiguously be classified into about 10 classes, each of which is relatively simple in form: lines, circles (filled or open), dots, arcs, zigzags, coils, spirals, and whorls, closed and open rectilinear forms (squares, triangles), and patches of opaque pen work. A rather more finely subdivided set of categories used to analyze some of the protocols is set out in Fig. 9.5.

The concept of a graphic primitive distinguishes a class of stroke like a circle, line, or dot that in a mature drawer is more ballistic or automatized, the product of a standard motor subroutine, and can be distinguished, for example, from a shaped contour whose form is built up as a relatively unique and continuously monitored form. I have found it useful to use a third category for devices that seem to lie between the two. These are somewhat regularized or stylized contours that I have called *motifs*. The more rigorous specification of what a motif is will be set aside for the moment while the distinction between primitives and controlled contour is explored.

In adult drawings there are some items (the stocking is an excellent example) that are invariably drawn as a wandering, special-purpose line. It is not simply a series of straight lines or arcs drawn while the pen is kept on the paper. A tent, by contrast, is almost always drawn by adults as an organized constellation of straight lines. It would be absurd to say that these straight lines are uncontrolled: They are anchored, oriented, and regulated in length to suit their representational function. Circles too are not completely prepackaged; they vary in placement, attachment, and radius. They are sometimes distorted in shape because the space allowed for them is too narrow or because they have to make contact with another element in a drawing. It is nonetheless sensible to see them as circles rather than controlled contours simply because variation from circularity is not intended to convey representational significance.

The same logic applies even more pointedly to "primitives" in young children's drawings. For young children, the distinction between the ballistic movement and a controlled one is often not the relevant issue at all. A typical preschool child may draw a circle or "straight" line inaccurately, haltingly, and with considerable effort of control. The critical distinction is not how smooth or automatized the action is. The issue is that mentioned above: To what end is the control effort directed? Is it primarily aimed at producing a version of a circle, a straight line, or an arc, or at manufacturing a "custom-made" contour? The sharp corners and discontinuities in a 3-year-old's circle are usually defects in construction, not special-purpose representational devices.

One complication is that when a child draws a hand or a glove as a continuous envelope, we would ordinarily class this as a special-purpose contour like the sock, but in many instances it might just as readily be seen as a succession of linked arcs, and the distinction becomes equivocal. When we examine the par-

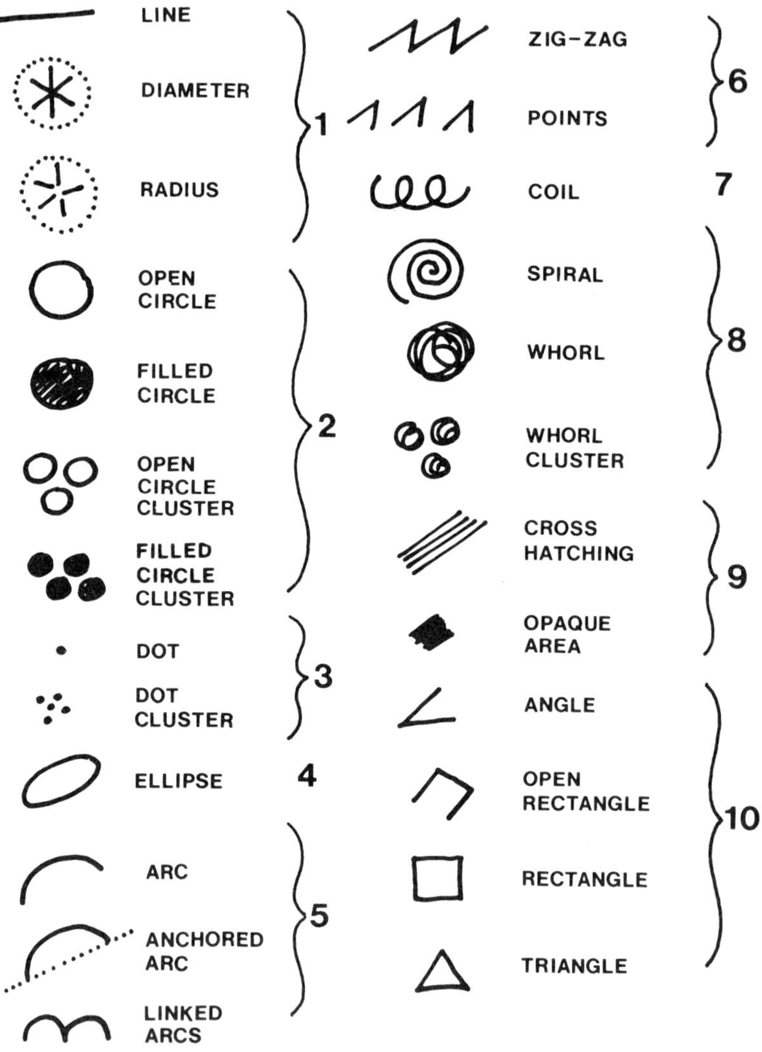

Fig. 9.5. 25 ''primitives,'' basic geometric forms used in children's drawings. They have been grouped into 10 broader categories.

ticular contours produced by the children in this study, we will see that there are a number of such particular issues about how and why contours of a certain form were produced. From a quantitative point of view, the gray area between contour and primitive should not be overemphasized, however. In practice, it is relatively easy to identify a large, indeed predominant, class of unambiguous standard geometric forms used in the young children's drawings.

Repetitive stylizations: the motif

Children (and adults) sometimes use repetitively a graphic unit that is neither one of the common primitives like a straight line, zigzag, circle, or whorl, nor a "one-off" contour. Usually such a device bears a detailed iconic relation to what it represents, as a contour does, but is repeated a number of times to depict the same feature. Common examples are when a child invents a special shape to represent the feet of a telephone, paddles for a boat, or the elements in the pattern on the skin of an animal. I think it is best to regard these simply as contours that happen to portray features of objects that are themselves repetitious. The idea of a motif is probably better reserved for items outside the normal range of simple geometric primitives, but like them are used for a variety of purposes. Arnheim (1964) quotes the case of a child who constructed a whole drawing from strokes resembling hearts. Such "motifs" occurring in our sample include hooked lines developed to represent wheels and then used for handles, or handle shapes used as pedals. One child used a shape like a crotchet variously to represent arms, oars, the legs on a television set, and wheels on a pram. Motifs in this sense are more complex shapes adopting the status of primitives for particular individuals.

There is another type of regularization that does not qualify as a primitive or as a motif because it is used to portray only a single object. For example, a particular curve is used only to represent hair, yet it may be modified in a wide variety of ways. It has clearly become a standard element in the graphic vocabulary, but with a variable "morphology."

Primitives as signifiers of a variety of signified items

We have been exploring the range of devices used by drawers to signify. The listing and counting of "types" and "tokens" unifies graphic elements geometrically and constructionally but suppresses the important differences between what they signify. The ability of a line to signify a wide variety of features of objects is widely remarked. Kennedy (1975) gives a nice capsule review in an anthropological and archeological context. Lines can represent the *boundary* of a flat surface like a table top or the *terminator* of a curved surface like the side of a glass. They can mark the inner *boundary of a cavity* like a mouth or a porthole, or can summarize a *two-edged object* like a bristle, a ribbon, a wire, a leg, or even a tree trunk. They can mark off *subdivisions of a region* corresponding to a difference in material, a discontinuity of form, a pigment boundary, or the edge of a shadow. When placed within an area, they can indicate the *reflectivity* of a shiny surface, its *texture*, or its *slant*. Dots in their turn can represent individual objects (flies or rain drops), excrescences (buttons, noses), cavities (nostrils, holes in a telephone receiver), texture, color, and so on. An opaque area can represent an object or distinguish one of its parts; it can convey opacity or color, distinguish contents from container, identify shadows, and so on.

Part of the task of signification is carried by the choice of geometrically appropriate primitives and their placement, but of course a good deal of the decoding depends on those questions of *critical contrast* between candidate objects to which I referred in the chapter on the simple representational drawing of adults: a circle containing four dots is a face in the context of a body, a button when it is on a coat, and a plate of peas when placed in the context of a table and cutlery. These "contexts," of course, may themselves be nothing more than lines, dots, circles, or more or less simple stroke configurations, so that each component acts as context for other components to aid us in "reading" the whole.

In most cases, this reading presents no problem. The equivalence between the form and juxtaposition of elements in a typical preschool child's drawing of a bicycle and the uniquely distinguishable form of the real bicycle it signifies make correct interpretation very probable. In other instances, such as drawing a light bulb, there is room for errors of interpretation not so much because there are other objects that could easily be confused with light bulbs, but because the use of a repertoire of primitives provides a too limited range of representational devices to handle the variety of contrasts in material and form in such an object. The line has to serve to represent the terminators of a thin glass envelope and of solid glass components, the boundary of a metal holder, the substance of supporting wires, filament, and so on. The line in this sense is both versatile and ambiguous, and the precise configuration of the component lines used to convey a distinctive shape becomes critical.

Signifiers and the signified

In one sense Saussure's (1974) characterization of language as a system of signification is inappropriate to drawings, for reasons already given: He stressed arbitrariness, whereas relations between drawings and what they signify are not arbitrary but iconic. (Even if one cannot positively identify an object from a drawing, if the drawing has any claim to adequacy one can at least say something about the object's shape.)

But the idea of contrasts in and between the domains of the signifier and the signified that Saussure stressed is both apt and useful. The ease or difficulty

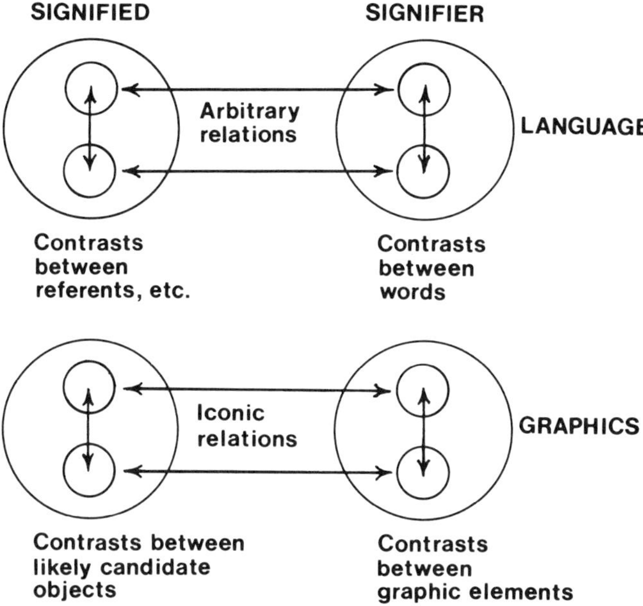

Fig. 9.6. Saussure saw language as a system of relations between differences. Each language used certain contrasts between sounds to signify contrasts between items that the words (arbitrarily) signify. An analog for drawing suggests that contrasts between graphic devices map onto contrasts between objects they represent. (A circle and an ellipse are in contrast and correspond to the contrast between ball and egg.) The choice of graphic device does not depend only on visual similarity, but reflects also what the task of disambiguation is within the domain of the signified.

adults and children have both in producing and in "reading" drawings depends to some degree on the contrasts and ambiguities between elements within the drawing itself and on the contrasts and similarities between objects that are likely candidates as the signified (Fig. 9.6). A circle would be a good signifier of a dinner plate if plates were the only round objects, but in a world of balls, moons, hoops, wheels, and a hundred other common objects with circular perimeters, there is, to say the least, a problem of disambiguation in the domain of the signified.

In terms of this system, the "primitives" are the contrasting elements in the domain of *signifiers*. The circle can represent an open eye, the arc a closed one, and for this purpose the arc is a better device than a straight line. The development and use of controlled contour and special motifs simply acknowledges the inadequacy of the gamut of standard geometric forms to handle contrasts and permit identification.

We are dealing here with another example of that rapid and unself-conscious calculation the drawer must continually undertake. The outcome of the calculation will be a product of a constellation of factors: First, the subject matter itself, whether it lends itself to representation as lines (like a fence or a telegraph pole), or demands a special contour (like a stocking or a pear); second, the "contrastive isolation" of the object (whether it has confusable relatives, as a ball has, or is as distinctive as a bicycle); and third, whether it is supported by an informative context or not, and this context may be both within the drawing (a rectangle on a sloping roof is a chimney) or extra-graphic (when we are giving directions, a complex street intersection can be represented as a cross).

Drawers are more or less efficient in marshaling these factors and will have to various degrees the resources and talent to meet them. With younger children, the calculation is by no means faultless, as most people will know who have watched a small child represent everything from a face to a pram, a boat to a shoe, a telephone to a pond, as an unadorned circle.

The reason I am pursuing these multiple factors that affect drawing strategy is to show that if we are tempted to regard the use or nonuse of special-purpose contour as some direct guide to graphic maturity or sophistication, we must realize that it can arise as much from the graphic task as from graphic competence. To quantify the balance among primitives, contours, and stylized motifs would be an exercise with limited rewards if it reflected little more than the geometry of the subject matter. It would be comparable to observing children paint scenes and trying to find out something about their "operating characteristics" by counting how many vertical and horizontal lines they produce relative to the oblique. If the subject matter comprises trees, fences, houses, swings, and telegraph poles, the number of horizontals and verticals will be high relative to the number of oblique lines, but this is a comment about the physics of the world and the technology of the environment, not the characteristics of the drawer. The same applies to the proportions of the various primitives used. When children move away from the widespread and relatively indiscriminate use of curved closed forms and begin using a range of primitives more flexibly and appropriately, semantics is likely to shape the frequency profile of types they use.

The multiple origins of contours

Contour is perhaps not an impeccable term for the controlled line defining a shape. We ordinarily associate contour with the external boundary of an object or the form of a surface. Although these are probably the most common items graphic contours represent, the category should also include single modulated strokes that by themselves represent objects, such as a plant stalk, a path, and a hairpin.

But this is simply a terminological question. More interesting is the question of what motivates contour and how it develops as a graphic device. The first point is that contour in drawing does not always result from a mapping of shapes in the external world (or memories of them) onto paper. First, we can make a distinction between *positive* contour in a drawing, where in the normal course of events one outlines a profile of a face, or draws the shape of a shoe or a brush, and *complementary* contour, where one draws a line around some existing elements. The children who draw an amoebalike outline of a human figure are producing positive contour, but if they draw a figure and clothe it, as they often do by tracing around what they have already drawn, they are executing what I call complementary contour. It may be internal or external. The clothing is external, as is the drawing of a fender and chassis line over a pair of car wheels. Internal complementary contours are rarer and are likely to be simply echoes of positive contours.

As I mentioned at the outset, contours can and most often do represent boundaries or envelopes of objects and hence will often be closed. Less often they constitute the object itself (like a tail, a hairpin, or a snake). Sometimes a line within a region is used to represent surface contour.

One might assume almost by definition that the production of a complementary contour would always and necessarily follow the construction of the form to which it is a complement, but in the children's drawings of common objects there seem to be occasional instances of anticipated complementarity. For example, some children draw the body of a tape dispenser with a curved line running around half the circumference of the tape spool. Sometimes this involved anticipation. Such cases occur when the dispenser has been drawn at least once with a round tape reel, and there is a conflict between breaking off from constructing the dispenser body to draw the reel, producing transparency or anticipating the shape.

Before I make some final comments on the development of contour use, let me draw attention to some features of contour that represent controlled responses to unplanned contingencies or seem to result from perceptual-motor difficulties. A trivial example of the first is provided by the child who mislocates a long crocodile on a short sheet of paper and has to manufacture a contour to make it fit. Not infrequently a line designed to fill a gap may have to detour to reach its destination because of poor anticipation or misjudgment of direction, Fig. 9.7(a) to (e). (The numbers i, ii, and so on in these figures indicate the temporal order of critical events.)

More interesting are the items that reveal failures to produce symmetry in contour where it is clearly intended. This is shown first in the lamp base of a child who negotiates one step in the boundary of an object but fails to produce the mirror-image step on the opposite side, Fig. 9.7(f). Scott (aged 5.3) had the

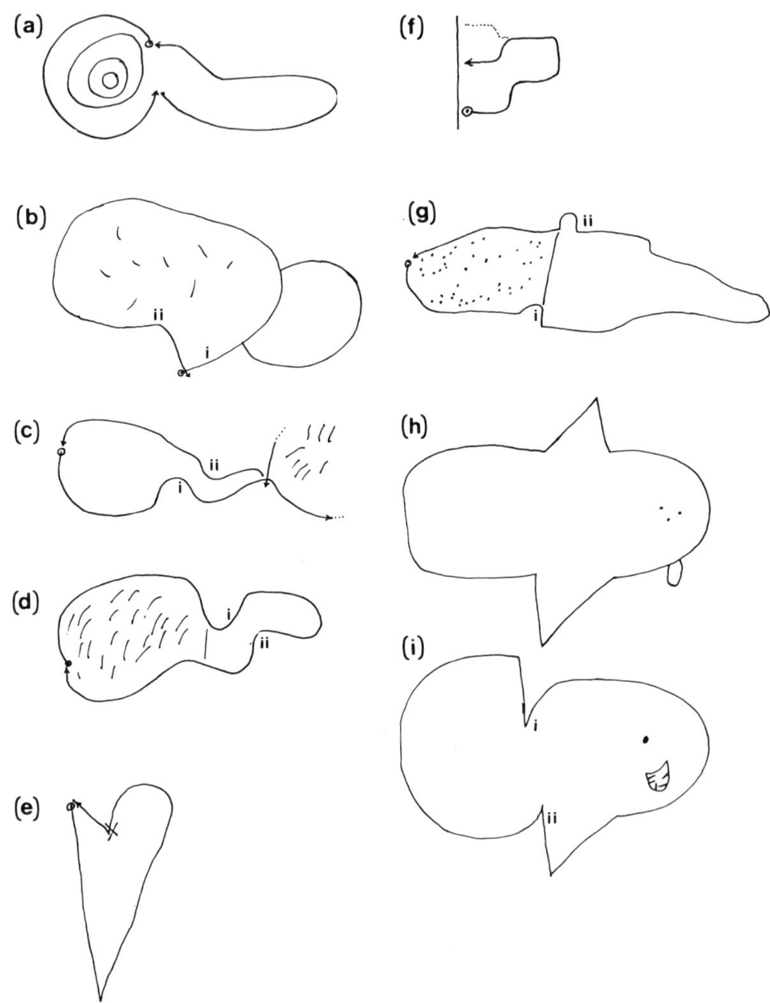

Fig. 9.7. (a) to (e): A series of items showing how simple miscalculation, difficulty with gap filling, and the estimation of the proper destination of part of a closed contour produce anomalous features. (f) to (i): Difficulties with the production of the slope and direction of mirror image contours.

same problem in drawing a brush, Fig. 9.7(g): The curves are parallel rather than opposed. Georgina (aged 5.4) had two problems [Fig. 9.7(h) and (i)] : First, she appears to confuse crocodiles with sharks; and second, although subsequent drawings showed she was aiming to equip her animal with matching fins, she produced an inversion on her first attempt. This is not simply a piece of clumsiness, but seems to be a systematic perceptual-motor problem that occasionally appears also in adult drawings.

There is also a type of perceptual contamination or "cross-talk" affecting contour production in which a shape is transferred from one line to another. Ai Hong (aged 5.10), in drawing the tape dispenser, quite properly makes its upper surface concave but does the same thing to the lower surface which, regarded from the same viewpoint, would be flat; see Fig. 9.8(a). (It is in fact drawn flat in all his subsequent drawings.) This transfer of geometry from one part to another is analogous to the way in which thickness sometimes translates itself into length, as in portraying the teeth of a comb, Fig. 9.8(b). There are in fact two features of the comb that elicit an anomalous reaction: the thicker members at each end and the two gauges of teeth. The breadth of the end pieces is translated into increased length, and the larger teeth are drawn longer when they are in fact wider (but of the same length), or are packed together more closely to suggest thickness when in fact they are more widely spaced. Another example is the use of the converse in color: A silver spoon with a black plastic handle is drawn as a black spoon with a white handle.

Most contours trace the boundary of one unitary component of an object – the body of the telephone is drawn as one region, the handset another. But there are exceptions of two contrasting sorts. The first involves making a contour that subdivides a unified object, as when a child draws a controlled line around the body of a crocodile and then tacks on a muzzle at one end and a tail at the other. The second violation of the structure of objects involves overinclusiveness of contour, as when, in Fig. 9.9(a), a child drew a line along the upper edge of a tape dispenser that incorporated the tape reel into the dispenser body, almost as if the whole device had treacle poured over it. Fig. 9.9(b) shows a line that defines the sky and the lower edge of the sun's disc. This also violates the natural separation of the two objects represented. This is perhaps more comprehensible in a sense than the agglomerated tape dispenser because it was the product of a frequently repeated routine. The sky and sun seem almost to have lost their representational significance and become like a standard border to the page.

Beginning drawers sometimes betray they have a problem in depicting shape that goes beyond a single graphic device because they produce not only a less than faithful version of an object's shape in their contoured lines, but duplicate this when they draw the same thing with various combinations of juxtaposed primitives. Fig. 9.9(c) presents a relatively rich example of this. The tape dispenser has a smooth curve to its upper surface, yet the child depicted it (as many did) with a contour that "kicked up" abruptly at the ends. On other days this same child heightened the ends of the dispenser by amendment. He variously added arcs, rectangles, vertical lines, or even patches of opaque pencil work to give the impression of local added height. It is very likely in a case like this

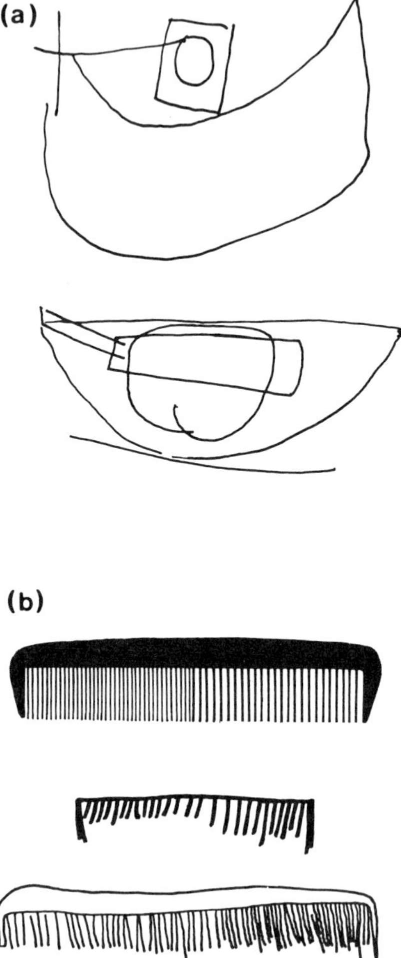

Fig. 9.8. Perceptual "cross-talk" or contamination in children's drawings. (a): The upper surface of the dispenser is curved and the curve is translated to the lower surface, which elsewhere is drawn flat. (b): Length and density of strokes are substituted for thickness in drawing a comb with teeth of two different gauges. The thickness of the ends of the comb is translated into greater length, as are the thicker teeth. (The model for the lower drawing had a broken left end.)

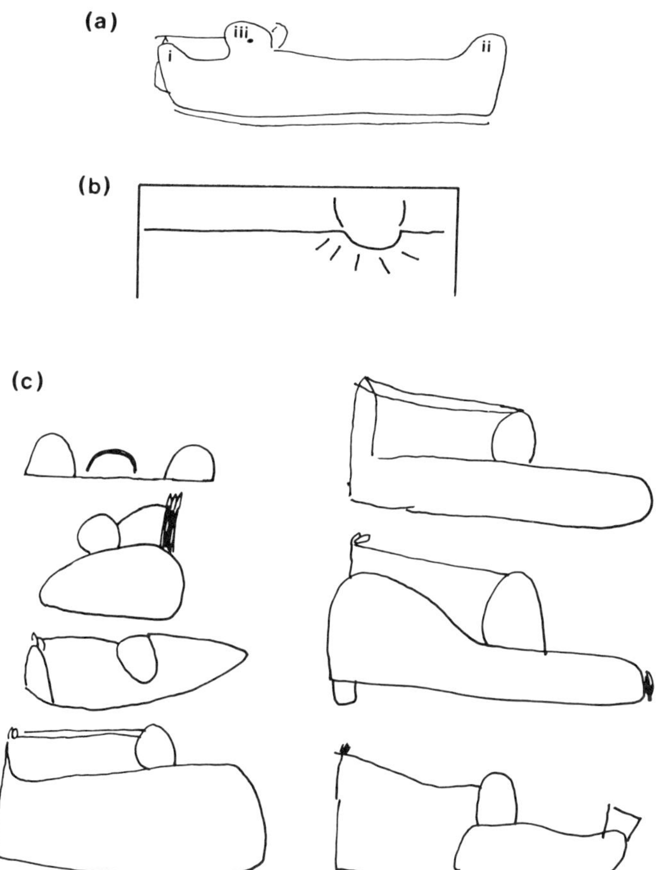

Fig. 9.9. (a): Overinclusive contour. (b): Boundary of sky and sun combined into single contour after frequent repetition. (c): A 5-year-old boy uses at least six separate devices to represent the upward curved shape of a tape dispenser: arcs, an opaque area, various contours, a single vertical line, and a rectangle.

that the drawer is reproducing not the shape of the dispenser itself, but the shape of an early graphic image of it, and doing so by a variety of means.

To review, contour in the work of 5- and 6-year-olds cannot be conceived of as a single unitary phenomenon. Some are positive, others are complementary embellishments on a skeleton of primitives. Some are preplanned, many are produced on a short-term ad-hoc basis. Some contours are little more than threaded primitives; sometimes they are modified or even precipitated by mis-calculation; sometimes the departures from good form seem to arise from fundamental perceptual-motor difficulties, including difficulties in preventing "cross-talk" between boundary shapes.

How does controlled contour develop?

It is not possible to give a full account of a transition from the exclusive use of simple circles and lines to comprehensive use of controlled contour on the basis of a longitudinal study that occupies only six or eight months, but it is possible to talk about the microhistory of the period, which for many children does include a changeover from one strategy to the other. First, it is important to note that it is not a one-way conversion process, because children switch backward and forward from cobbling together a shape from simple elements to drawing a special-purpose line.

In the protocols of the young children, we can detect the actual evolution of contours of the various types described: (1) Children draw continuously what was previously separate, but are simply threading from primitive to primitive. (2) This procedure sometimes progresses to a true special-purpose contour. There are a few cases of an extremely labile, wandering line representing a complex shape that had as precursors simple combinations of lines and circles. (3) A line may be produced first as a complementary contour and then become an autonomous outline without a skeleton. (4) Children may sometimes move to contour as a "journey" around an object before them or some internal quasi-visual memory of it, showing little reliance on a "bridge" from primitives. (5) Finally, they may begin with a very simple version of an envelope or contour and substantially upgrade it in subsequent drawings.

Handling spatial problems

The principal themes of the foregoing material on the structure of children's drawings have been how elements are selected, how they are constructed, and how their compilation is ordered. I should like to turn now to one further important aspect of structure, the semantic integration of components within drawings. This deals with such issues as how children create and organize elements to portray physical arrangements like occlusion (the overlapping arrangement of items in space), how they deal with physical elements embedded in plane surfaces like the bristles on the face of a brush, or how they organize the portrayal of an object whose components are best visualized from a variety of different viewpoints.

These issues carry the inquiry into an area of practical graphic problem solving that is intimately tied to particular subject matter, and for this reason is as boundless as the range of objects and events in the world that could be drawn.

After all, one could walk into any one of a thousand factories and find hundreds of special-purpose objects that would present the vernacular drawer with graphic problems. On the other hand, this particular constellation of problems does not derive simply from complex or exotic subject matter, but from a crucial and widely recognized feature of all drawing: the problem of translating a three-dimensional world into a picture in two dimensions.

This is one of a cluster of problems arising from the nature of the drawing medium. An analogous difficulty derives from the fact that drawings are better adapted to representing momentary events than events in time, or rigid stationary objects rather than those that move. It is also better suited to portraying objects with distinct boundaries than those that are fuzzy or amorphous, or objects whose identifying features are outlines rather than contours or textures. It is significant that for the purposes of this study of children's graphic development I had automatically chosen a set of relatively rigid static and stationary objects, and this in turn makes it easier at an empirical level to concentrate on the one major systematic problem that such objects present, that of the handling of their spatial properties.

Occlusion in children's drawings

First some comments on the matter of *occlusion*, which refers to the overlapping of the boundary of one object by another. The issue was explored in an earlier chapter that dealt with how adults portrayed pairs of objects in front of or behind others. Several of their tactics were described: object separation and boundary contact, intersection and overlap (transparency). That taxonomy can now be slightly amplified and applied to the methods used by children. We deal first with complete occlusion. We found that adults never completely omit occluded objects in the drawings, and this is largely true with children.

A few years ago, Dr. Penny Jools and I asked primary school children to draw "a boy hidden behind a wall." Some children simply constructed the figure and drew the wall elements over it. Some drew the boy above or beside a wall. A few drew the wall edge-on, with the boy to one side. (This was not a widely favored approach, probably because walls are not prototypically displayed in this way.) Most children allowed some part of the boy's anatomy (usually the head) to show at the edge of the wall.

In this we have the operation of the equivalent of Grice's (1975) conversational maxim on quantity: Include all separate items on the agenda of the drawing. There seems to be a reciprocal undertaking that one does *not* show occluded material which is an intrinsic part of an object unless there is a special reason to do so. Hence, we do not normally draw the engine in a car, the core in an intact apple, or the contents of a closed cupboard unless the pragmatic context explicitly demands it.

I will shift attention at this point to the portrayals of the one object drawn from life that included a partially concealed element – the reel in the tape dispenser. Perhaps because it was repeatedly inspected and because of its peculiar structure, it yielded a greater richness and variety of approaches than the imagined objects that involved occlusion. The critical characteristic was, of course, the location of the tape reel in a recess in the dispenser body. Seven separate devices were used to represent this feature, plus some "hybrids." They are listed below and illustrated in Fig. 9.10.

(a). The object is represented in the conventional side elevation. A semicircle representing the upper half of the reel is anchored to the upper boundary of the dispenser body.

(b). The reel is drawn as a complete circle but displaced upward, either tangential to or separate from the dispenser body.

(c). The whole reel cuts across the boundary, producing "transparency."

(d). A gap or indentation is formed in the envelope of the dispenser to accommodate a circle, spiral, and so on representing the reel.

(e). The complete reel is enclosed within the body of the dispenser. This seems often to result from a so-called orthoscopic approach to the object. The term *orthoscopic* was used by Bühler (1934) to refer to the juxtaposition within one drawing of elements each of which is portrayed in its most characteristic or visually informative perspective, so that a table top might be drawn as a rectangle and the legs in side elevation, a glass drawn with straight sides, a flat bottom, and a circular top, and so on. Hence the dispenser may be drawn viewed from above as a region with the tape reel drawn within it. The reel, however, is depicted in side elevation as a circle or whorl. Some children had to distort the circular outline of the reel to fit it into the region representing the dispenser. In another instance, the circle was radically flattened to have it fit into a narrow strip representing the dispenser's top surface. Ai Hong (aged 5.10) drew a rectangle representing the cavity outside the body region and located a circle within that so that there were three changes of perspective, from body to cavity to reel. All these procedures have in common the reel represented as a full "circle" within a surrounding boundary.

(f). The visible half of the reel is drawn as a semicircle but located within the dispenser body, so that the point at which reel and body make contact is represented simply by the alignment of the free ends of the semicircles.

(g). Half the reel is depicted as in (f) but is anchored to the *lower* boundary of the dispenser.

Various hybrid versions tell us something about the mental operations involved in handling this representational problem. Frequently the tape reel was drawn as two concentric circles – the perimeter and a core. One hybrid version had the perimeter as a half circle, but the core drawn as a complete circle. This was either displaced upward to clear the dispenser boundary or cut across it. These represent mixtures of strategies (a) and (b) or (a) and (c). Alternatively, the core is displaced upward while the perimeter is transparent, as in (b) and (c). There

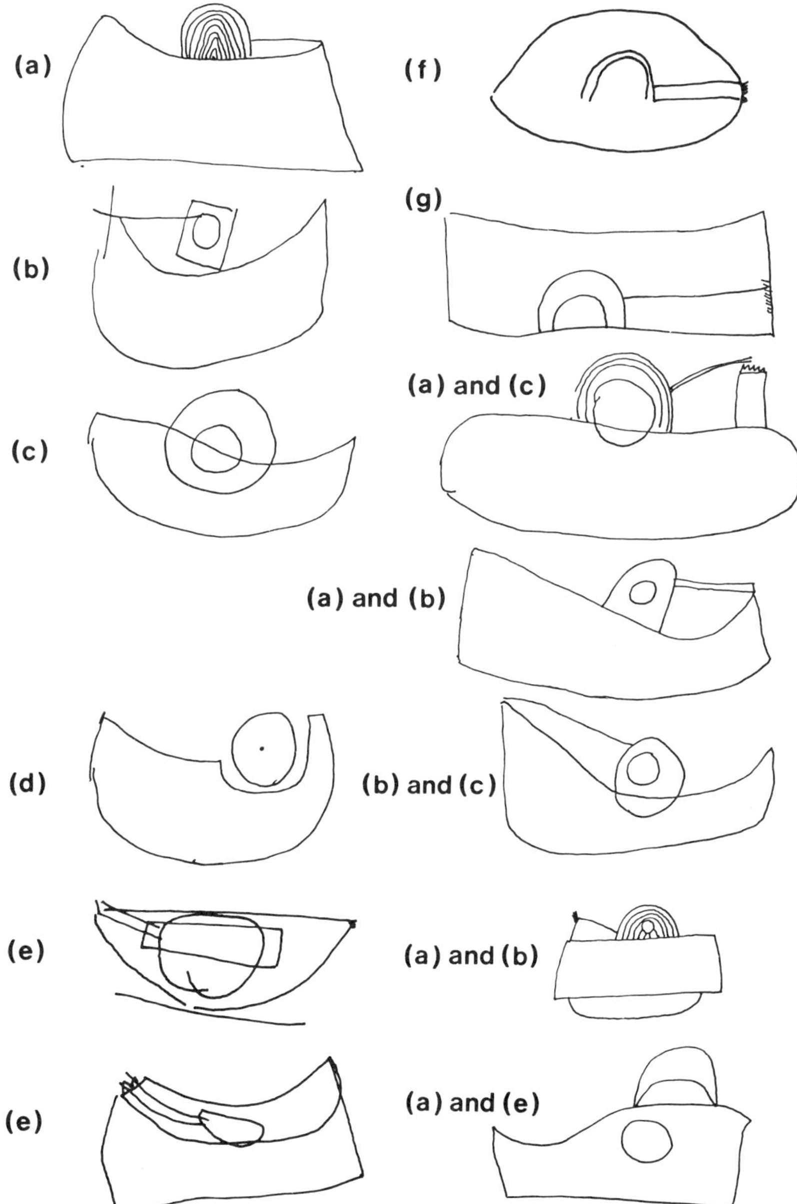

Fig. 9.10. Strategies for representing the spatial relations between a tape reel and dispenser. The numbers refer to descriptions in the text. The last five drawings are "hybrids," including two basic strategies juxtaposed.

is a case where the tape is detailed as a sequence of concentric semicircles, with a complete core located embedded in and cutting across these lines (Fig. 9.10). There is even a case where the reel is represented twice, once as a pair of semicircles and once as a full circle within the dispenser body. Furthermore, within a short series of drawings children may utilize three or four of these devices sequentially.

When I first drew up a list of strategies, it seemed possible to put them into two classes: those like the semicircular representations of the reel and the interrupted outline of the plastic body that seemed to indicate the children were aware of the spatial problem, and those incorporating circles, transparencies, and so on, in which they were not. But this view that drawing simply reflects awareness cannot prosper in the light of the various hybrid forms and the appearance of both classes of strategy in the same drawing, or indeed the rapid alternation between one type of approach and the other in a series of drawings by the same child. It is probably safer to assume that most children of this age recognize the problem but give different priorities to one or the other of the two elements, integrity of form or spatial overlap, and oscillate between the two.

When I was describing adults' use of various devices to represent occlusion, I pointed out that it was only when circumstances forced them to do so that they allowed the boundaries of opaque objects to cross ("transparency"). Children do this frequently. It may be a question of contrast. As I have said, drawers tend to avoid using devices that have their own representational significance, and perhaps for adults more than children, boundaries that cross have a representational significance (that is, actual transparency) to which children are less sensitive. (The test of this would be to expose children to pairs of real transparent objects and to see if they then reduced the amount of boundary crossing for nontransparent pairs.)

Surfaces represented as open regions

As I mentioned earlier, the devices listed in this analysis of the tape dispenser are applicable to other subject matter. A quick review of 100 drawings of the baby carriage and rowing boat provided examples of almost all the strategies mentioned. In both the baby carriage and boat drawings, there were one or two versions in which only part of the figure (such as the head) was drawn within an open region representing the carriage or boat, an arrangement directly analogous to the semicircular tape reel located in the center of the region representing the tape dispenser.

Although this procedure of locating an element in the center of an open area may seem rather exotic, it has a very common analog in other drawings, the brush in particular, where the majority of children produced an outline representing the head of the brush and filled it with independent strokes representing the bristles. In a very large number of cases, these strokes were drawn upward from the base, contrary to preferred stroke direction, as though the children were anchoring the bristles to an imaginary surface. Not all children were tolerant of this situation; a few avoided placing the lines freely in space and anchored them around the periphery of the brush.

Orthoscopic representation

The third issue relevant to space – the variation in viewpoint – has already been dealt with in passing. There are some classic examples in the drawings of the tape dispenser of features drawn from different angles combined together. There is evidence here, as elsewhere, that this "orthoscopic" approach is coded at the level of remembered shape and not remembered motor sequence, since the forms are preserved while construction strategy alters, and children assemble and reassemble the configuration in different ways on different occasions. This process of coding information and using it at a later time will be the main theme of the following chapter, which uses the same corpus of repeated drawings that we have been analyzing and discussing.

Coordination of representational devices

Orthoscopic representation could be classed as a confusion and a failure of consistency of view by the photographic literalist. Most commentators on children's drawings rather admire it as seeming to represent an escape from the tyranny of the fixed viewpoint and a triumph of sense and imagination. Both views are overdrawn, since the one assumes that the fixed viewpoint is necessarily the best, and the other assumes that children have assessed the merits of the fixed and the variable viewpoint and have decided on the second. It is more probable that they simply have not been very attentive to the possibility of consistency.

Another variety of anarchy found in children's drawings is just as fruitful of graphic curiosities as orthoscopic representation. When there exists a complement of primitives (lines, spirals, circles) and when each is capable of representing a variety of features of objects (a line represents the edges of a rod or the rod itself), there is the issue of the coordination of the choices within a drawing. One might expect, for example, that if an adult draws a human figure with "stick" arms she will also draw stick legs, not legs with double boundaries. Further, if an adult wants to put stripes on a pole, she usually gives the pole thickness; if she wants to portray a hole in an object, the object is normally drawn as a region and the region will normally be large enough to incorporate the representation of the hole. There are exceptions to this even in adult drawing, the most common being the "stick figure" in which the head is a region (a circle), but the trunk, which is in reality broader than the head, is drawn as a line. Another example is a fur coat drawn with a continuous boundary with short lines representing hair within it, instead of the outline also being composed of short lines. But these are mild aberrations compared with the lack of coordination occasionally found in young children's drawings.

I refer here to a special class of coordination, that which applies at the level of the line. A child may draw a human figure as an amoebalike region with excrescences representing arms and legs, and later add regions to make the limbs more prominent. Here the devices may be redundant, but the elements that are combined are of one type (regions). When the added limbs are single strokes, the devices are no longer coordinated. The phenomenon is best illustrated by examples: Fig. 9.11(a), for example, shows a drawing of a hammer. The upper part shows the head with the striking surface to the right and "claws" to the left, all represented as regions (notwithstanding that one is an open region!). The handle, by contrast, is a single line, and at the bottom is the round end of the handle, which had a circle and dot engraved on it. This is drawn as a region. Fig. 9.11(b) shows a similar mix: a hose drawn as a single spiral, the opening at its end as a circle from which water issues. In Fig. 9.11(c) we have a brush with a hole in the handle: The handle is a line, the hole is a broad dot superimposed on it. Fig. 9.11(d) shows a footbridge supported by vertical piles, all drawn as regions. The concrete stairs that ascend the side of the bridge are drawn as open rungs (arrow). Fig. 9.11(e) shows a staircase that begins as a line, transforms itself into regions, and then continues as a line.

These mixtures do occur in adult drawings, as I have said, and are found particularly when people are illustrating something with speech accompaniment. One draws a map showing a main road as a double line. The cross streets are quickly sketched as single lines, an important junction with double lines again. An increase in speed, a drop in the level of precision, and often the accompanying dialogue all signal this inconsistency as a matching of detail to the emphasis in the communicative task. This is, in fact, no different in principle from what the child may be doing. A single line is enough to show the length of coiled hose; when an opening is needed, one changes to a different register. What differs is the degree of self-consciousness about the process. Adults do not normally produce such blatant lack of coordination in their standard representational drawing, and if they use it in more functional contexts, they often acknowledge the departure from the canon of consistency. The young child more likely works in an ad hoc fashion without any compulsion to coordinate.

The topic of coordination is no trivial matter when one moves from vernacular to skilled professional performances. Even the most cursory examination of the

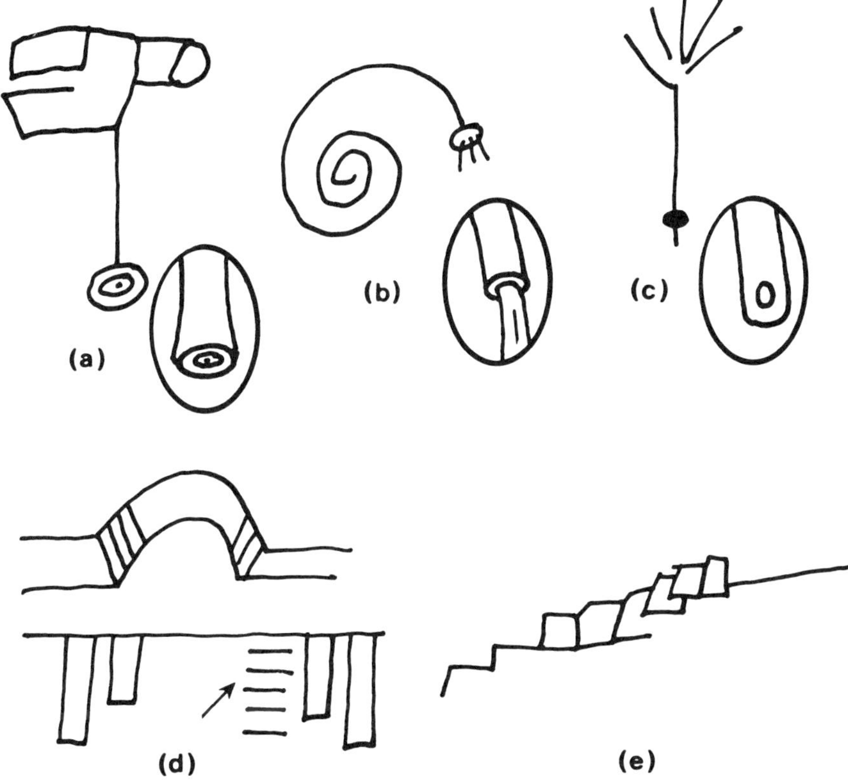

Fig. 9.11. Lack of coordination of representational devices in children's drawing. (a): Embossed circle on base of hammer handle. (b): Hose. (c): Brush with circular hole in handle. (d): Footbridge drawn as regions, with free-standing lines representing stairs. (e): Stairs represented as a mixture of lines and regions. The "canonical" version of the first three objects is shown within the ellipses.

styles of representation in a book like that by Ivins (1958) shows not only the ingenuity used to achieve consistency, but the highly sophisticated analysis that would be needed to specify the tight coordination of linear and textural devices used by artists like Daumier, Goya, or Dürer. It is not that each restricted himself to one line or one textural device, but rather that each moved systematically and judiciously over a carefully chosen range. It is in these matters that graphic analysis comes closest to the concept of a grammar, although it is a grammar incorporating a large component of mimetics and sensibility.

10 Children's repeated drawings: How are innovations coded?

Two illustrations in Eng's *The Psychology of Drawing* (1954) depict an assemblage of dolls drawn by a girl of 5.11 years. Most of the dolls wear cloaks, which Eng says have their origins in an error that became stylized into what she calls a "formula." There are no details given of the construction process beyond the fact that in the initial drawing a basic triangular female figure was accidentally elaborated by two long sloping lines that were later "discovered" by the child to represent a cloak.

A close examination of the dolls drawn 3 and 10 days after the initial accidental creation of the cape motif reveals that the child used at least six different construction strategies to produce what are visually rather similar figures. Fig. 10.1(a) and (b) show the relevant parts of the two drawings, and below in Fig. 10.1(c) are diagrams that expand the microstructure of the figures to show the various procedures.

Eng does not comment on this feature of the drawing, and when the variability first caught my attention, I assumed that if it was a real effect (as opposed to an error in reproduction, which seems unlikely), it surely represented a graphic oddity. Yet these illustrations now seem to crystallize very well what I wish to document more fully – the production of similar and distinctive graphic products by a variety of different means.

Consistency of appearance in sequences of drawings

First I want to establish the reality of distinctive personal approaches to representation by individual children. The first two examples demonstrate the identifiability of drawings produced by the 5- and 6-year-old Sydney children whose work we have been analyzing. The first series (Fig. 10.2) shows whole objects; five series of 10 drawings of a tennis shoe. The same type of family resemblance can be seen in Fig. 10.3, which shows a *detail* of a drawing, the spring assembly of the paper punch. In each instance, it would not be difficult to sort the drawings fairly accurately into sets corresponding to the particular children who produced

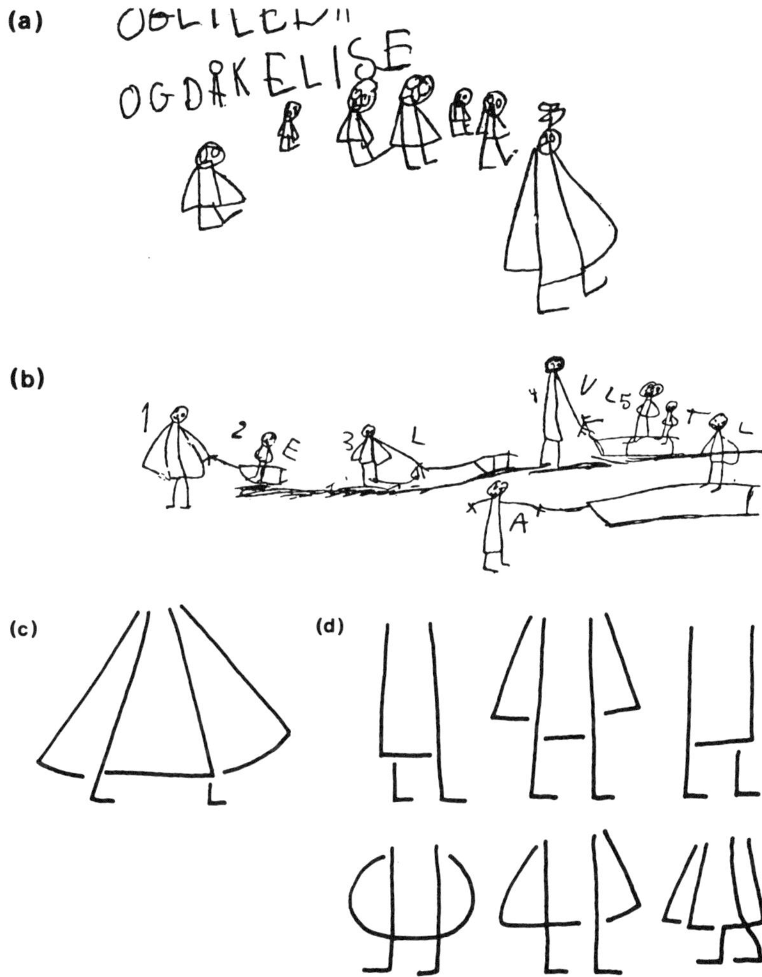

Fig. 10.1. (a) and (b): Facsimiles of portion of Fig. 65 and all of Fig. 68 of Eng's (1954) book on children's drawings. The drawings of dolls by a girl aged 5.11 years show a variety of production strategies within the same drawing. (c): Diagrammatic representation of the first female figure to be drawn by the child who produced (a) and (b). The "cloak" was, according to Eng, an accidental product of drawing two extra lines beside the body and was incorporated into the doll drawings soon afterward. (d): Diagrammatic representation of six different structures to be found in the doll drawings. These drawings suggest that a form accidentally produced becomes a visual schema later produced by different means. [(a) and (b) used by permission of Asbjørn Eng.]

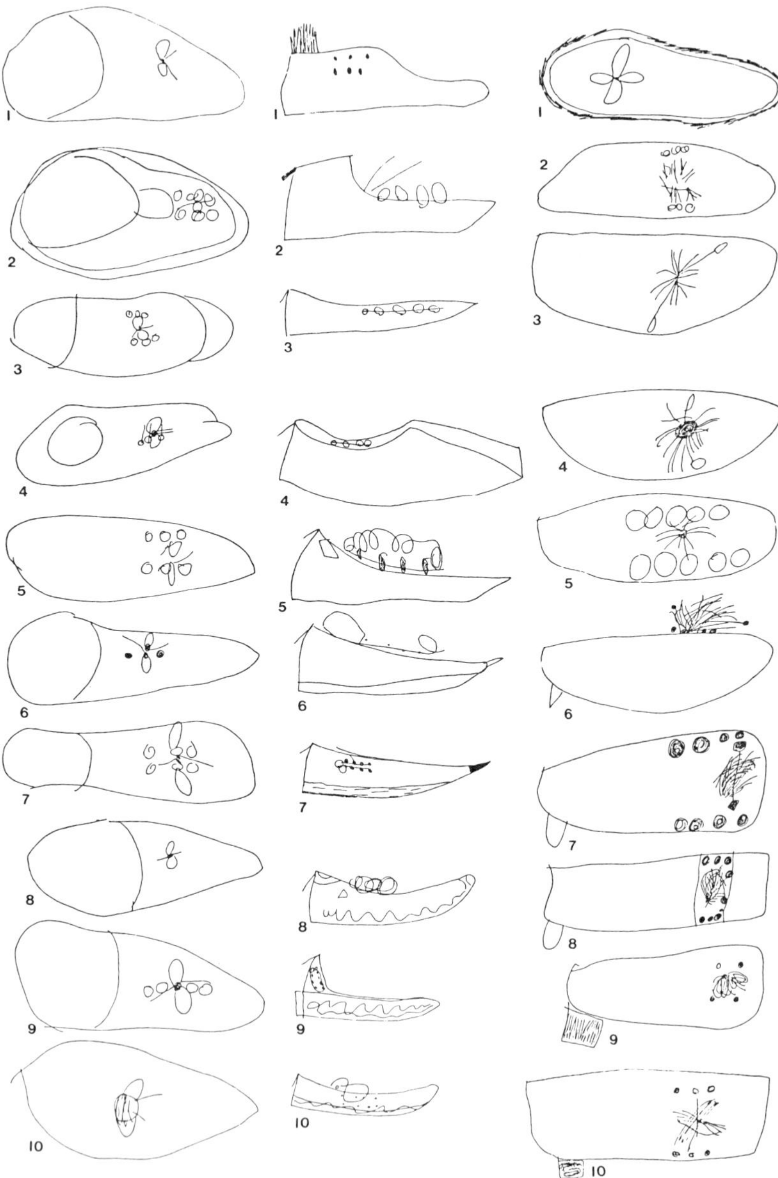

Fig. 10.2. Ten successive drawings from life of a canvas tennis shoe by six children. In spite of certain changes in structure and detail, the approach of each child remains quite distinctive.

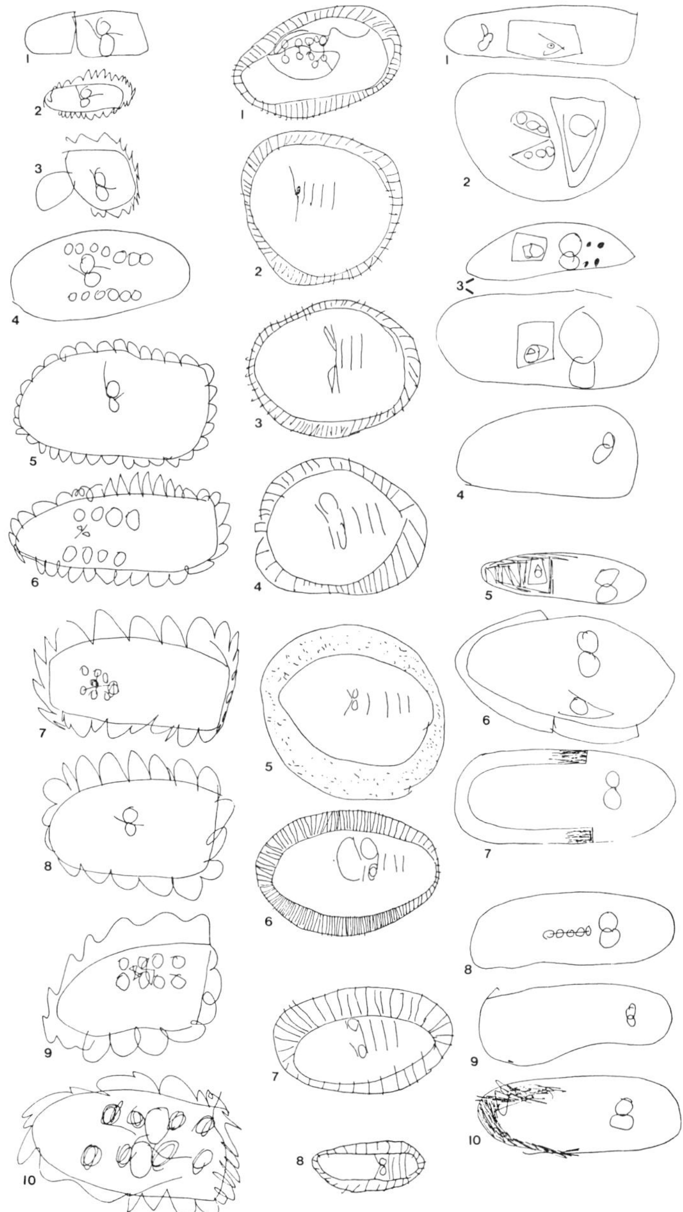
1
2
3
4
5
6
7
8
9
10
1
2
3
4
5
6
7
8
1
2
3
4
5
6
7
8
9
10

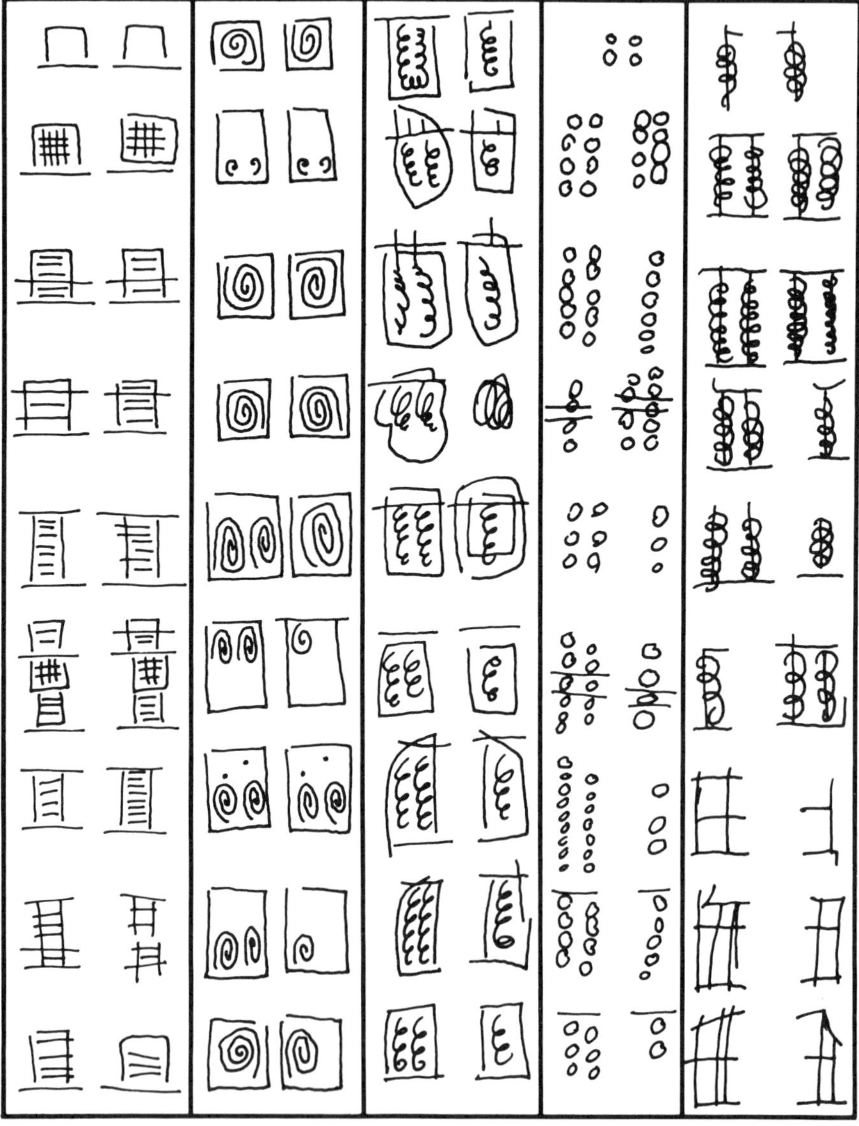

Fig. 10.3. Each column shows nine versions of the spring assembly on a paper hole punch drawn by each of five children aged 5 to 6 years. (The assemblies have been reproduced closer together than in the original drawings and slightly stylized by the author to indicate some of the structural variations in the way the assemblies were drawn by the children.)

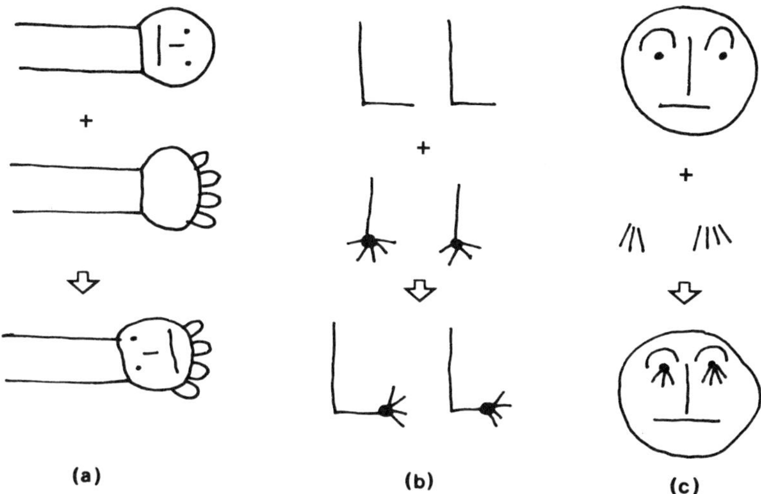

Fig. 10.4. Redundancy in children's drawings resulting from the convergence of two different graphic devices. (a): face with line for mouth *plus* teeth to make crocodile head. (b): Lines representing feet combined with dot and radiating "toes." (c): Open eye motif combined with eyelashes to portray sleeping.

them. Even with material that is more heterogeneous than this, children are frequently found to be moving to and fro among a number of versions. This applies at every level, from overall structure to small details. Although in many cases it appears that a child has adopted a quite fresh attack on the task of representation, different themes in drawings do not remain compartmentalized. Close examination quite often shows cross-fertilization from one drawing in a series to another, with features and devices juxtaposed or blended. In some cases this process brings together into one drawing two different versions of the same part of the object, so that we get the type of redundancy shown in Fig. 10.4.

The same family resemblance between drawings in a series is obvious in the paper punch drawings of a boy aged 5.11 shown in Fig. 10.5. The shape of the base plate, handle, spring assembly, triangular paper guide, horizontal axle, and so on is relatively consistent. Further, the formal constraints on stroke construction and order apply: The line delineating the base starts most often near the top left and runs counterclockwise, rectangles are drawn from a top-left start in 19 cases out of 22, triangles usually begin from upper corners, left rectangles are most often drawn first and before the spirals they enclose, most arcs run from left to right, and when in pairs most are drawn from outer to inner, and so on.

These are the continuities and the regularities. Let us now review briefly the other side of the issue. A superficial inspection of these 11 pictures reveals some variation – for example, in the number of springs present or in the form of the

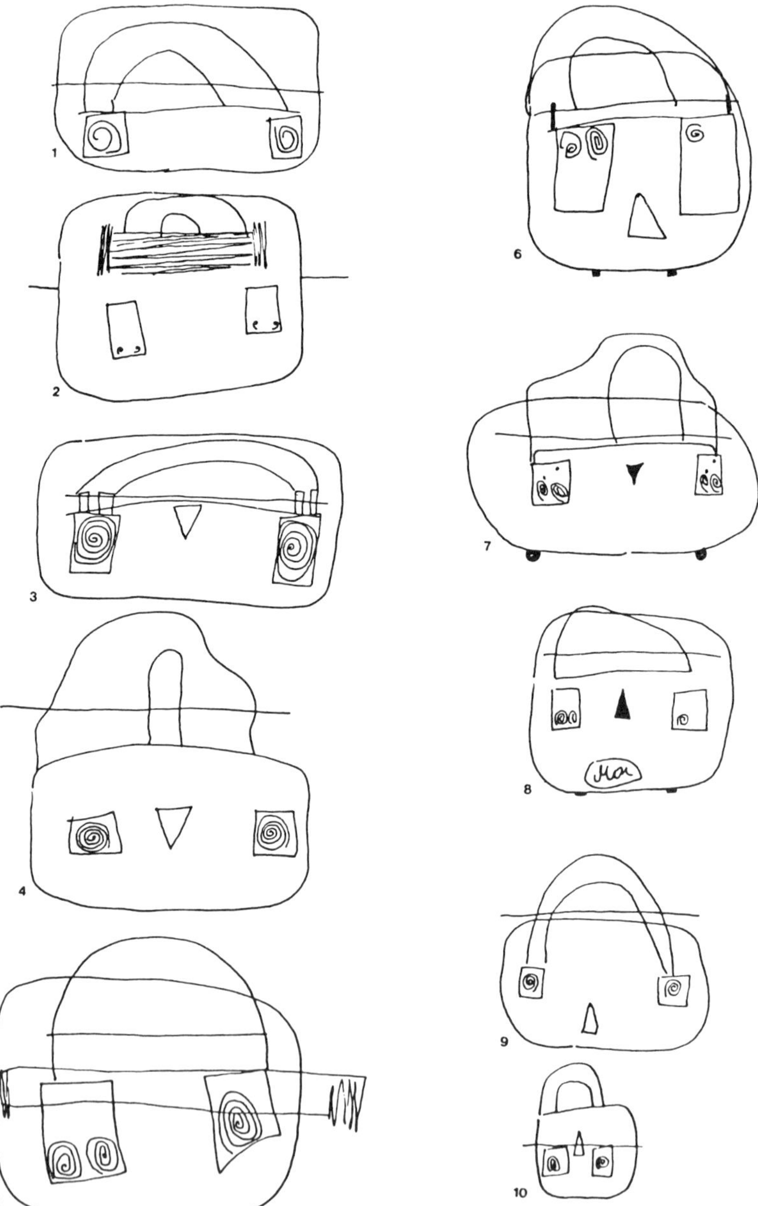

Fig. 10.5. Twelve drawings of a paper punch drawn over a 9-month period by a boy aged 5.11 years. In spite of a certain family resemblance between these drawings, there is an immense amount of variation in structure and in production strategy.

curved handle, which is sometimes a double line, sometimes a single line, sometimes a plain arc, sometimes a contour. But a thorough examination reveals that the variability is much more pervasive. Indeed, this series of drawings, which is above average in consistency, nonetheless varies continuously and simultaneously on almost every feature and structural characteristic it possesses. Not only does the handle vary in shape and change from a single to a double line, but it is sometimes placed entirely within the general frame, sometimes completely outside, and sometimes bridging it. The handle terminates on a single bar, on a double, on four punch dies, on the rectangles containing springs, or on two narrow stems. The springs themselves vary from drawing to drawing not only in number and size, but in direction of rotation and starting point. The springs and the rectangles that contain them are drawn in seven different orders in 11 drawings. Although on average the arcs making up handles obey general rules, there are in fact four strategies of order and direction among the eight instances of double lines. Even the small central triangle appears and disappears, point down, up, down, up, down, successively. The base, although most often drawn counterclockwise, changes direction five times in the series.

What this rather obsessive chronicle reveals is that the drawer is quite heavily influenced by formal constraints, but at the same time he never locks onto a standard routine of production. What we will do in the rest of this chapter is try to make some sense of this mixture of order and disorder within and across drawers.

Salience and order

If we are looking for some principles of order that extend beyond formal principles, the most likely candidate is some dimension of importance or salience. This involves a switch from geometry to semantics, so it seems sensible to begin our analysis with an object – the bicycle – whose parts are easily recognizable and usually clearly separable from one another even in the drawings of 5- and 6-year-olds.

There is available a corpus of 200 drawings (20 children repeating the bicycle 10 times from memory). If frequency of appearance can be taken as a rough indication of salience, what is the order of frequency of features? And what does it tell us about construction? Counting features produces this list:

Feature	*Percentage*
Wheels	100%
Frame	99
Handlebar	91
Handle support	74

Spokes	73
Seat	58
Seat support	47
Hub	40
Handgrips	27
Pedal	12
Mudguard	9
Bell	9

There are other minor items: basket, lamp, sprocket, chain, ornamental ribbons, and so on.

If these are the "frequencies of mention," how do they relate to the "*order* of mention"; that is, the place in the compilation process where the item typically lies. Fig. 10.6 plots mean position in construction order against frequency of appearance. The wheels and frame are virtually universal and appear earliest; items like cranks, pedals, sprockets, and bell are least common and appear late.

Although this way of displaying the data does show a systematic relation between how common a feature is and how early it is drawn (and reflects such formal constraints as left to right progression), it does not really come to grips with the dynamics of construction. It treats the drawing process as though children simply lay down features here and there on a page as one might make a list, with salient features coming to mind first and being invariably present, and less salient items being late and unreliable. When we repeat this process with a second object, the tape dispenser (Fig. 10.7), we find that the frequency/order relationship is much less striking or consistent, with a group of items of low frequency of appearance being constructed relatively early in the drawing sequence. The key to understanding the true significance of this relationship requires us to consider not only salience of features, but the structure of both drawing and object. To make sense of construction by both children and adults, we need to recognize a principle that is part geometric and part semantic, the principle of accretion.

Types of accretion

I have adopted the general term *accretion* to cover any mechanism that builds new elements onto old. It is to be distinguished from anchoring, which is just one way of accreting. When we draw a conventional sun the rays are accreted to the disc, but usually only those to the bottom right are actually anchored to it in the sense that the pen starts its movement there; those to the top left we might say are *attached*, beginning in space and making contact at their terminations. Likewise children may draw a bicycle and add a rider, but they do not

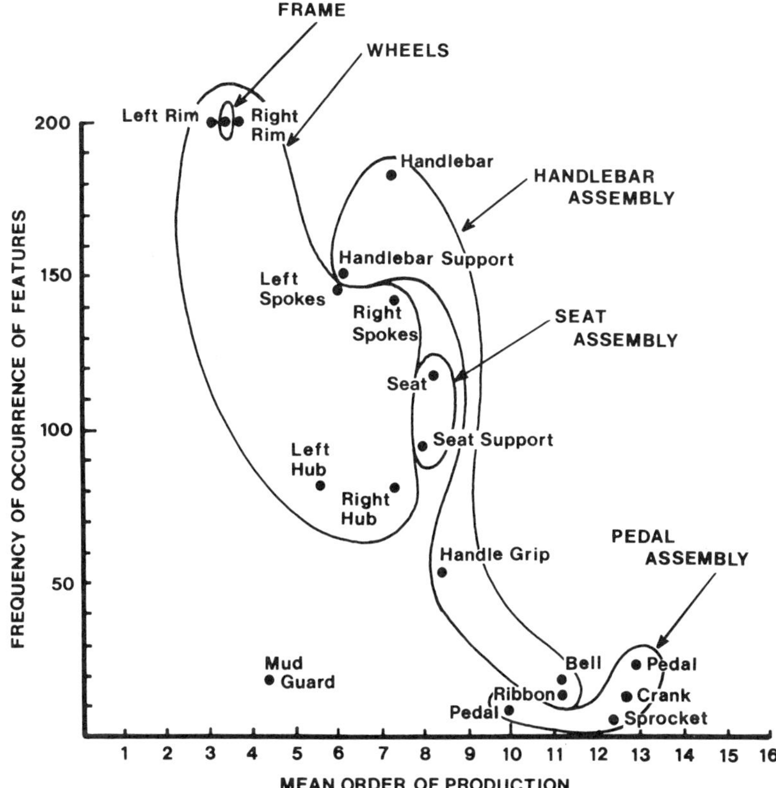

Fig. 10.6. The relation between overall frequency of appearance of features of a bicycle and the temporal order in which the features appeared in the individual drawing sequences. This figure represents data from 20 5- and 6-year-old children repeating the drawing 10 times. Each feature is labeled, and features forming subsystems (frame, wheels, seat assembly) are enclosed within boundaries. Left and right occurrences of features like wheel rims, hubs, and handlebars are plotted separately.

necessarily begin it by drawing upward from the seat. Again, they are accreting but not anchoring.

The third and rather less common mechanism is *conformity;* that is, adding new elements in a set relationship, usually physically close, to those present. For example, a dot may be placed at the center of a circle, a line drawn parallel to another, an arc made to follow closely the circumference of a circle. All these are accretions by conformity. It may even be useful to specify other types of accretion that do not involve actual contact, as when one draws a pair of wheels or a line of strokes in an open space (seriation) or fills a region with a cluster

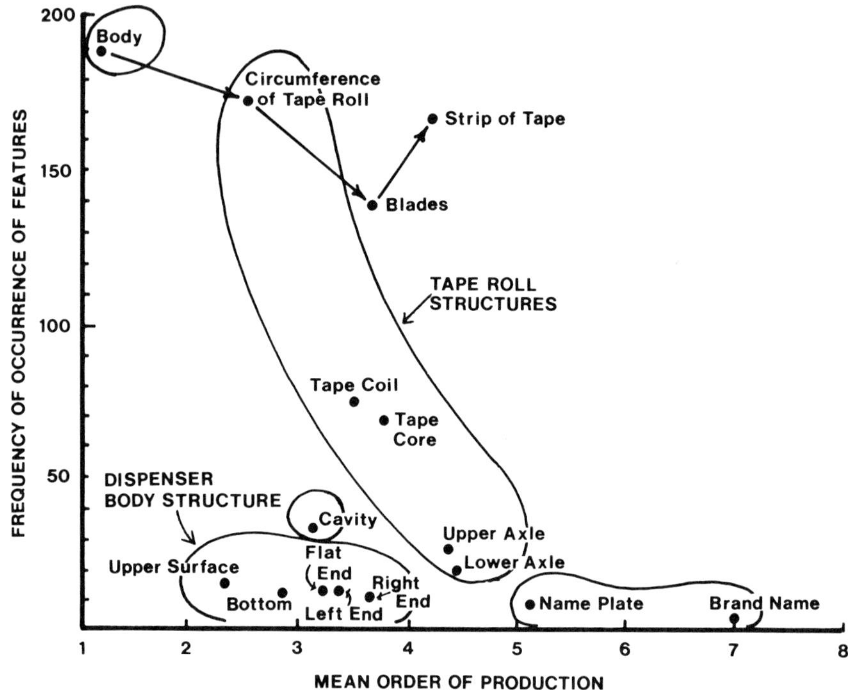

Fig. 10.7. The relation between frequency of appearance of features of the tape dispenser and average order of appearance. Data from 200 drawings by 5- and 6-year-olds. Features are labeled, and five subsystems are surrounded by boundaries. The arrows indicate a common sequence for the minimal portrayal of the object.

of dots (aggregation). The thing all these drawing actions share, and which I have called accretion, is a process of steady outward growth from what has already been drawn, a process so natural to us that we find it hard to think of likely alternative strategies.

This accretion process in drawing has its roots partly in the structure of objects. After all, we usually mean by an "object" something that coheres. From a geometrical point of view, birds sitting in the branches of a tree are as much part of the tree as a bell, lamp, and basket are of a bicycle; but we tend to organize them differently in our minds. In the case of the bicycle, both the object and the drawing have a "core" – the frame and wheel rims. If we select a drawing with a rich range of features, we find that some of these elaborate the wheels (mudguards, hubs, spokes), and others form one part or another of the handlebar, the seat, or the pedal subsystem (these have been outlined as clusters in Fig. 10.6).

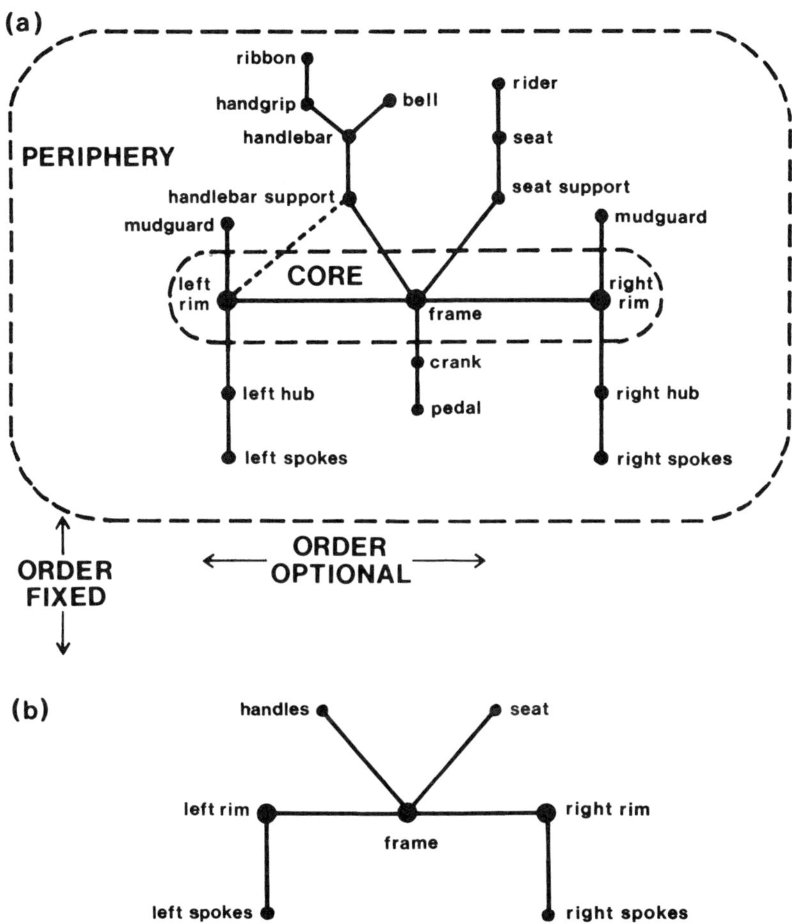

Fig. 10.8. Connection diagrams for the bicycle. Network (a) symbolizes a detailed drawing; (b) shows a minimal representation. The structure contains a "core" of wheel rims and frame and a periphery of side chains. Accretion progresses vertically away from the core. Selection of features horizontally or obliquely is optional. [The dotted line in (a) indicates that the handlebar subsystem may arise from the wheel or from the frame.]

Connection networks for drawings

In Fig. 10.8(a) this structure of core and periphery has been visualized as a network. This particular network summarizes a relatively detailed drawing of a bicycle. Fig. 10.8(b) symbolizes a more rudimentary ("minimal") bicycle. Note that in the first version many of the features form *chains*. The handlebar system, usually originating at the frame (but occasionally from the front wheel) makes up a vertical sequence – handlebar support, handlebars, handgrip, to ribbons or bell. The seat system branches from support to seat to rider, and so on.

In addition to the question of salience and the issue of how far down the hierarchy of detail a particular drawer will go, there is the issue of what such a structure allows and what it limits with respect to drawing procedure. In constructing these networks, I have contrived to have chains of features running vertically so that one can "read" where their movement is optional and where it is constrained. Drawers may vary their orders by moving horizontally or obliquely in these diagrams, but along the purely vertical dimension they must move only outward from the core. They rarely if ever move directly backward along the chains attached to the core. This is simply a way of stating and visualizing what was said earlier: Drawers accrete – they do not often draw remote elements and then fill the gaps.

We can now be more definitive about the basis of the relationship between frequency of appearance of features and their position in the order of construction. First, note that the bicycle (Fig. 10.8) has a number of extended "side chains" and that these vary in salience in a consistent way. The side chains ensure that when they are present, supports for handlebars are drawn before handlebars, handlebars before handgrips, and so on. Salience determines that handlebar assemblies appear before seats, which appear before pedals.

An object like a tape dispenser presents a different picture. There is a general, if weaker, relationship between overall frequency of features and their order of production (Fig. 10.7). The main exceptions are a cluster of features that relate to the main body of the dispenser which are relatively uncommon (none appears in more than 10 percent of the drawings) but which appear early. This is *not* an artifact of some children doing very simple drawings; quite the reverse. These features appear only in drawings with considerable detail. Connection networks diagrams for this object appear in Fig. 10.9.

In the elaborated drawings of the tape dispenser there is a complex "core" that children tend to complete before they progress to the other subsystems. Again, nobody moves backward down the chains of attachment or inclusion. Any apparent reversals in order within the frequency-order plots are due simply to the range of complexity of detail across subjects (since these plots represent lumped data). The "minimal" dispenser shown in Fig. 10.9(c) contains one core element (dispenser body), and drawers usually progress from tape to blades to tape strip (arrows, Fig. 10.7). If the tape roll itself is elaborated, this also follows a predictable sequence: perimeter, coil, core, axle.

Perhaps the most elaborate chains of accretion from the current body of data are found in the drawings of the light bulb. Figure 10.10(a) provides a sketch of the object and names its parts. Figure 10.10(b), (c), (d) show representations

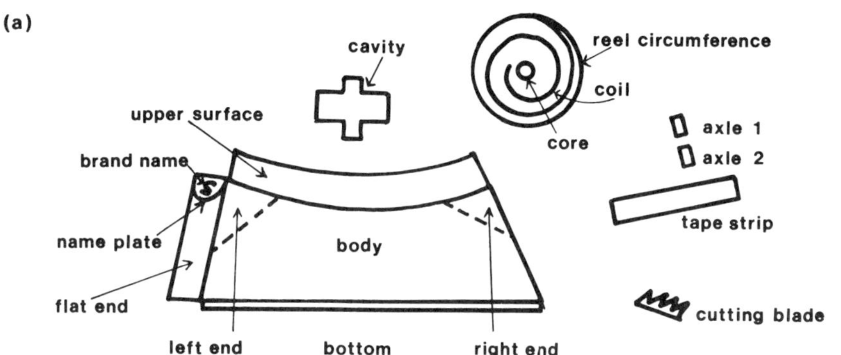

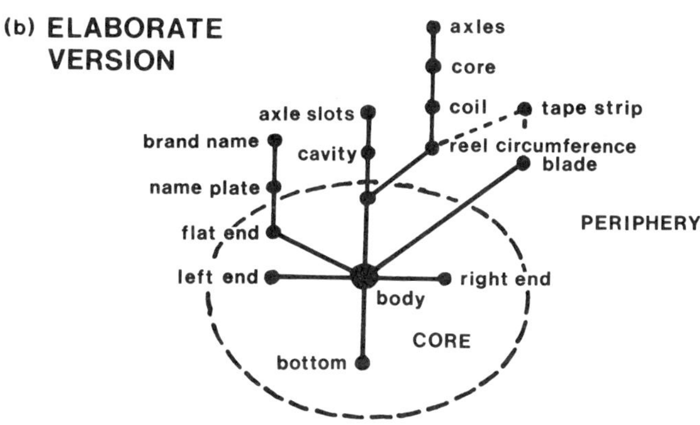

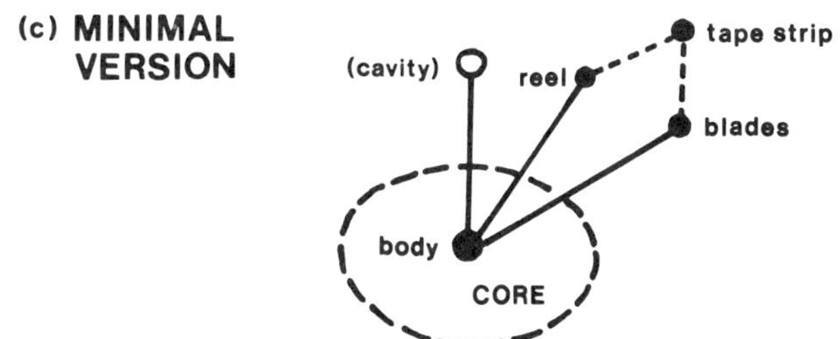

Fig. 10.9. Exploded diagram (a), and two connection networks for the tape dispenser. The core of the elaborate drawing includes a cluster of features to which various side chains are attached. The minimal version is shown in (c). It includes one optimal feature (open circle). Dotted lines indicate that the strip of tape is anchored or attached to both reel and cutting blades.

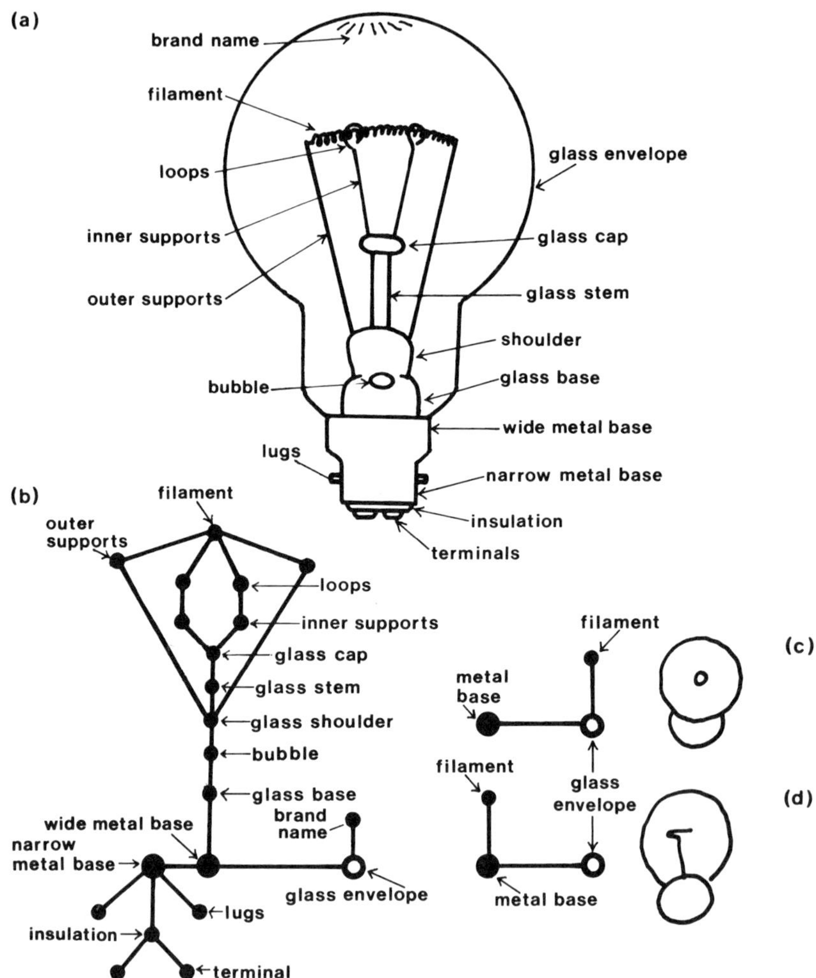

Fig. 10.10. (a): Sketch of clear light bulb, with features labeled. (b): Connection network for an elaborate drawing. Metal base and glass envelope comprise the core. (c) and (d): Networks for two simple drawings, one with the base attached to the glass, the other with glass attached to base: (c) has a filament as an inclusion; (d) has it attached to the base. (There is no necessary correlation between the latter two variations.)

of connection networks, one elaborate and two simple. Here the idea of a "core" remains appropriate, since the metal base and the glass envelope are invariably present, and elements are either built out from the common boundary between base and glass or are inclusions within the latter.

We are now in a position to examine in more detail a set of drawings of this object that reveals the anatomy of change across a series of drawings. The material was produced by a girl who at age 6.4–6.10 was one of the older subjects, but about average in graphic sophistication. Her original 12 versions of the lamp are shown in Fig. 10.11, and Fig. 10.12 shows network diagrams for each of her drawings. In the latter figure the progress down the page corresponds generally to the actual week-to-week order in which the drawings were produced, but they have been arranged horizontally to emphasize certain important structural themes.

There are at least seven repeated graphic themes in these lamp drawings. Each has been visualized in Fig. 10.12 by a numbered outline that surrounds certain linked features in the network diagrams. To indicate what is meant by a theme and how they appear and reappear in various combinations, I have listed the first six below (the numbers in brackets indicate in which drawings the theme appears):

a. The metal base forms a closed region to which both glass envelope and the filament system are attached [1, 2, and 6].
b. The metal base is represented by two juxtaposed regions [1, 2, 3, and 9].
c. The filament assembly comprises one region, with two concentric regions attached to it [1 and 11].
d. The filament assembly is represented by two regions attached in a sequence out from the base, with a third region surrounding them [3, 4, 6, 7, 8, and 9]. (In drawing 3, three additional components are added to this configuration.)
e. The base is represented as a rectilinear region crossed by parallel strokes [4 and 11].
f. The base is subdivided in two by a partitioning line and elaborated with lugs [7, 8, 9, and 10].

I do not believe these common themes are simply arbitrary groupings imposed on essentially random drawing elements. They are sufficiently complex and distinctive to be seen as real units, especially when viewed against the background of other children's versions of this object. Enumerating them in this way reveals that *the whole process of depicting the lamp is a mosaic of graphic devices developed and mobilized in various combinations throughout the sequence*. In one case (drawing 9), two independently motivated devices for subdividing the base of the lamp co-occur: two juxtaposed regions and a single region subdivided by a partition, yielding a redundancy of the sort mentioned in the last chapter. But generally the topology, although simplified, is faithful to the object. Indeed, the fundamental logic of the organization of boundaries and regions is concealed

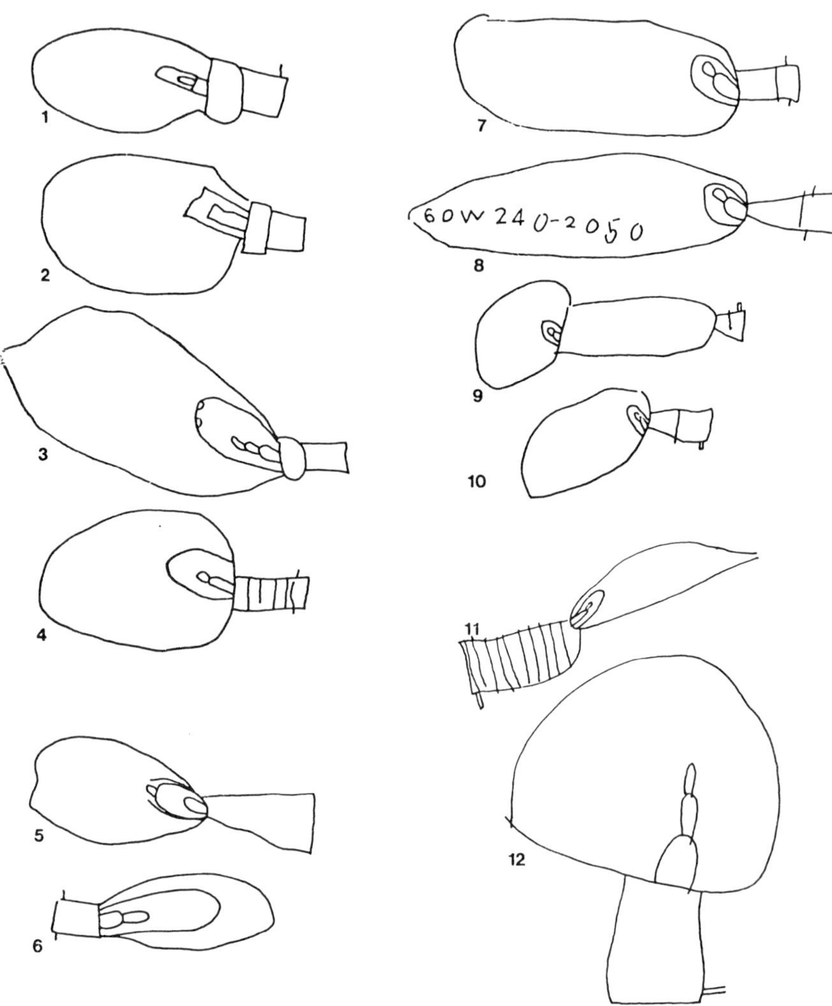

Fig. 10.11. Tracings of 12 drawings of a clear light bulb produced by a girl aged 6.4 years. The symbols on drawing 8 represent a small imprint on the round end of the lamp. (A photograph of the Australian version of Mr. Edison's invention is displayed in the previous chapter, and the author's version in Fig. 10.10.)

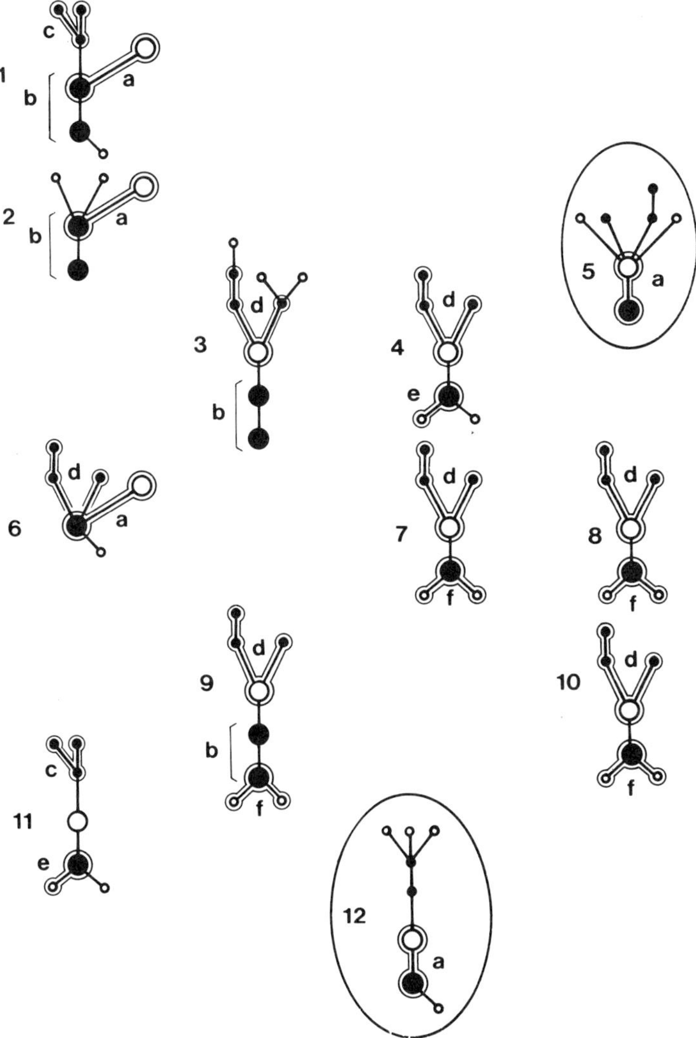

Fig. 10.12. Connection diagrams of the 12 drawings of the lamp shown in Fig. 10.11 arranged vertically in order of production. The lines around certain features identify recurring themes. The letters refer to items listed in the text. The glass envelope is shown as an open circle for ease of recognition. The set of drawings can be seen as a mosaic of themes. Drawing 9 includes two mechanisms for portraying the taper of the metal base. The circled diagrams represent more divergent representations.

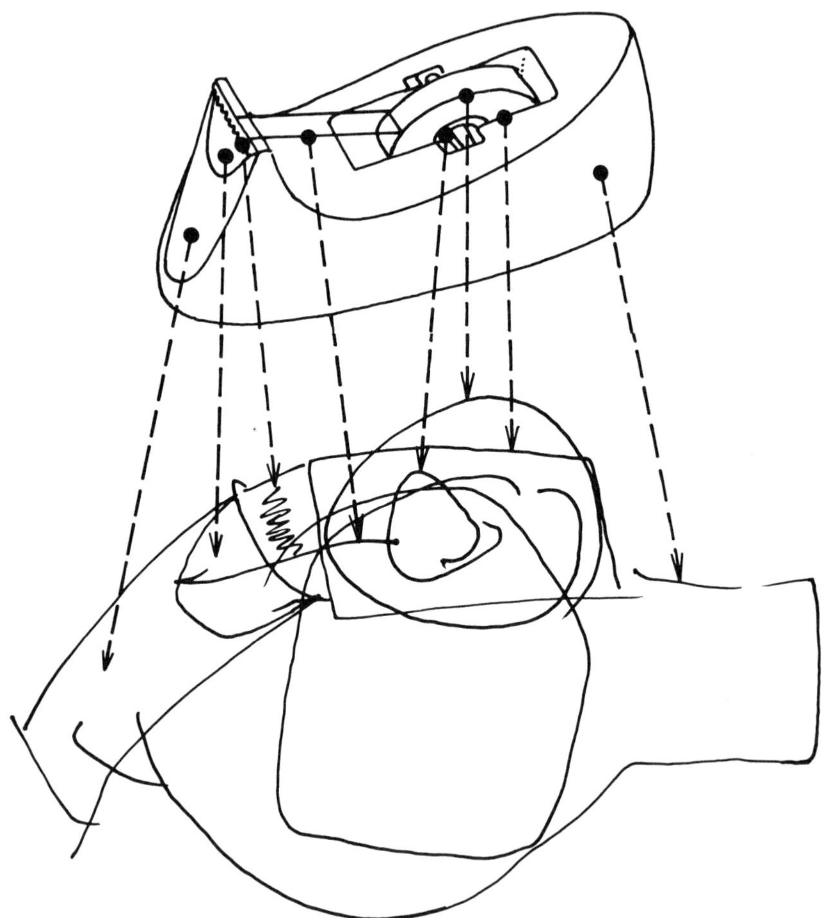

Fig. 10.13. This maze of lines (bottom) represents a tape dispenser drawn by a 5.3-year-old boy. Examination of earlier drawings by the same child indicates that the various lines each represent parts of the dispenser, and that the poor line control conceals a relatively complex representation.

from the viewer to a certain extent by the apparent looseness of control over line in the original drawing. In certain cases, this waywardness of line is so exaggerated that without the opportunity to examine the earlier history of the drawing in preceding versions, one would simply assume the child is producing barely organized scribble (see Fig. 10.13).

Variation at the level of microstructure

We can take this analysis of themes and variations one stage further by examining the microstructure of the girl's performance. One theme in these lamp drawings recurred six times in the series and appeared quite stable. Here at least one might suppose we would find evidence of a standard motor routine. Fig. 10.14 shows the filament subsystems for 12 of her drawings. The diagrams in Fig. 10.14 are topological simplifications of the originals, but unlike the network diagrams of Fig. 10.12, they show stroke order and direction. They too have been reordered horizontally to show the alternation and recurrence of different filament arrangements. Close examination of these diagrams reveals that in spite of the topological similarity among the six items, there is almost as much variability in microstructure as can be imagined. There are four different orders of construction among the six drawings and at least five different patterns of rotation of the curved lines.

This situation of variability in microstructure repeats itself in each of the dozens of drawing sequences analyzed. Fig. 10.15 shows the orders of construction of the lower sections of 100 bicycle drawings (10 successive drawings by 10 children). The core elements – left wheel rim, frame, right rim – are shown as larger circles, and below each rim symbol are smaller circles representing the hub and spokes. A filled circle indicates where the drawing began; the successive steps in the production of features are shown by the lines joining them. Dashed lines indicate when the sequence has moved away from and returned to the seven basic wheel structures. The dominant impression from these charts is of constant change. Since there are 10 drawings in each sequence, there are 9 transitions from drawing to drawing for each subject. Even if we leave out changes due to the omission or addition of features (hubs and spokes), there are changes in strategy in 86 percent of all these transitions. Four children changed their strategy from drawing to drawing on every occasion, and when there are "runs" of two or three similar patterns of construction, this is often because there are only three elements involved.

Even amid all this variability there are the customary stable features: 98 percent of all these drawings started within the core, and in almost half the core is completely formed before going out to side chains (hubs, handles, and so on). The principle of accretion and conformity is strongly observed. Within the 27 drawings in which both hubs and spokes appeared, in only four instances was there reversal of order. (One subject, not included here, regularly produced reversals, but was using a pattern of diagonal strokes across the diameter of the wheel and adding a hub at their intersection.)

Can we summarize the impact of these various stabilizing forces? If we take a hypothetical set of six elements, there are 6! (= 720) possible orders. But if we apply the principle of a core of two elements, a left-to-right progression within it, and a constraint that retrogression along two side chains is proscribed, suddenly there are only four possible orders, as Fig. 10.16 shows, and it is this more limited (but real) residual scope for variation that is exploited.

On the other side, certain conflicting constraints work *against* consistency of attack. One formal constraint (proximity) prescribes movement from an element

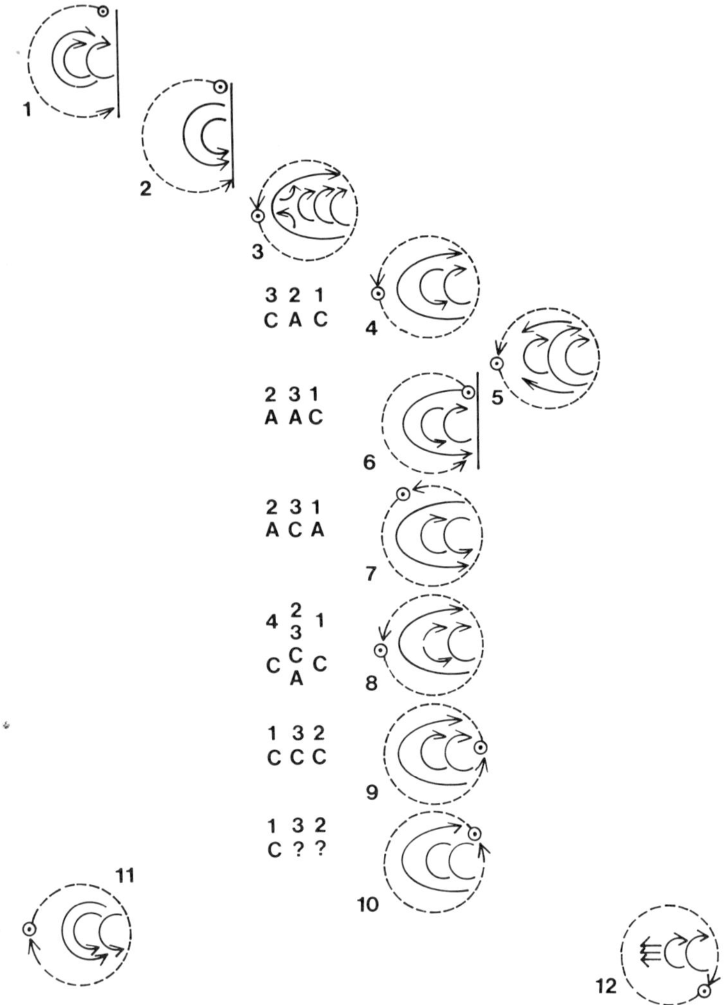

Fig. 10.14. Topology of the lamp filaments assemblies. The original drawings are in Fig. 10.11. The solid straight lines indicate part of the base, and the broken circles the glass envelope of the lamp. Drawing 6 has been reoriented with base to the right for ease of reading, and the original shape of all lines has been suppressed in favor of standard curved lines indicating order, origin, and direction of all strokes. The original order of drawing week by week is preserved in the vertical order. Horizontal order divides the drawing topology into six families. The values in column 3 indicate the order and direction of movement in the "stable" configurations in column 4: (c) is clockwise; (a) is counterclockwise. (Coding for drawing 10 was incomplete.)

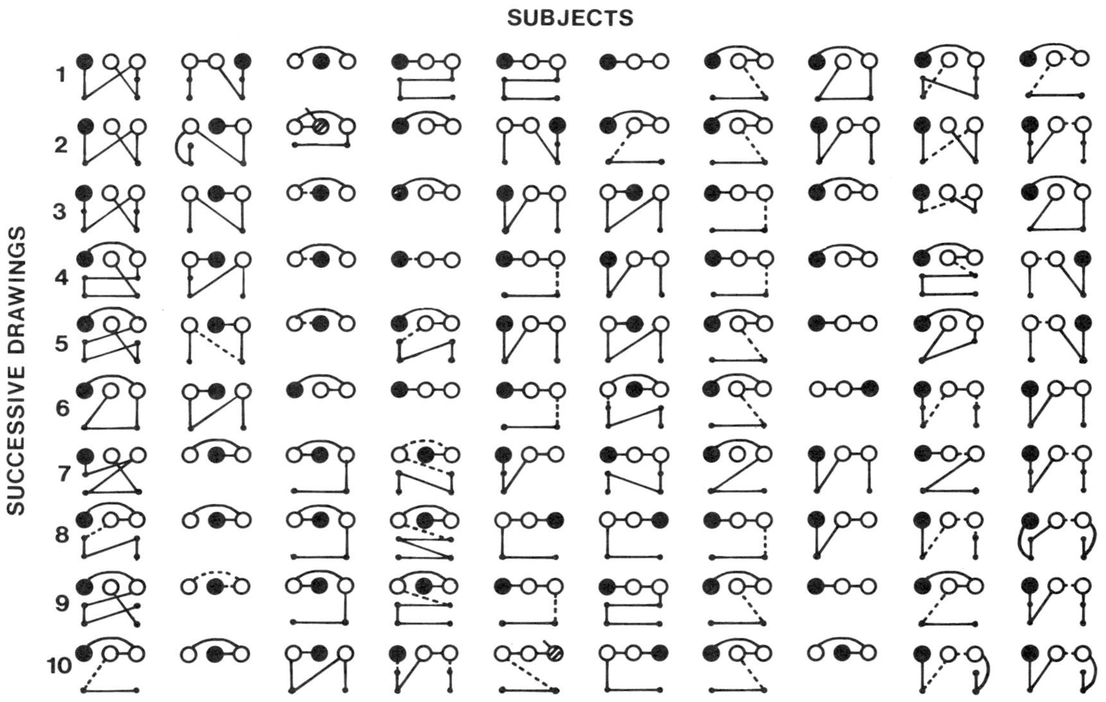

Fig. 10.15. Order of construction of wheel assemblies of bicycles across 10 successive drawings by ten 5- and 6-year-old chidlren. Seven features are included. The large circles represent left wheel rim, frame, and right rim. The points below the rim symbols are the hub and spokes. Filled circles indicate where the stroke sequence started, and lines show progression. Dashed lines indicate that the child interrupted the production of wheel elements to draw features elsewhere and returned. Of all transitions, 86 percent show a change in strategy of production.

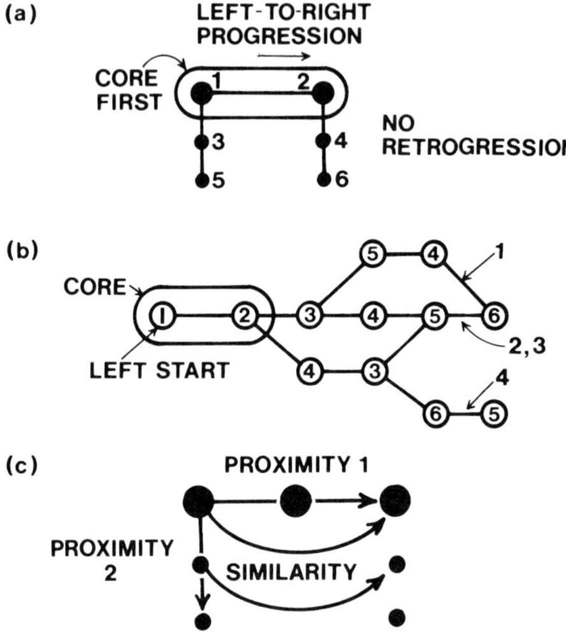

Fig. 10.16. Mechanisms that restrict or promote variability of drawing sequence. (a): A set of six features in a hypothetical drawing are organized into a core of two features and two side chains of two features each. To this are applied certain constraints: The core is to be completed first; it is to be constructed left to right; and no movement is permitted back along a side chain. (b): These restrictions combine to reduce the scope for variation from 720 possible sequences to 4. This is the residual variability a drawer unconsciously exploits. (c): Two executive constraints, proximity and similarity, prescribe movement in three contradictory directions in a seven-feature drawing. Such conflict promotes variability of attack.

to its neighbor in space. This would favor progress serially from left wheel rim to frame to right rim, but also movement from rim to hub to spokes, as in Fig. 10.16(c). A second constraint favors elements of the same kind being constructed as a group. This favors production of two rims before frame and both hubs before spokes. These conflicting pressures undoubtedly contribute to the fluidity of the approach.

Deliberate variation

It is perhaps appropriate to deal here with the theoretical possibility that all this variation in strategy is not a product of failure to store or recover details of graphic procedures and conflicting pressures to work in different ways, but is a triumph of memory for these details on the part of the children. This notion would suggest that the children interpret the instruction to do a "better" drawing as an instruction to vary it at the level of production routines, and that from week to week they observe and store their starting points, stroke directions, sequences, and so on so as to produce what they believe to be the required variation. This phenomenon, if true, would in some ways be more interesting than what I believe to be the actual case. It would require all subjects to make the same (not very plausible) misinterpretation of the task from the outset, and to store procedural information at several levels across all the objects drawn to guide the implementation of that misunderstanding. It is not impossible, but it is certainly improbable. It is much more likely that they simply fail to store or recall the details of production.

The idea that local form is ephemeral is of course a commonplace in language. Studies like those of Jarvella (1971, 1973) and Johnson-Laird (1981) show that unless it is difficult to transfer information into semantic memory (because it is incomplete or because the meaning structure is ambiguous), the surface form of language is ordinarily lost quite quickly. In the case of drawing, neither adults nor children could report even a few seconds after they had drawn an object how they proceeded. They needed to repeat the process slowly and with deliberate effort to recover the information.

The source of graphic individuality

If children do not store information about the order in which they work, how do they achieve the consistency of style we have documented? The similarities among the drawings of a single child could result from (1) a standard translation procedure from object percept or memory to graphic scheme, or (2) remembering the form they previously produced, if not the construction routine (Fig. 10.17).

It is important to recognize the difference between these two possibilities, both of which I think are relevant. Both operate at a level before actual constructional "readout"; that is, they are not production schemas in the sense of a prescription of stroke order or direction or anchoring, because these all vary. One hypothesis suggests children have some structure of an object's appearance in their minds that is more or less "real," which they repetitively translate into action using whatever means of graphic implementation they need and neither noting nor utilizing any details of this implementation to modify subsequent performances. The other alternative is that they solve the object-to-drawing translation problem once and implement it, and when they return to the task again, they remember the solution and use it to drive a new implementation sequence.

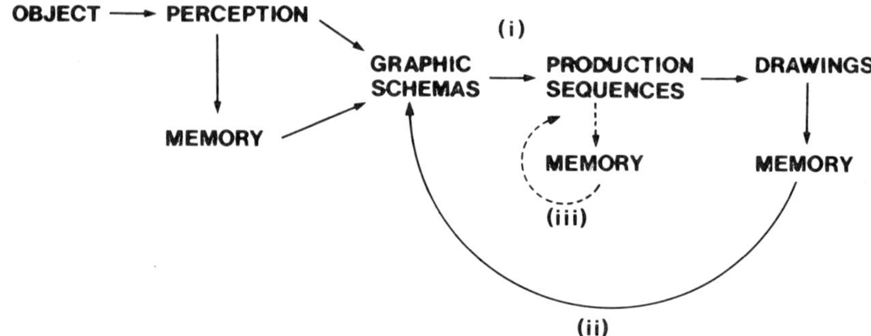

Fig. 10.17. Sources of graphic consistency. In producing a succession of drawings, children may read out repetitively from a more or less complex and diverse set of graphic schemas (i); and they may augment these from the experience of producing drawings, remembering their earlier products (ii). The possibility of remembering past production routines (iii) is not well supported by the evidence.

We can return to the verbal analogy for a moment. If children witness an event or are told a story and have to recount it more than once, they may simply call up the original memory. Their accounts may vary because the readout process is not bound to duplicate the events exactly, but there may be a certain sameness to their accounts both because they are based on the same memory and because the same complex readout facilities are being used. Alternatively (or in addition), they may tell the story once and on telling it a second time remember the way they structured the gist of the account and particular incidents on a previous occasion. In neither case will they necessarily store and recall the surface structure of their previous utterances.

The parsimonious view would be that all the variability and continuity in drawing could be accounted for by supposing that the representations of objects (percepts and memories) are rich, or that the readout process is very versatile, and no reference need be made to feedback from previous production or products. I do not find the idea plausible, but parsimony is frequently lined up against believability, and evidence is a good arbiter.

Happy and persistent graphic accidents

Frequently one sees in a child's (or an adult's) drawing a predicament that calls for an ad hoc solution. A child may draw a human figure, put an umbrella canopy over its head, and then find that the umbrella handle has to be distorted to bridge between canopy and hand. If that distortion now appears when the umbrella's context no longer demands it, we have good circumstantial evidence for the feedback process. If furthermore it is constructed by a variety of production processes, we have evidence that the feedback process is visual and abstract rather than a motor program built on earlier motor routines.

Unambiguous instances of these accidents that persist are not particularly abundant, but they can be found. All the examples that follow are taken from the protocols of the 5- and 6-year-old children we have been discussing. The first piece of ad hoc graphic engineering I will report appeared at least three times. Children were asked to portray a man rowing a boat. Boat, water, and man are themselves no problem for 5- and 6-year-olds, but coordinating the oars with hands, boat, and waves does present problems. A boy aged 5.9 drew a figure with stumpy arms, Fig. 10.18(a). He had earlier drawn the oars protruding from the sides of the boat and had to bridge the gap between figure and oars with supernumerary arms. This compromise construction persisted through a series of drawings, while at the same time the orders of construction varied widely.

There is a phenomenon in children's drawings I have dubbed the "Cheshire cat effect." It involves the proliferation of elements simply to be consistent and complete. (Tenniel's Cheshire cat had a long but narrow mouth showing thirteen teeth.) If a child draws a wide mouth and begins with one or two narrow teeth, she has to vary teeth size, leave the sequence unfinished, or end up with a grin like a picket fence. In drawing a tennis shoe, a boy aged 5.7 laid down an elongated rectangle toward the toe across which he began to draw lines representing the lace. Because the first couple of lacings were drawn close together and he maintained consistency, he ended with 12 lace crossings. Two drawings later, a similar set of lines appeared *without* the elongated rectangle that gave rise to the proliferation in the first place, and to complete the paradigm these strokes were drawn in a different order and reversed stroke direction, as Fig. 10.18(b) shows.

Fig. 10.18(c) shows an outboard motor drawn by a boy aged 5.8. It begins as two regions, one L shaped (that is, with a "step"). After one or two repetitions, this configuration became elaborated into a veritable pyramid, the number of steps proliferating. At the same time, the construction techniques altered fundamentally from two regions to an outline, back to a stack of regions, and finally again to an outline. A girl aged 5.6 drew the frame of a bicycle as a short rectangle, then extended it into a longer shape with a second rectangle to form two regions, Fig. 10.18(d). In two subsequent drawings the frame continued in its new form as a pair of adjacent regions, but at the same time the technique of production diverged radically. Another girl, aged 5.6, drew one bicycle wheel larger than the other and added a vertical line above the smaller circle to make the frame horizontal, Fig. 10.18(e). This marked a new departure based on a piece of graphic ad hoc repair work. The vertical became a regular feature of

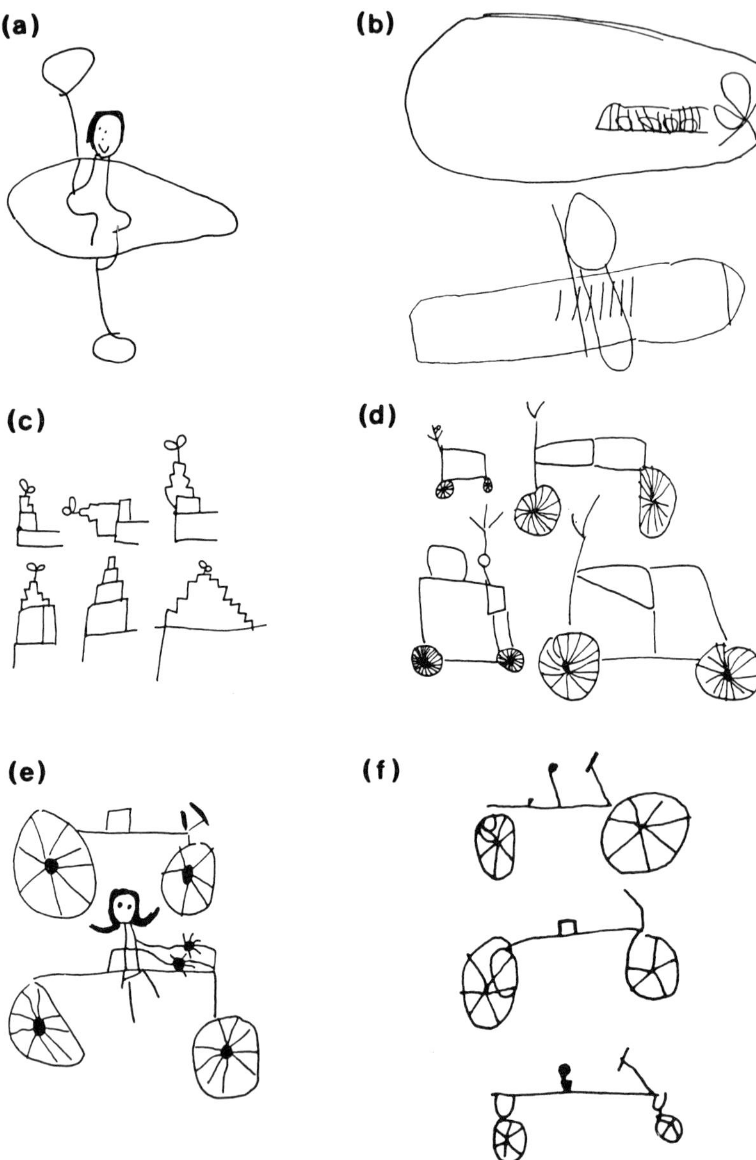

Fig. 10.18. Graphic devices developed in the course of representing objects that persist, often when their original motivation is no longer present, and are produced by a variety of means. These provide evidence of feedback from past drawing efforts and show that themes are stored as quasi-visual schemas and not just as production routines. (Details in the text.)

the bicycle structure, and it too was realized in different ways. A boy (5.8) drew one bicycle wheel as a very small circle but corrected it with a larger circle superimposed on it to match its partner, Fig. 10.18(f). This theme was then built into several subsequent drawings and became two small half circles to which the wheels were attached.

These errors or compromise devices that grow out of graphic predicaments are by nature ephemeral. When they persist at all, they become solutions without problems, and like a biological variation that has lost its primary function, they are bound for inevitable extinction unless they somehow become useful in a new context. Nonetheless, they provide us with necessary formal substantiation of an otherwise purely intuitive feeling that drawings grow from visual memories of past drawings (or drawing intentions), as well as from the primary object they signify. The accidents also confirm that these memories are visual rather than procedural.

Reviewing the variables

This completes the treatment of successive drawings by children. On the whole, I am not making strong claims that the drawings of 5- or 6-year-olds are governed by constraints and principles fundamentally different from those of adults. I find myself echoing all sorts of forces and even sources of difficulty we encountered earlier in giving an account of the work of the untrained adult.

I should like to sum up simply by enumerating the major constraints and influences I have called on in making this analysis. The issues cannot be categorized neatly into hermetic compartments: drawer, subject matter, task, and so on, because most of them express relationships between and among these items. The level of detail emerging in a drawing, for example, involves a complex intersection of general pragmatics, specific task demands, the nature of the object and its contrast set, the load of manipulative and planning effort the medium demands, and the drawer's skill, resources, and style. If we begin, however, by placing the drawer at the center of a constellation of relationships with the medium, the subject matter, the audience, and the task, we can identify this minimal set of forces:

1. The drawer faces a medium that is two-dimensional, largely atemporal, static, and linear. It imposes strict limits on amendment, so that devices used often preempt others.
2. In working on this medium, the drawers even at an early age display certain pervasive operating characteristics: preferences for movement, starting, ordering, paper contact, end control of strokes. They must exercise judgment in planning and organizing execution to achieve adequacy and accuracy with economy of effort.
3. Drawers accumulate a certain repertoire of graphic devices and a capacity to

generate new ones. They show a strong tendency to proceed by accretion rather than dispersal of elements. They seem to suffer severe limitations on visual storage and in the ability to draw and at the same time maintain their internal representations. They seem largely amnesic for or at least indifferent to past executive performances; they experience certain sensory-motor confusion and tend to lock onto established graphic plans. Their capacity to innovate is often surprisingly limited and commonly takes the form of later embellishment rather than early restructuring. Graphic change tends therefore to evolve as a mosaic of established practices and occasional innovations that are alternated, juxtaposed, and blended.

4. Drawers have to come to terms with the general pragmatics of graphic expression and communications (quantity, quality, relevance) and to absorb certain expectations about consistency of viewpoint and the coordination of graphic devices that can be combined together in a single production.
5. The drawer has to assess what the audience needs, expects, and assumes; what is given, what is new; what support each element gets from local internal and external context; and what support the whole project can get from accompanying dialogue.
6. The subject matter (say, an object) carries its own structural characteristics: the type, complexity, and salience of its features; the profile of detail; its structure, including the hierarchical arrangements of its parts; their pattern of connectedness. Concrete objects in particular introduce problems of form, occlusion, and the prototypicality of faces presented to various viewpoints. These have to be registered by drawers in ways that are relevant to graphics and intersect with their preferences and distortions. At the same time, each object has to be related to the features of other candidate objects both generally and for the task in hand.

Such a listing cannot substitute for the fuller discussions that preceded it, but at least it serves as a reminder that drawing must be regarded as a complex system. And it is a system that demands an active, problem-solving, planning, and sometimes compromising drawer.

It remains now to extend the discussion by one more step: to move further away from the context of the laboratory and the school and get a glimpse of what the vernacular drawer draws and what effect relating drawings to a social context can have on graphic structure and production.

11 The pragmatics of everyday graphic production

In an earlier chapter I described how unquestioning (and obliging) both adults and children are when they are asked to produce drawings. They fulfill the request much as they would add a column of figures put before them or type "The quick brown fox. . . ." By contrast, if you ask them to provide a recipe, tell a joke, name a hotel, or describe their feelings, all but the most acquiescent will ask for the pretext. There are two reasons: Knowing the task in hand helps them to frame their response, but more important, in everyday life these pieces of behavior are not identified as pedagogical performances but social acts, and to produce them without a motive is anomalous.

Drawing in everyday life

In this final chapter I wish to take drawing out of the investigative-pedagogical frame and to ask three questions: (1) What sorts of functions do drawings serve for the ordinary person in a middle-class Western urban setting? In language, one refers to "speech acts" (Austin, 1962; Searle, 1969), and there is no reason why we should not try to identify "graphic acts." (2) How is the graphic act embedded in ongoing affairs: Does it typically appear by itself, or is it usually part of a broader action that includes speech, gesture, and so on? (3) Finally, how is the execution of the graphic performance affected by its social function and by its integration into a broader communicative scenario?

Functions of drawing

There are no universal answers to these problems of pragmatics. I have been collecting data from informants in Australia about their everyday use of drawing, mapping, copying, and doodling, and I will report some of the results, but one must recognize that like semantics, the pragmatics or use of drawing strongly reflects the social and cultural milieu, not some regular feature of the mind. Even in our highly technological society, we encounter a proportion of people who virtually never draw. This may seem mildly surprising, yet there are clearly millions of people (indeed could one say the majority of the world's population?) who never draw at all. The practical base of drawing seems to us minimal: pen, pencil, crayon, brush, paper. Occasionally these materials are provided specifically for drawing, but most often this is only a secondary use. They are almost always writing materials used for drawing as a subsidiary function, and that immediately restricts the practical base of drawing. It is limited not only to the literate, but to the literate producer, the writer as opposed to the reader. (In this discussion, I am neglecting for the sake of the main point those who make marks on the ground, trace patterns in sand, or decorate walls by one method or another.)

Even when resources are on hand, the subject matter and motive for drawing are likely to be quite local. For example, my inquiries in Sydney have shown that among middle-class adults, producing sketch maps is high on the list of domestic graphic acts, but a high volume of spontaneous map drawing is not likely to be found in a small rural community. It is predicated on several obvious circumstances: a literate population, wide dispersal, mobility, and a contact pattern neither very frequent nor entirely new. In this sense, the distribution of graphic acts has to be assayed region by region and from one subculture to another and is contingent on certain facets of the social life of which it is a part.

Speech act and graphic act

Let me briefly explore the parallel between drawing in social life and speech act theory. The mainstream development of speech act theory concentrated on a few conspicuous cases of social interactions in which speech was as much a social action as any other physical performance. To say "I arrest you" is not any less a social act than grabbing someone by the collar. The prototypical speech acts were requests, promises, and such institutional performances as pronouncing people married or ships commissioned. These are the examples most students and most introductory texts quote.

From its inception, however, workers have recognized that there is a vast range of speech acts. Fraser (1975) recently published a taxonomy comprising over 300 different acts in 14 general categories. One could be excused for thinking that the best way to take a census of speech acts is simply to edit a thesaurus somewhat. Indeed, Austin himself made the comment: "...going through the dictionary...in a liberal spirit, we get a list of words of the order of the third power of 10" (1962, p. 149). This is not because speech act theory got out of hand, but rather because speech comprises perhaps the largest single category of human social action. Furthermore, we have come to recognize that the simple declarative that describes or announces is no less a social act than lodging a complaint or proposing marriage.

When one extends the theory to graphics, two things emerge. First, that it is possible in theory to carry out a good proportion of speech acts with drawings. One could court a lover by drawing a heart, insult a police officer by drawing a pig, place an order in a hardware shop by drawing a hinge, or even sack someone by drawing a boot. The main reason we don't do most of these things hardly needs stating: Speech or even writing does it faster and more reliably. Having tried to shop for shoe polish, order hard-boiled eggs, and find the route to the railway station in foreign countries with the aid of drawings, I can testify personally to their shortcomings as an exclusive channel of communication. When we lack language or occasionally when we must be silent or wish to convey a message surreptitiously, we may substitute a drawing for speech. But in most cases the choice of graphics is simply because for a specialized purpose it is more explicit, economical, or eloquent than the alternatives available.

As I hinted earlier, we are not obliged to treat speech acts and graphic acts as strict alternatives, since they usually complement one another. If I indicate my needs for a special item of hardware with a drawing, I don't ordinarily walk into the store and silently thrust the paper at someone. My experience trying to buy insect repellent and shoe polish in Asia by this method revealed that there were at least two problems (leaving aside questions of courtesy). First, neither of the products is in itself easily recognized from a drawing, and so one has to draw mosquitos, shoes, brushes, and so on; and second, these drawings do not explicitly convey the idea "I want to buy." One does not fully appreciate the economy and precision of speech until one tries to illustrate events, functions, and transactions without it. Drawing may be well suited to portraying objects and even systems, but it has serious problems of specificity when it comes to expressing social transactions.

Public actions and private processes

Speech act theory emphasizes the communicative aspect of language. (I mean communicative here in the broad sense to cover not just the transfer of descriptive propositions, but all types of social influence.) It is significant that the term used is *speech* act rather than *language* act, because there are some important things we do with language in the absence of speech, notably certain aspects of thinking. The involvement of speech usually means we are "going public," and so by definition it involves *social* action. (Nonsocial speech, talking aloud to oneself, is popularly regarded as aberrant – a sign of loneliness if not madness.)

Had the field been defined as "language acts" rather than "speech acts," we should perhaps have had some even more broadly based taxonomies that take in all the private mental manipulations, social and nonsocial, that are carried

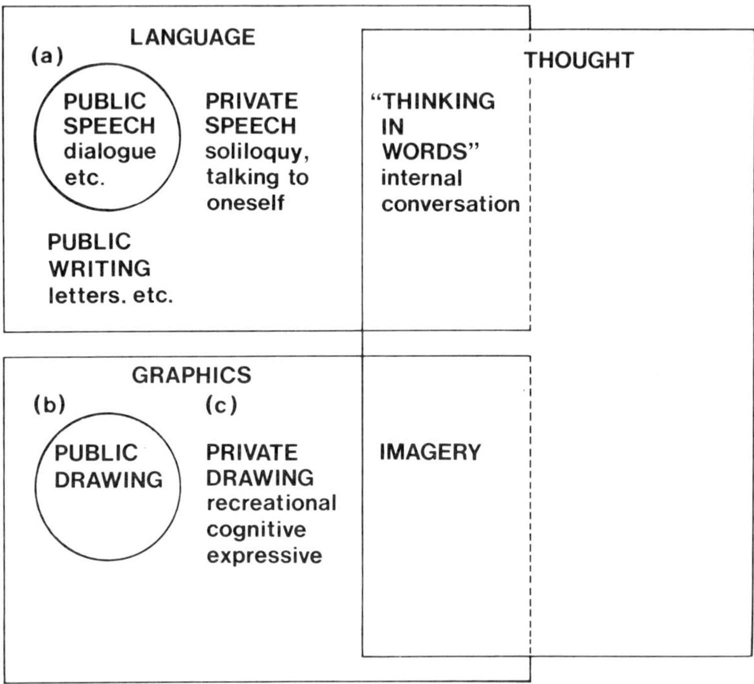

Fig. 11.1. Speech acts (a) encompass the social or public use of spoken language. "Graphic acts" (b) might be similarly restricted to the production of maps, diagrams, sketches, and so on to communicate with others, but this would not deal comprehensively with all graphic activity, since it would exclude the drawing done without an audience, usually for recreational, cognitive, or expressive reasons (c). "Language acts" that extend into private speech and internal dialogue would provide a better analog for broadly defined graphic action.

out through language (Fig. 11.1), and this in turn would provide a broader and more adequate base for talking about graphic acts.

Although this discussion may seem rather scholastic and theoretical, it has its origins in empirical reality. Although many "graphic acts" are social (such as map drawing), a substantial number of reports are of drawings or diagrams that are not produced for an audience either at the time they are executed or later. They are in many cases simply instruments for organizing thought. I will provide further examples later, but let me quote three instances now: A man is planning to line the ceiling of a basement room and makes himself a sketch to see how he can best utilize standard plywood sheets; a woman is listening to a description of a badminton court over the telephone and draws the court as the description unfolds; a woman feeling depressed produces drawings of herself in a pit or with dark shading around her head and shoulders, "...to express to myself exactly how I felt."

There are no intrinsic features here that define the boundary between the public and the private in terms of subject matter and style of representation. Any one of the three drawings mentioned above could have been produced with and for an audience, but they were not in fact communicative. The first two are more reasonably regarded as an extension of the internal imagery system (and a testament to its limitations). Because the man cannot keep a picture in his head of an irregularly shaped ceiling while he juggles various arrangements of rectangular boards, he produces a working space on paper in which to manipulate and store them. The woman is using a drawing as a way of accumulating and integrating successive items of information about the court she is sketching. The third example, that of the woman drawing symbolically how she feels when depressed, is not cognitive but represents a case of what Karl Bühler (1934) referred to as the expressive function of images. As she was recounting the incident, the woman experienced some difficulty in articulating why she made the drawings beyond saying they helped her to understand better how she felt. She was emphatic that there was no audience either present or anticipated, and there was not enough content in each to represent a "readout" for cognitive purposes. One might almost describe the drawing as an elaborate visual sigh.

Recreational drawing

Let me extend the examples to a more common category of private, noncommunicative drawing. Subjects "doodle": They draw faces and geometric forms, they construct friezes around regions, fill in the areas within printed letters, run their pens around staples; they draw moustaches and blacken the teeth on photographs. We could call this recreational drawing, the graphic equivalent of humming or singing to oneself. Most people caught doing it "disown" the activity; they crumple the paper or make discounting remarks of the sort they might use if they were caught talking to themselves. Within this "graphic humming" there are "tunes" of various levels of sophistication, and in an area that extends from banal, motiveless repetition to virtuosity, people have to do some work in establishing and advertising the relation between their performances and their pretensions.

The same spectrum is found in everyday writing: Setting aside the unambiguously communicative writing of notes and letters, there are private performances like diaries and the jotting down of random thoughts. There is perhaps some ambivalence about the public-private status of this behavior too; there may be half-formed intentions or fantasies that the private actions may become public, and this applies also to some "private" drawing. Sophisticated doodlers often do not resent a little eavesdropping, provided they can disavow their pretensions. There are some nice examples of finesse involved in allowing someone to glimpse what one produces in the instant before it is destroyed or disowned. There are also some interesting lines to be drawn between creative doodles, recreational sketching, and artwork that revolve around effort, permanence, and display.

Surveying everyday graphic output

My approach to the problem of what people draw outside work and study situations has been direct. Sue Koenig and I have simply asked informants to recall an actual incident in which they had to draw something: a map, a diagram, an object. We asked them as far as possible to reproduce it as it was originally drawn. They were asked a series of questions: What was the drawing for? What was the situation in which it was produced? What relation was there between drawing and conversation? What was the source of drawing materials? Who was present? For whom was the drawing produced? Was it sent or taken away? Finally, did the drawer regard it as adequate for the purpose for which it was constructed?

This interview was carried out with 50 subjects, some of whom were university students, but most of whom were adults in the 30- to 50-year age range visiting the university on an Open Day. On the basis of their replies, I devised a questionnaire that set out 25 different categories of everyday drawing, map making, plan construction, sketches of clothing, and so on. After a review of the outcome, I should like to make some more detailed comments on map making and the graphic portrayal of time. The informants were 56 women and 30 men. The modal age was 19, and they ranged from 18 to 53 years. They were first-year students in a university, with a substantial proportion of mature-aged students. The instructions on the main part of the questionnaire said: "I am not interested in drawing, graphing, diagram-making associated directly with university study or any other kind of education or work." (They were asked separately about graphics in these domains.)

Beside each of the 25 categories listed were three time slots: the past 7 days, the 3 weeks preceding, and the 11 months prior to that. Within these spaces, the informants were asked to place a symbol for each drawing they remembered doing in that period. A circle with a cross within it indicated that the drawing was private – not done for an audience. If the drawing was made with an audience present, the size of the audience was represented by a number within the circle in place of the cross. If the drawing was done with no audience but was sent or given to someone (in a letter, a note to a tradesperson, and so on), an arrow was drawn across the circle with a number indicating how many people received the drawing. A miscellaneous category was included, although it was little used. A space was provided for a sample of any doodles regularly produced, and there were questions at the end about work, study, training and artwork, and about the portrayal of time.

The sampling of three periods of time allowed us to check on the accuracy of recall or reporting, since on average there should be, for instance, more than 40 times more entries in the final 11-month column than in the first 1-week column. Of course this was not the case, although on items like doodling, which was very common and very frequent, more than half the informants indicated that they did more over the year than they could reasonably report. On the whole, the female informants seemed more conscientious in reporting than the males. (This can be inferred from the fact that they often marked all the null entries with a symbol, that they included more gratuitous information, and that the number of entries in the longer time periods was closer to what might be expected from extrapolation.)

The first question we can ask of the data is whether males or females are more prolific. If we overlook the possible relative underestimate of male output, the volume of drawing is almost precisely the same. (Because there were almost twice as many females as males in the sample, all figures quoted for females have been adjusted proportionately to those of the males in the text and tables to permit direct comparisons.) As a group, the females placed entries 399 times in the various cells of the questionnaire, and males 395. The data were divided according to whether the drawing was done with or without an audience, and again the sexes were virtually identical, with private drawing slightly more common than drawing for an immediate or future audience (females: 205 private, 194 public; males: 205 private, 190 public). Table 11.1 shows the 25 items of the questionnaire arranged in order of frequency of report, and Table 11.2 shows the same for males. In both cases, a separate rank-order is provided for private and public drawing. With the exception of doodling, which females on the average report distinctly more often than males at all time slots, the order of items and the quantity of output is remarkably similar across the two groups.

Among the items high in the private drawing category are a number of "recreational" or expressive items: doodling, drawing imaginary people, defacing or elaborating pictures in publications, copying illustrations, drawing animals, doing drawings that express feelings. There is a second group, less common but still important, that seems to involve personal planning: drawing parts of houses, constructing house plans, sketching clothing and hair styles, making up timetables and flow charts.

Among the drawings produced for an audience, making a local district map is most common for both females and males, and drawing a map at the scale of

Table 11.1. *Frequency of reports of various public and private drawings, female adults*

	Private		Public
66	doodling	21	local district map
20	deface pictures	20	sketch clothing
16	draw imaginary person	14	puzzle or game
16	express own feelings	14	amuse child
13	sketch clothing	13	house plan
10	puzzle or game	11	draw real person
9	portray time	10	large area map
8	draw animal	10	doodling
7	sketch car, bike	9	half house plan
5	copy illustration	9	teach child
5	sketch hair, makeup	8	deface pictures
5	draw real person	6	jewelry
5	flowchart	6	sketch hair, makeup
4	jewelry	5	draw imaginary person
4	half house plan	5	flowchart
3	house plan	5	express own feelings
3	furniture or appliance	5	sports area, court
2	small part of house	4	draw animal
2	large area map	4	sketch car, bike
1	local district map	4	copy illustration
1	mechanical device	4	help child to draw
0	sports area, court	3	furniture or appliance
	(amuse child)	3	small part of house
	(teach child)	1	mechanical device
	(help child to draw)	0	portray time
205		194	

Note: $N = 56$. The values have been adjusted proportionately to make them comparable to the smaller group of males.

the state or larger is also common. There is a cluster of items that are necessarily public associated with children which for both males and females go in order: amusing children, teaching or helping with homework, and less common, helping children to learn to draw. Some items we normally think of as private like doodling, defacing pictures, drawing imaginary people, and so on are sometimes produced with an audience, as I suggested in the earlier discussion.

Certain patterns in the data pick up the differences in female and male activities and styles. For example, males and females draw items of clothing as a private activity quite commonly and to about the same degree, but the females do so more than six times as often as males as a public performance. Exactly the same

Table 11.2. *Frequency of reports of various public and private drawings, male adults*

	Private		Public
46	doodling	20	local district map
23	draw imaginary person	19	doodling
18	express own feelings	16	puzzle or game
16	deface pictures	12	draw real person
11	sketch clothing	10	house plan
10	draw animal	10	amuse child
10	small part of house	9	large area map
10	portray time	9	deface pictures
9	puzzle or game	9	teach child
8	draw real person	8	express own feelings
7	copy illustration	8	half house plan
6	sketch car, bike	7	sketch car, bike
4	large area map	7	sports area, court
4	house plan	7	flowchart
4	half house plan	6	draw animal
4	furniture or appliance	5	draw imaginary person
4	mechanical device	5	portray time
4	sketch hair, makeup	4	small part of house
3	sports area, court	4	mechanical device
2	local district map	3	sketch clothing
1	jewelry	3	furniture or appliance
1	flowchart	3	jewelry
	(amuse child)	3	help child to draw
	(teach child)	2	sketch hair, makeup
	(help child to draw)	1	copy illustration
205		190	

Note: $N = 30$.

pattern applies to the sketching of hair styles. Men and women do it privately to the same extent, but only women do it with an audience. The reverse applies to drawing cars, motorbikes, and bicycles. Although it is as much a female as a male activity in private, men do it more often with an audience.

Both women and men draw plans of houses or substantial parts of houses, and these are at least twice as often drawn for an audience as for themselves (females: private 7, public 22; males: private 8, public 18). But when we consider small construction details, these are more commonly drawn by men and most commonly as private activity, presumably as a background to maintenance work, and so on. I have calculated the ratio of the two types of drawings (public versus private) for the two sexes to crystallize some of these patterns (Table 11.3). The

Table 11.3. *Percentage of drawing reports that were private as opposed to public, female and male adults*

	Female, private		Male, private
100	portray time	88	copy illustration
76	doodling	82	draw imaginary person
76	draw imaginary person	79	sketch clothing
76	express own feelings	71	doodling
71	deface pictures	71	small part of house
67	draw animals	69	express own feelings
64	sketch car, bike	67	portray time
		67	sketch hair, makeup
57	small part of house	64	deface picture
56	copy illustration	63	draw animals
50	flowchart		
50	furniture or appliance	57	furniture or appliance
50	mechanical device	50	mechanical object
45	sketch hair, makeup	47	sketch car, bike
42	puzzle or game	40	draw real person
40	jewelry	36	puzzle or game
39	sketch clothing	33	half house plan
31	draw real person	31	large area map
31	half house plan	30	sports area, court
19	house plan	29	house plan
17	large area map	25	jewelry
9	local district map	13	flowchart
0	sports area, court	9	local district map
0	help child to draw	0	help child to draw
0	teach child	0	teach child
0	amuse child	0	amuse child
	Public		Public

25 items are ordered from those that are predominantly private through a group that are equally often solitary and public to those that are predominantly or necessarily social.

This brief review of some of the findings strongly supports two of my earlier observations: First, that the graphic output of any social group will to a large degree mirror their general sociology and psychology. Patterns of activity (drawing maps to direct people, entertaining or educating children, constructing or reconstructing houses, planning timetables, and so on) determine much of the content of public drawing and a certain amount of private drawing among this middle-class group. The other main outcome is that there is at least as much private as public drawing. Some of the most used categories are largely private recreational activities: doodling, defacing, drawing faces, copying, sketching, doing puzzles, and there is a certain amount of graphic work that involves the organization of thought at a private level.

Perhaps one of the surprising items was the frequency of drawing to express feelings, including communicating to others. It is possible that drawing a face or a figure is an acceptable way to overcome shyness about conveying emotions – a piece of graphic "face work" in a double sense. Drawing under such circumstances becomes an "off-record" method of communicating (Brown and Levinson, 1978), a way of expressing something the receiver can choose to accept or ignore and the drawer can discount if necessary, a sort of graphic "throw-away line."

How contingent drawing is on its material base is suggested in occasional comments on questionnaires about where and when informants draw. Private recreational drawing is common wherever paper and pencil are usually at hand – at the business meeting, in the lecture hall, and at the telephone.

This small survey deals with predominantly domestic graphics, since it excludes all graphic work connected directly with work or study. Informants were instructed to include only items that were peripheral to their main job – for example, drawing a map to direct a messenger or using pen and paper to illustrate a point in a meeting were acceptable, but not the plan drawings of an architect, the technical drawings of a machinist, the flowchart of someone in computing, or graphs and diagrams drawn for university courses. In a separate section of the questionnaire informants were asked what professional or serious recreational drawing they did and whether they had any graphic training beyond school. The great majority reported that the only graphic work they did that was not ephemeral was done at school or in connection with university courses.

The distinction I am making between "ephemeral" and "serious" drawing has already been alluded to. It is, of course, rather contentious but at the same time important to any assessment of how graphically productive a community is. Perhaps the important dividing line is between drawings that are admired or are meant to be admired for their virtuosity and that are displayed and/or change hands for that reason. Another significant element is whether the producer of the work seeks or expects the approval of strangers rather than acquaintances.

Of the 56 women, 4 reported that they sketched, produced watercolors, did screen print designs, or "designed posters when asked." Two drew as a background to craft work (pottery, jewelry making). Three said they did a little desultory sketching; 4 others said they used to draw but had stopped. The situation was very similar for the males. Three-quarters simply said they did no graphic work outside university courses. One said he drew regularly, four said "very occasionally," and four others said they used to paint or draw but had stopped. (Three of the four were 18 or 19 years old!)

This survey is no substitute for a proper assay of graphic work in the community generally, but I doubt if it underestimates the general level of activity. The sample is probably at the more productive end of the range – young, urban, middle-class, some with teacher training, many of the women moving into tertiary education after other attempts to move away from exclusively domestic routines. Sometimes if we visit local art exhibitions at which amateurs show their works in cities like Sydney we get an impression of widespread and vigorous creative activity, but my estimate would be that it is the product of a small fraction of 1 percent of the adult population. This is not to downgrade its social or cultural significance; after all, if we were to take any other single activity, whether it be active sport participation, music making, dancing, opera going, even church going, a hard-headed calculation of the number of current active participants in relation to the total eligible population would rarely exceed 1 or 2 percent in any single case. (In one Australian city, one sporting event each year regularly attracts 100,000 spectators. This is slightly more than 2 percent of the city population.)

My informants gave occasional explanations about their lack of activity (or their declining activity), and it could be summed up in two phrases: lack of time, lack of talent. I think talent is perhaps more critical than time, but talent is itself relative to social forces. Most of the "domestic graphics" I have been reviewing are the products of minutes or seconds of work. Producing graphics with more pretensions is usually demanding of effort, and it is characteristically solitary effort, the popular stereotype of the gregarious, bohemian artist notwithstanding (Getzels and Czikszentmihalyi, 1976). So the emphasis tends to fall on the product rather than the performance, and nothing about the sociology of art in our society favors the outpouring of competent but unexceptional original graphic products. It is an extraordinarily elite activity, and even among the small band of practitioners it is highly stratified. Quite a proportion of them could be described as a disaffected rump of rather low morale and fragile self-esteem. I am not alleging that the situation is less hospitable in my own city or country relative to others; my estimate is that it is a widespread phenomenon wherever visual arts are part of high culture. I simply mention it here to emphasize that to understand grassroots graphic productivity, one has to pay as much attention to Bourdieu, Berger, and Raymond Williams as to technical reports on the psychology of perception and skill.

The charms of doodling

I should like to return from this momentary excursion into the graphic stratosphere to reflect briefly on the humble doodle. I have to confess a strong distaste for the word because it further trivializes one of the few moments of graphic play. I asked my informants to supply me with examples of doodles and should like

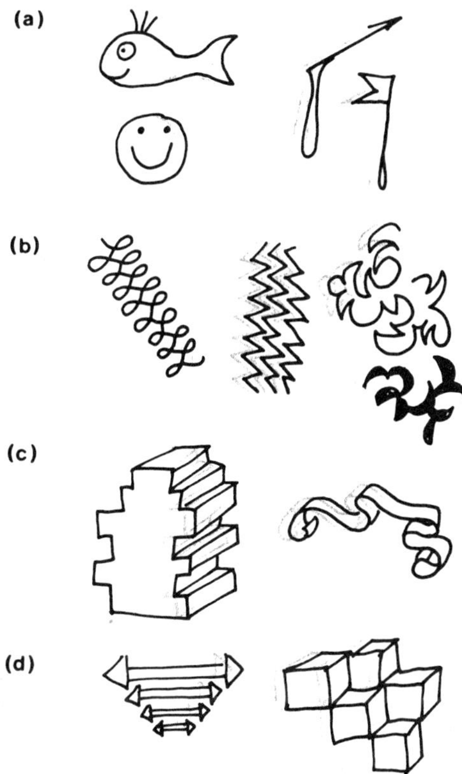

Fig. 11.2. Typical doodles reproduced by adult informants.

to reflect on one recurring property, recursiveness. I divide doodles in two ways in terms of their repetitiveness. Some doodles are one-off items that are not repeated from occasion to occasion. Others, like a "smiley" face or perhaps the mascot of the local football team may be drawn over and over again by one person. Internally, however, these items are not repetitive or recursive, whereas a very large category of doodles may be likened to the products of a "graphic engine." In other words, there is a routine of various degrees of complexity that generates the doodle. One simple but common example is a line that progresses like a braid, forming opposed loops and continually reversing curvature, as in Fig. 11.2(b). This braid may have a secondary structure that loops about on the page or forms borders around other forms. Fig. 11.2(c) shows a rectilinear form embroidered in depth. This is sometimes done with curved lines to produce a scroll-like form. Often a single closed figure is accreted in two or three dimensions as in Fig. 11.2(d), or two or three forms alternate, or forms increase or decrease in size and proportions. Some doodles are of a very low level of complexity, simply repeating a single motif or changing in a single dimension such as length or orientation. Others are more complex and probably demand a degree of focal attention.

I referred to the idea of a "graphic engine." This is a concept that is more widely applicable than just to doodling. One of the key features of graphic work is, of course, that it represents the accumulation of the traces of serial action. There is a popular idea that artists necessarily have a fully developed conception of their work in their heads, and production is simply the technical readout of that representation, not dissimilar in principle to a carpet weaver working from a pattern. But of course in much visual art the development is to a certain degree unpredictable; artists can almost be likened to spectators of the cumulative effects of their own actions. I believe that repetitive doodling represents a minor version of this spectacle of the buildup of residues of action, with the doodler adjusting in a more or less complicated way the form and parameters of the "graphic engine" or production system.

Questions of cognitive difficulty

The social and pragmatic forces that shape the output of a group of everyday drawers do not operate alone; they intersect with the intrinsic difficulty of the graphic tasks themselves. Certain graphic acts are relatively concrete and direct; others are abstract and in various ways cognitively demanding. We are, in fact, dealing with a spectrum of possible performances: the sketch, the plan, the map, the diagram, the chart. Of course, each one may be more or less ambitious, but in their very nature and definition we find a number of distinct transitions as we move across the spectrum. A review of these transitions may explain first, what vernacular drawers do or do not produce, and second, what the general public may be expected to decode.

To anticipate a little, I believe there are two important transition points, one that divides the spectrum between sketches, maps, and plans (which are often produced) and diagrams and charts (which are rare). The second breaking point is between the more concrete and the more abstract diagrams and charts. This transition marks the point on the spectrum of graphic work at which popular media cease to offer graphic representation for interpretation. As one might expect, more abstract diagrams, graphs, and charts tend to appear only in professional publications.

Sketches, maps, and plans

Consider first the distinction between sketches on the one hand and maps and plans on the other. Although there are some standard codes, more or less esoteric, associated with professional map and plan production, the key feature that marks maps and plans off from sketches is the high viewpoint. Maps and plans are sometimes very economically drawn, but so are many sketches. The nature of the economies, as Gombrich (1972) points out, is tied to their use. We include or omit various features for the purpose at hand. Atmospheric conditions appear in weather maps, but are not included on route maps. Contours may be present on a military or a hiker's map, but are usually omitted from street or political maps.

Nonetheless, the main substance of maps and plans preserves what Gombrich terms "iconicity"; that is, a coupling of space and form in the map with that in the area it represents. It is the relative or absolute loss of iconicity that marks off the diagram and chart from the sketch, the map, and the plan, although as we will see there is no distinct boundary that defines what is iconic and what is not. Perhaps the cautious thing to say is that one expects iconicity in maps, plans, and sketches and should not be surprised to find it lacking in diagrams and charts.

Maps versus plans

What is the difference between a map and a plan? There seems to be a criterion of scale: the map of Africa, the plan of a house. Yet we have to come to terms with the reversal of this in the distinction between the plan of the city "versus" the map of the exhibition. One can have both a map and a plan of either one.

Maps and plans were two of the most common products of everyday drawers, and in naming them the distinction was clearly one of function, of actions to be taken. People draw maps to direct movement and draw plans to organize action affecting structure. That people usually need directions about movement only when they are moving about on the scale of streets and suburbs and on the other hand only have the privilege of altering things on the scale of rooms and houses means that function and size are confounded: big areas and movement for maps, small areas and changes for plans.

Abstract diagrams and iconicity

Let us now move to the other end of the spectrum for a moment, from what people regularly draw to those things we would not expect them to interpret, let alone portray. This move takes us over the boundary between sketches, maps, and plans and well into the territory of diagrams and charts.

It is difficult to exemplify an abstract diagram that will be easily accessible to all readers of this book for the reason that is at the heart of the discussion: It is just abstract diagrams that tend to need specialist audiences or the labor of explanation and interpretation. A diagram of a feedback control system is an example that recommends itself to me, simply because each year I have to try to explain it to undergraduate classes. The simplest version has an input and output, a detector, a feedback loop, a comparator, and so on. The classic prototype is a temperature control system where "output" is actual temperature that has to be adjusted toward the desired state, which is the "input." So the initial impulse to regard the input as the place where you pour in the oil and the output as the place where heat emerges is hardly appropriate. Also, a feedback loop is not a diagram of a state of affairs or even a single event; it diagrams a continuous process that produces changes over time, but does not illustrate the changes it produces. All in all, it is not the sort of diagram that a canny editor would publish in a newspaper or popular magazine, for two reasons: (1) It requires more explanation than most casual audiences are prepared to accept, and (2) if they do pay attention to it, they will usually try to map it onto a physical arrangement in space and a single event in time and find themselves quite off target.

Contrast the control system diagram with an abstract example that *does* appear in the nontechnical literature: a chart of the hierarchical organization of a company or government department. The test of its iconicity is to ask if it would be useful as a map to find the office of the vice-president. In a company with a very literal view of "room at the top" it might almost work, but essentially it maps authority, not space. The reason it is readable enough to be used by the general public is that although it is abstract, it is familiar and usually simple. It plots a single relationship of superior to inferiors over and over and follows them down in a consistent cascade. Let us consider as a third example of an abstract diagram or chart the genealogical tree, which Gombrich classifies as essentially relational rather than iconic. There are two related devices we can look at. One is the family tree that describes the relations among a particular set of people; the other is the kinship diagram that shows the general pattern of relationships for a culture or subculture. In either case, a number of dimensions – marriages, generations, siblings, gender – make them potentially more complex than a company hierarchy, which represents a single relationship of authority.

If we consider the most common fragment of a tree, the immediate family of two or three generations, our reading of it is made easier by the fact that although it is formally defined in an abstract way, at least in our society it does reflect certain spatial and temporal features of the family it describes: spouse is juxtaposed with spouse, offspring are adjacent and linked. A specific family tree is much more likely to be reproduced or read by a member of the lay population than a kinship structure of the same type for pragmatic reasons. But even a kinship system or fragment of one is not inaccessible, for although it deals with general categories rather than particular persons, we probably think about it in terms of an example or prototype. So it is not so purely "relational" in practice as it is in theory, and for this reason not by any means beyond the power of an ordinary person to read or even produce.

The psychological conversion of the abstract to the concrete may be seen in some of the diagrams and charts that occasionally appear in the media: the portrayal of the distribution of the national budget, the fate of the cash paid for a glass of beer or wine, the sources of oil or the pattern of its consumption, the makeup of the political vote, the comparison between the strength of the armed forces of two countries. Nobody believes we could translate these diagrams quite literally into the physical form or location of checks, cash, oil, voters, tanks, ships, infantry, and so on. Yet all these are imaginable physical objects and can in theory be aggregated, so again, in a loose sense some iconic traces persist. In many cases it is simply a matter of translating area on a page into volume: a region of a drawing of an oil drum represents the quantity of oil from the Persian Gulf states, and so on. In other cases we relate size and numerosity, as in the case of ship silhouettes representing navies, and here one could take the additional step of visualizing the navies actually arrayed against one another at sea. The fact that such imaginings are often rather unrealistic does not disqualify this as an example of iconic representation.

The main points I am pursuing are these: (1) That iconicity is in my view a powerful force in determining what ordinary people will produce or be expected to interpret, (2) that because of the possibility that certain abstract ideas can be translated into concrete terms and dispersed things aggregated in the imagination, it is hard to draw a clear boundary between what is iconic and what is not, and (3) that iconicity is only one of a complex array of properties that favor or inhibit our use of diagrams. If we find it easy to draw a diagram of our immediate family relationships, we do so in spite of the multiple variables involved and because it is concrete, familiar, important, and limited in scope. If we fail to understand (let alone produce) a diagram of a feedback control system, it is not just that it maps only in an obscure way onto physical reality; it is complex, unfamiliar (not to say arcane), and represents not just an object or event, but a continually changing process.

I should now like to revert to a consideration of one of the mainstream items of production, the map and some of its close relatives, including the representation of time.

Orienting maps and plans

The first body of data on maps and plans that I collected addressed the question of whether people used different strategies to represent outside space (courtyards, quadrangles, streets, squares) and inside space (rooms, corridors, halls, foyers).

I began with drawings produced by some of my colleagues and was struck by the sometimes unusual orders and starting positions used in their production. These, in turn, seemed to stem from how the maps were oriented, and I began to try to isolate the determinants of such orientation. I collected maps of their homes, asking them to indicate such data as the slope of the land, the direction of the local railway station if there was one, which way they drove to and from home, where the center of the city lay, the nearest main road, and so on. I also related their sketch maps to the local street directory, which operates on compass coordinates. None of these external landmarks, routes, or coordinates bore a consistent relation to the orientation of the drawings.

The solution to this problem came first by asking the members of my family to draw a simple map of the house of a friend living near the harbor foreshore. Although there were only four people, there was some consistency: The two adults drew the house with the street above it parallel to the upper edge of the page; the two children drew it rotated 180 degrees, with the street below it. The house in question is on the high side of a street overlooking the water. Adults visiting the house normally remain inside looking out toward the harbor; the children are usually outside in the street or the foreshore park and reported themselves to have been looking back toward the house when they visualized it. It therefore seemed that in order to predict the orientation of a map, one would have to establish how people are "facing" psychologically when they set out to draw the map, and further one must assume that they will represent the area as if they are facing up the page.

The first confirmation of this came from asking staff members to draw a map of a house familiar to them all located in a cul-de-sac. Without exception, they drew the street vertically up the page, with the blind end at the top and the house on the right. When asked where they felt themselves to be psychologically, they all reported that they were walking along the cul-de-sac toward the house. I then returned to the drawings of the university. I had 34 staff members draw a sketch map of the offices they occupied, keeping a record of the actual location of the room, where they customarily sat, and where they were physically located when they made the drawing. Fig. 11.3, which summarizes the results, shows the various floors in one of two adjacent buildings. In each, all the rooms opened onto an axial corridor. The black arrows indicate the orientation of the drawings. (It points to the top of the page on which they drew.) The shaded arrows show where the subjects were facing when they drew the plan. In all but four cases, this was at their desk in the room. Plain arrows show the orientation of the seat they normally occupy for those four who did their drawings outside the room. The outcome is further summarized in Fig. 11.4(a), which shows the orientation of the maps with respect to compass points. Fig. 11.4(b) shows the map orientation with respect to the main corridor, and Fig. 11.4(c) shows the relation

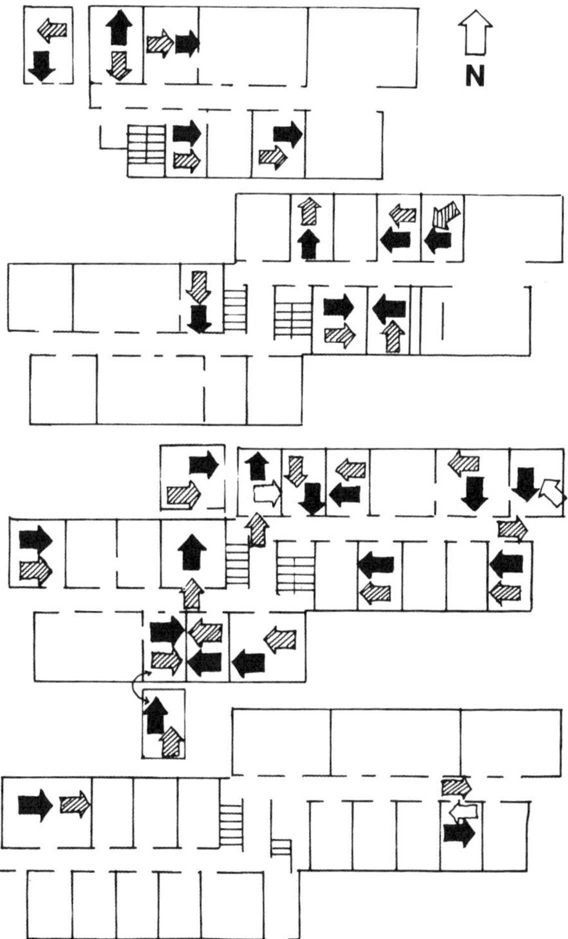

Fig. 11.3. Plans of various floors of one of two office buildings occupied by informants who drew sketch maps of their rooms. The black arrows indicate the direction corresponding to the top of the drawings. Shaded arrows show where subjects faced while drawing. Plain arrows show normal seating orientation of subjects who were not in their rooms while producing the map.

between orientation and the position of the drawer. The latter relationship is clearly the dominant one, and this outcome has subsequently been confirmed over and over again by informants describing recent mapping efforts. They almost invariably oriented the maps on the basis of their facing within their house, shop, street, and so on.

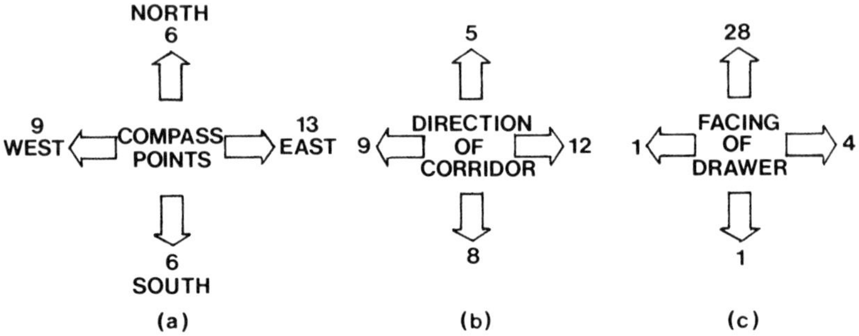

NORTH 6
9 WEST COMPASS POINTS 13 EAST
6 SOUTH
(a)

5
9 DIRECTION OF CORRIDOR 12
8
(b)

28
1 FACING OF DRAWER 4
1
(c)

Fig. 11.4. Relationships between orientation of maps on the page and (a) compass directions, (b) location of main corridor, and (c) position of drawer while producing the map (usually in their normal seating position).

In the early stages I had asked people where they felt themselves to be when they drew maps. It took them an appreciable time to answer the question, and I began to suspect that they were in fact reconstructing their orientation from the maps rather than the reverse. This is why in Fig. 11.3 I have documented where people were actually facing rather than where they reported themselves to be psychologically. When they did answer the question, some said they felt themselves to be "in that room," or "in the room at my desk"; others said they pictured themselves above the room looking down into it. I shall return to this issue shortly because it is not possible to understand the situation for any individual subject in terms of a single unitary viewpoint.

The outcome I have described of orienting plans and maps with the drawer looking up the page is, of course, consistent with the way people handle maps and street directories both as readers and producers. When we tackle a route involving turns and landmarks, we typically rotate the map to correspond to the way we are facing. Automobile clubs provide maps of common routes precisely on this basis and courses in simple mapmaking conducted by the military or scouts prescribe that the map be drawn up the page away from the drawer. Whenever there is anything more than a minor change in direction, the map has to be broken; continual compass bearings are added so that a unitary map can be reconstructed from the vignettes.

We can now return to the structure of the drawing process. To understand where on a page a person will typically begin a map, one has to coordinate at least five factors: (1) What is the point of departure (a railway station or main highway for visitors to a house, the house itself for those departing)? (2) What is the goal? (3) Does the drawer find it natural to work from the departure point? (Occasionally drawers work backward from a destination.) (4) What is the psychological orientation of the drawer at the starting point? (5) What is the general direction of the goal in relation to that orientation?

Drawers may well begin a sketch map not at the normally favored 11 o'clock position, but at the bottom right corner of a page if, for example, they are drawing outward from their home, if they orient themselves in the position of the departing guest walking toward the street, and if the destination is toward the left and forward of that location. (We assume, of course, that the drawer displays some graphic foresight. False starts are not uncommon, and people often sit staring at the page, rotating it to and fro before they begin.) Such a starting position low on a page may, through anchoring constraints, lead to a succession of awkward stroke movements. But the semantics and pragmatics will usually dominate the situation because of the cognitive difficulty of rotating the map with respect to the psychological trajectory, and because such maps are often drawn as an accompaniment to speech and are tailored to the needs of the audience as well. The audience is, figuratively speaking, side-by-side looking upward along the route with the drawer.

The principle of psychological facing applies to many locations and objects. Players drawing a squash court put the "front wall" at the top of the page; the theater is drawn with the stage or screen at the top, or if it is the stage itself that is portrayed, the footlights and audience are at the top. Although I have not put it to the test, I should expect players to draw plans of tennis courts or pingpong tables with the net horizontally across the page and nonplaying spectators to draw it laterally. When my informants drew a place setting for a meal, the plates and so on were at the lower edge of the rectangular table top. Beds and baths, fireplaces, upright pianos, stoves, sinks, telephones, and typewriters when drawn from above all have their fronts facing down the page.

In all these cases, the drawing involves two separate points of view, just as in map and plan drawing. First, because in all these instances we are talking about *plans*, the viewpoint of the drawer is directed downward from directly above the object being drawn. Simultaneously, the plan is oriented as though the subject were in front of the object looking horizontally forward. As I mentioned earlier, drawers will nominate one or the other of these "facings" when asked. Nobody, in my experience, has volunteered a statement about a dual viewpoint, although it is logically necessary. It also seems to me that of the two viewpoints, that of the drawer facing upward toward the object or upward into the space of a room is the more direct and intuitive, and those who identified the viewpoint as being from above looking down seemed to be giving a more formal academic response to the question of viewpoint.

Clark (1973), in his early review of the language of space, distinguishes *intrinsic* and *extrinsic* fronts. The intrinsic front of a car, a ship, or a cow is the part that leads when the object moves. The intrinsic front of a static object is defined ultimately by our sensory or motor interaction with it. The intrinsic front of a clock is the facet we look at, the intrinsic front of an armchair is the side by which we enter. The *extrinsic* front is that facet of an object nearest the speaker, the hearer, or even a third person. ("It was right in front of the tree, but they still didn't see it.") What is drawn facing down the page is the extrinsic front or the intrinsic front of static objects, because the observer is an essential element in these specifications. When people draw objects like cars or boats in plan, objects whose intrinsic fronts are defined by their movement, they will usually depict them laterally, not front down. Even a trumpet, whose "front" (such as it is) is defined by where the sound emerges, will face laterally (or even with the bell upward as though the drawer were the player). The "front" of a slide projector is the surface with the lens. This will not normally be drawn downward because we are visually oriented not to the lens, but toward the surface toward which it faces or the side from which it is viewed or operated.

All these aspects of psychological viewpoint and the definition of "facing" affect the basic organization of everyday drawing. They are partly representational issues. We find it more natural to portray objects in orientations in which we normally interact with them. At the same time, it is pragmatic. We automatically portray things in a way that will be easily read by those with whom we are interacting. It is quite usual for drawer and audience to move their heads if not their bodies so that they share the same orientation to the page as the drawing is executed or explained.

Time in diagrams

The language of time depends heavily on the language of space (before June, on the weekend, in the winter, through the year, down the centuries). Clark (1973) points out that we use two contrasting metaphors: (1) We move through time (through the day, next week, up to lunchtime, 10 minutes from now, past 6 o'clock). (2) Time moves toward us (the coming winter, night follows day, bring the appointment forward, Christmas comes before New Year). Fig. 11.5 illustrates the two analogies.

In my interviews with people about their drawing in everyday life, I routinely ask how they typically represent time. The most common reaction is to say that they cannot remember doing such a thing. When the question is put hypothetically, informants usually have no hestitation in producing a scheme of one kind or another. Two or three people, regarding the task as a challenge to their imaginations, tried to develop a divergent approach. One drew time as a horizontal series of overlapping ellipses; another drew a horizontal wave running across the page; a third drew a figure something like a histogram, with blocks

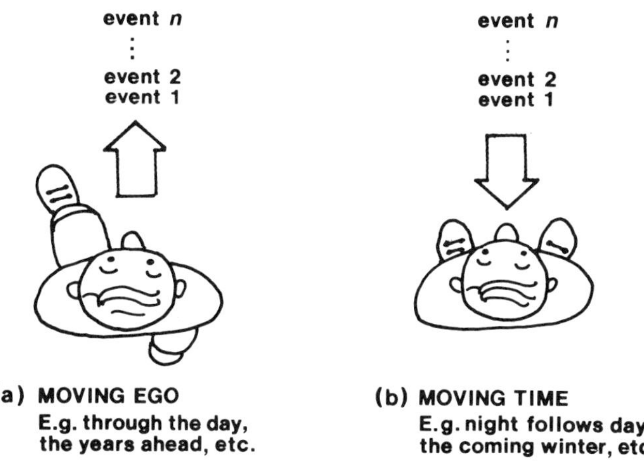

Fig. 11.5. Spatial analogies of the passage of time. In (a) we move forward through time; in (b), time moves toward us.

or bars side by side across the page each representing a month, and their height suggesting how busy he was at each stage of the year.

The more common approaches fell into four categories, in descending order of frequency: (1) the "time line," a horizontal line with either an arrowhead at the right or short horizontal lines defining the ends. The direction of time's arrow was always left to right, and there were the usual marks and divisions that one might expect identifying hours, or meals, months, or holidays. Most informants proposing the time line were happy to adopt the same device for the day, week, and year, although one or two changed to a matrix for the longer periods, presumably because they felt that a single sweep across the page might not accommodate all the detail they might want to enter. (2) The vertically organized list was the next most common device. Sometimes the vertical array was simply a list of dates; in other cases, it qualified as a graphic display – a line, a series of short horizontal strokes or blocks. In all cases, it was arranged downward from early to late. It will be recalled that the spatial analogy prescribes the reverse order, but no subject proposed that, nor would they entertain the idea when it was put to them. (3) The third most common representation was a matrix resembling a diary, timetable, or calendar, with larger time units down the left and smaller units horizontally (days as a vertical list, hours across the top). (4) One or two subjects drew a clock face divided into segments.

Although few subjects could recall using any of these devices in real life, they generated them quite readily and expressed clear preferences. Three or 4 of the 35 subjects stated that they would *never* use a time line and identified it with (male) technical occupations. I made a quick review of some of the popular scientific and historical periodicals (*Scientific American*, *La Récherche*, *L'histoire*) and found that the preferences of the people I had interviewed were echoed in the graphic work. The principal difference was that the horizontal arrangement, although common, did not often take the form of a simple time line, but was almost always part of a graph in which time was the independent variable, plotted from early to late on the horizontal axis. (The only occasion I found time on the vertical axis was when its place on the X axis had been preempted by space.) The left-to-right convention, of course, conforms to the Cartesian precedent, which in turn probably had its source in the Latin writing system.

In the periodicals, time is represented vertically less than half as often as horizontally. There are two types of vertical time scales: the recent short epoch of months and years, and geological or cosmological time. I will deal first with the longer scales, which show much more variability than the shorter periods because there are two salient reference points, the present and the beginning of geological time or the birth of the universe, and there are two ways of assigning numbers, one simply going forward from zero at the beginning to, say, 2×10^{10} years at the present, the other calling the present zero and using negative values back to -2×10^{10}. Neither is consistently tied to a top-to-bottom progression. Even the geologists seem uncertain whether time's arrow should ascend or descend. We sometimes bubble upward from a magma or trickle down from a cloud of ionized hydrogen! For short time spans, on the other hand, time's arrow is consistent. It always descends from past toward the present, from January to December, from 1900 to 1978; like the people I interviewed, it reverses the spatial analog.

Should we assume from the two sets of examples that the spatial analogies are linguistically robust but psychologically weak, that in the temporal domain we talk space but do not think it? This explanation encounters problems, not the least of which is the patent fact that people will quite readily display time in space. (In American Sign Language time is indicated by movements toward and over the shoulder, future forward, present at the body, past behind.) When my informants produce a time line moving horizontally left to right, they will place themselves on that line near the left-hand end, facing right. They find it inconceivable to do the reverse, showing that thinking is committed to the spatial analogy of moving through time.

I pointed out earlier that to understand spatial representation in plan or map drawing one must use *two* viewpoints, that of the person looking down on the environment from above and that of the same person located within the space. Likewise, when informants draw a horizontal time line with themselves within it they are adopting a viewpoint perpendicular to the transverse movement, and at the same time they place themselves within the frame looking into the future,

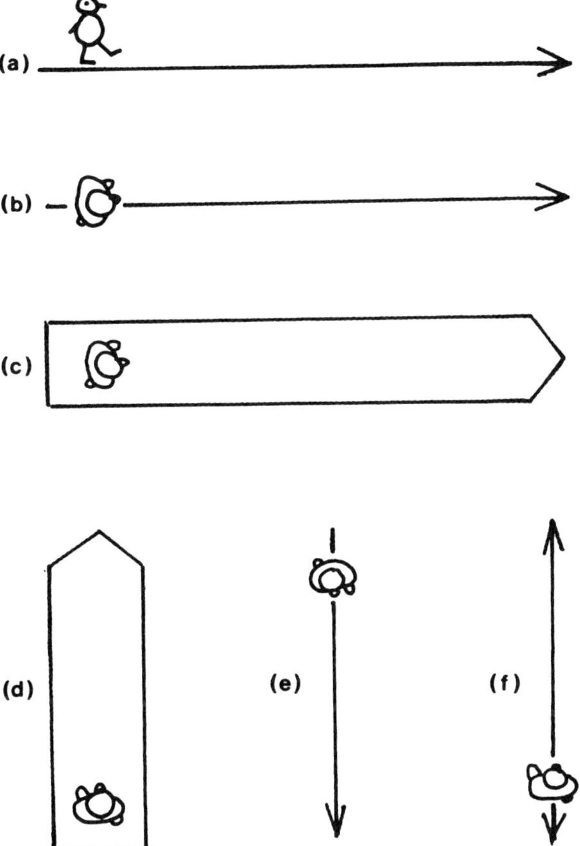

Fig. 11.6. (a): Adult informants place themselves at the left facing right when asked to locate themselves on a time line. (b) and (c): Common responses when informants are asked to represent themselves in time "in a plan view." When asked to show the plan vertically, informants may look "up the page" (d), produce a "lists" orientation (e), or produce a representation in which the passage of time and their facing within it is inconsistent (f).

as in Fig. 11.6(a). This is analogous to someone drawing himself running from left to right. What people do *not* do is spontaneously adopt a plan or map view of time. This is because it is characteristically seen as one-dimensional. If you ask a subject to translate the transverse view of time into a plan, the most common response is simply to tip the line "on its side," drawing a line, Fig. 11.6(b), perhaps drawing a horizontal strip, Fig. 11.6(c), with the person drawn in plan looking to the right. If they are then asked to arrange it vertically, they face a conflict – first to obey the principle of looking up the page, which places later events above earlier, Fig. 11.6(d), or conversely to arrange time as a list downward from early to later, which is consistent with normal list structure but requires the person to be looking down the page, Fig. 11.6(e). Internally contradictory representations, Fig. 11.6(f), are not uncommon.

This analysis, which claims that the linguistic space-time analogy has psychological reality, is also consistent with the findings of Bowerman (1982), who showed that even at the age of 3 or 4 years, children start implicitly to recognize the spatial analogy and coin new temporal phrases using spatial terms not present in the adult language.

A return to space

Once we have recognized that the plan view is not a natural way to visualize time, we can crystallize a salient fact about plan and map drawing: that it is a response to a technical problem which has its roots in the natural arrangements of objects in the physical world. When someone "draws a house," it is quite common for that person to produce a plan. Sometimes these plans show the influence of technical drawing precedents and sometimes the versions are more naive, but in either case we are inclined to say that they have adopted the architects' conventions. I will not recapitulate my earlier objections to the term "convention," but simply observe that the architect and the less sophisticated drawer face the same problem: Objects in the world are spread thinly and tend on the whole to sit side by side. Everywhere one looks, one finds objects that are "one-deep" – free-standing and occupying their own floor space. (A study or office where this book is being read is perhaps an unrepresentative example because the items within it are typically small and light and space is at a premium, so they are often placed in stacks and piles, and extra "floor space" is created in the form of drawers and shelves.) But in representing objects in less crowded situations, a conflict arises between the virtues of the lateral view that often represents the most typical face of individual objects and the plan view that avoids occlusion and displays both horizontal dimensions optimally.

This conflict is resolved in three ways: (1) To represent laterally. This is almost universal for items that spread horizontally like runners on a track, vehicles on a road or bridge, houses on a street, or events in time. (2) To represent in plan or as a map those arrays whose horizontal two-dimensional relations are important. (3) To preserve both, either by the use of an oblique viewpoint or by combining a lateral view of objects with a plan view of space. Three examples from outside the area of vernacular drawing spring to mind. The first is the perspective of the classic primitive painter, who arranges space up the canvas and displays each object frontally on this surface. The other two examples are closer to pragmatics: the standard representation of the chessboard, with the board in plan and the pieces in side elevation, and the tourist map of monuments and public buildings, with the streets in plan and the buildings drawn as we view them. This mix could be described as an example of the orthoscopic in adult drawing.

Given the obvious advantages of such a display, it is surprising how rarely it appears in the everyday drawings of my informants. I do not believe that this is because they were obsessed by the need for a consistent viewpoint. The only examples I found were some stylized boats and waves to identify a bay and some side elevation views of trees in a plan of a garden. No subjects drew their houses, railway stations, schools, or shopping centers in this way. These were always simply a rectangle or a cross. The reasons for this distribution can be tied to questions of effort and identifiability. A tree, a wave, or a boat are generic rather than particular. A plan form (a circle, a line, or a lenticular shape) would not easily identify them, whereas a line for a trunk and a triangle for a sail disambiguate the forms quite economically. On the other hand, to represent one's house in literal detail as a particular identifiable building rather than simply as a site demands considerable graphic skill and disproportionate effort, and every informant simply identified the various buildings either in speech, by a street number, or very occasionally with a written word.

This complementary distribution of plan and side elevation according to item portrayed illustrates very well the inadequacy of a purely representational analysis of drawing studied in a conventional research context. Drawing in everyday life is not a matter of executing a pure graphic product. It is oriented toward cognitive, emotional, or communicative use. In the latter case, it is embedded in a context of mutual understanding of what can be assumed between drawer and audience, and is supplemented not only by the speech that provides part of the substantive message, but also by the speech, gesture, and modulation of the executive process itself that communicates about the communication. I will conclude with some remarks about this byplay that I have called the ''prosodics'' of graphic execution.

Prosodics and thematics

When I was exploring the role of semantics in drawing production, I pointed out that there is no buffer between meaning and the final actions of drawing execution, so when one steers a pencil around a curve, one may be representing directly the form of some object, or in making a stroke in a certain direction, portraying movement in the real world. On the other hand, when one is moving the pencil across a page in a wavy line or skipping it across to make a series of discontinuous marks, it cannot be taken for granted that these actions *are* representing forms in the world, because they may be conveying information about one's attitude to the subject matter. For example, one informant reproduced a map of two or three city blocks and added to it the trajectory of her journey to a certain shop. The line showing her path begins as a broken line and becomes continuous, indicating that one should not pay much attention to the exact route until it comes within a block or two of the destination. This message about the *status* of the representation could have been conveyed by a finer line or one drawn more carelessly. Such devices, by which the basic representational material is modulated in the process of production, seem to me to be analogous to prosodics in spoken language, whereby various attitudinal states toward the subject matter are expressed by changes in the sound stream.

There are two sides to prosodics (and paralinguistic features) in spoken language. One deals with the actual types of modulation, changes in pitch and pitch range, in loudness, duration, pausing. These physical characteristics are identified as the primary marks by which prosodic features are identified (Crystal, 1976), and from this base it is possible to extend the exploration into what they convey, which in Crystal's analysis means the "...attitudinal effects being signalled...." These attitudinal or emotional states include such things as being "irritated," "precise," "amused," "disapproving," "conspiratorial," "questioning," and so on.

Because in drawing the same graphic devices can be used (1) to represent, (2) to express attitudes about the topic, and (3) to communicate about the performance itself, it is impossible to isolate a series of devices or properties of line used in drawing and to claim that they *uniquely* signal dismissal, concern, emphasis, and so on. This is one of the several points at which the linguistic-graphic analogy cannot be taken very literally. If one does choose to work from the physical devices (rather than the functions) end, it is necessary to proceed by the method of "progressive exclusion" described in the opening pages of Chapter 1. This involves assigning formal or semantic significance to whatever actions or features one can and then searching for a motivation for the residue. In the example given this is not so difficult, since the change from a broken to a continuous line could hardly represent the actual mode of progression of the informant along the street, so we immediately see it as a comment on the interpretative status of the line. Furthermore, public performances like map drawing are commonly accompanied by speech and gesture that help further to identify the significance of various levels of structure within the performance.

An alternative procedure is to turn the problem on its head and begin from inferences about motivation and work backward to identify the prosodic devices being used. Since what I am trying to do is to open up the field of analysis with an impressionistic "first approximation," I am using whichever of these routes I can find, sometimes leading in from oddities of procedure to infer messages and sometimes searching in the accounts accompanying drawings and maps to see where emphasis lies and then seeking the graphic devices used to fulfill the

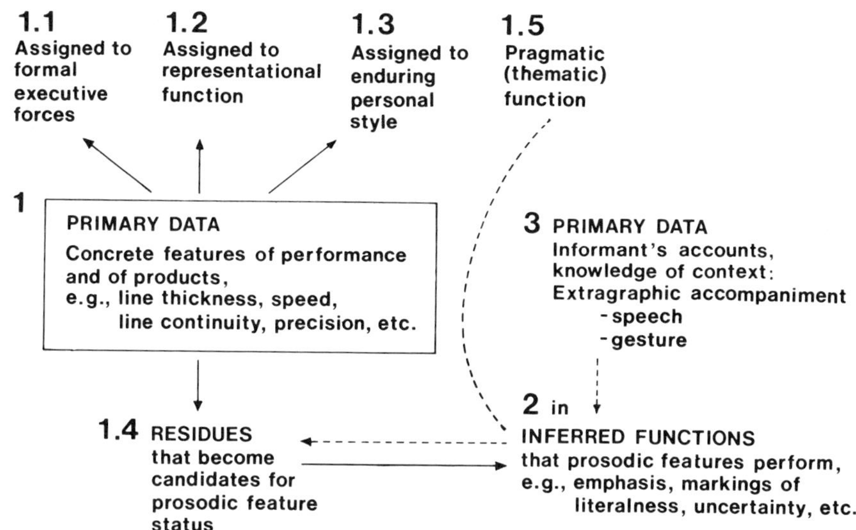

Fig. 11.7. Inquiry strategies for establishing the correspondence between graphic devices and "prosodic" functions in everyday drawings. Some features are assigned to nonprosodic functions like representation. The residue is assigned to prosodic functions. Broken arrows proceed from reports by informants and other clues to function and lead to a search for corresponding prosodic and thematic features within the drawing process.

need. What this yields is a heterogeneous array of devices, some of which, like line thickness, continuity, and strength and precision of stroke, are modulations on the actual production process and are clearly analogous to suprasegmental aspects of spoken language.

But this reverse analysis also throws up all those *thematic* mechanisms, like the basic order in which things are done, which in language are closer to textual analysis. I have tried to illustrate this situation in Fig. 11.7. We can start in this diagram at one of two places. The first is in the box marked (1) whose contents comprise certain concrete features of drawing and drawing production, such as those listed. Because none of them can be assigned uniquely to "prosodic" function, we have to parcel out some of them to executive constraints (1.1) (such as ordering due to end control of lines). Some are assigned representational function (1.2) (for example, a broken line drawn down a street could portray lane markers). A further parceling out connected with stable personal style is necessary (1.3). The residue (1.4) comprises the candidates for prosodic analysis, and from this residue we move to examine functions (2), which include things like emphasis or signals about literalness of the interpretation or the tentativeness of the detail.

The dashed lines in Fig. 11.7 represent the complementary strategy. The primary data here are not the functions themselves (2), but data from the accompanying dialogue and gesture and comments the drawer makes to the investigator about the history, context, and intentions associated with the drawing and parts of it (3). From this we can make certain inferences about emphasis, tentativeness, and so on. These in turn invite us to search for or inquire about the devices that express them.

The path from function does not lead only to mechanisms like line thickness and precision, but diverges into the whole thematic structure and pragmatic sequencing within the drawing (1.5). By this I mean the way in which the whole point in making the drawing contributes to the way it unfolds: "Here is the bay, and there is the jetty." "This is the house; this is where the new extension is to go." "This is the room; here is where we need electric outlets." "These are the foundations; here is the metal shielding I want; there are the walls that sit on it." "This is where we are facing now, and our path goes this way. . . ." The whole area resonates with the terminology of thematics: given and new, frame and insert, theme and rheme.

This division of the path from a single functional source toward "prosodics" and "thematics" is exactly as it should be. The two topics in both graphics and language are densely interrelated. In language, this occurs at both the sentence and discourse level (Bolinger, 1972, 1975, Halliday, 1967). (I have never found it obvious how to translate the distinction between sentence and discourse into the graphic domain. Is the drawing of a piece of clothing a word, a sentence, a paragraph? But from the present point of view it is not critical, for neither thematics nor prosody necessarily honor sentence boundaries in the linguistic domain.) For graphic analysis, all we need to note is that the actions being performed by a drawer are structured by the social act being carried out and that this structure of content and order is elaborated by prosodics; and further that it is often supported by extragraphic communication, the speech and gesture that accompany it. So, for example, the drawer constructs the frame with quick strokes, inserts the critical data with slower, clearer, and more precise lines and movements, and at the same time points at and comments on its significance.

The background of personal style

I have not made a formal empirical study of personal style, but before I describe a few of the "prosodic" devices and their functions, I should explore the important issue I have mentioned above, stable personal characteristics.

If we are trying to "read" variation in line thickness, sketchiness, precision, completeness, speed of movement, and so on as local or immediate contrasts, it is necessary to discount stable variations across informants in these same variables. Crystal reflects on the issue in the context of speech analysis: "Voice quality is . . . the permanently present person-identifying 'background' vocal effect in speech . . . distinguished from speech by a different set of parametric values which are never utilized for purposes of communication" (1976, p. 124). This treats the individual background level as a standard (a sort of "DC level" in electrophysiological terms), against which local variation is evaluated. This is a convenient encapsulation of the problem, but neither in graphics nor in language is it reasonable to reduce this simply to two levels, the permanent, nonsignificant and the local, immediately significant. There is a variable number of levels, each with its own extent or duration and each with varying degrees of semiotic value. To begin with, in graphics there are basic manipulative approaches to the medium, the grip drawers typically use, the degree to which their drawing movements use proximal or distal joints. Some subjects systematically engage wrist and fingers, others extend movement back to elbow, shoulder, and trunk (Connolly and Elliott, 1972). There are differences in scale (simply how big people make their drawings), in the basic types of graphic units used, in speed, in care. There are differences in the force subjects can and do apply, their use of firm, flowing line versus feathered, hesitant, tremulous, or overdrawn lines. Some highly competent performers are adept enough regularly to produce quite elaborate drawings without appearing obsessive or contravening "conversational agreements."

Some of these stable qualities may be independent of communicative intent, but it is not safe to assume this. People may be trying to say something about themselves or reflecting their own self-evaluation, even though they always work in much the same way. When one sees an unimportant local sketch map meticulously laid out, produced by much active paper turning and body reorientation, the streets quickly, neatly, and completely labeled, it is not entirely a question of competence; the drawer does seem to be delivering a message to herself or to others, notwithstanding that the performance is likely to be repeated over and over on different occasions. But if we know that this is the typical approach of the person, no matter how trivial the pretext, we do not read the precision as a pointer to local emphasis.

At a stage lower down, we may have a drawer sustaining a certain style and level of attention for the duration of one drawing. A householder reproduced for me a very elaborate drawing of a construction detail for a tradesperson because he wanted the job done with more than usual care. One informant reproduced a sketch plan of building allotments that she originally drew up as part of a campaign to get local government action on a drainage problem, and even when showing me what she had done, it took her 15 busy minutes to complete it. This was not because this was to be the engineer's technical specification; but it was intended to convey something of the intensity of feeling and the urgency she felt about the problem, first to the authorities and then to me. The graphic approach was the equivalent of writing across the top of the submission, "I am not easily put off." This was *not* a matter of permanent style; the same informant produced a quick sketch of a time line in a few seconds in the same interview session. The drawings of details of dress designs that three or four informants produced were done in an entirely different style from the "drawings of common objects: a dress." Outlines were produced with carefully placed short hatched lines rather than bold strokes. There were two reasons for this stress: to produce a more accurate contour, and at the same time to deliver a message about the level of fine detail a viewer might be expected to recover about the nuances of neck and sleeve shape, and so on.

As I reported earlier, informants were asked whether they had an audience present or were sending or giving the drawing to someone. In the cases of clothes drawings by women there were audiences present, and the actual drawing actions, their timing and precision, carried the message. Bolinger (1976) describes how when one writes, the emphasis must be shifted to a different code from that used in face-to-face dialogue, and in graphics we find examples of work for a remote audience where care is coded conspicuously in both quantity and quality of the product. One informant showed me how he had carefully sketched drawings of house extensions in plan and elevation, all produced in a fine meticulous line. He said he had made a set of six of these that he recently presented to his wife for comment. He added wryly that this studied gesture of consultation did not prevent her shortly afterward from becoming his ex-wife, and there was a clear implication that the care in producing the drawings carried more than construction information.

Although these cases sometimes cover an extended time span, they have carried us from the domain of enduring personal style into the arena where constructional practice is used to convey information beyond the representational content. It would be reasonable to classify this modulation of care as part of the prosodics of drawing in the sense that it conveys attitudinal information through the shaping of the production process, even though the modulation does not apply unit-by-unit within the drawing itself.

Attitude, emotion, and graphic act

Before proceeding to examples of these more fine-grained shifts in approach, let me comment on the use of the term "attitudinal content," which I have borrowed from the intonation literature. One has the impression that linguists who began at the phonetic and phonological end of the linguistic spectrum have made a series of cautious concessions to function, and the admission of "attitude" and "emotion" must once have seemed radical if not slightly corrupt to people who saw language studies as "general" at the level of the proposition. But when one does a quick assay of functions of intonation, for example by extracting terms from the index of Bolinger's (1972) collection of papers, one finds that along with emotional terms like "annoyance," "awe," "boredom," "contempt," and "cordiality," there are others like "accusation," "command," "complaint," "dismissal," and "interrogation" that are clearly in the spirit of speech act theory, and as far as graphics is concerned, this seems to me altogether more congenial territory. Modulations of graphic production of the sort we have been exploring are either graphic social acts themselves or contribute to graphic social acts. The man who gives the tradesperson a meticulous drawing is issuing a request for a meticulous job. The ex-wife of the house-plan drawer seems to have received some mixture of a reproach and a plea along with the prerogative of choice. The woman who drew her face and then drew over the head line after dark line of shading to express her depression was incorporating in the monotonous repetitive action something more than the dark area itself could provide.

Interactive relations between features

I should like to complete this section with a brief review of some of the fine-grained prosodic modulations of output. There is not enough material for any sort of adequate systematic taxonomy of devices and functions. Among the 50 or 60 protocols of everyday drawing available to me from interviews there is not a rich supply of material, but the drawings do at least provide the flavor of the relationship between device and function at the microlevel and show what level of analysis is demanded.

I have already quoted the example of the pathway that began as a fragmented line and changed to a firm one. This conversion is common, although the direction of change is not always the same. In local map drawing, a main thoroughfare may be drawn as a strong line or as a double line, and half a dozen rough single lines are then drawn across it to suggest an approximate number of minor cross streets. When an important road junction is reached the rate of production slows, lines are more distinct and more carefully laid down, more attention is given to orientation. This is not simply providing critical information to aid recognition. It is a form of stress and is often accompanied by appropriate gesture or comment. One of the signs of stylistic informality that is found in the unimportant lines is the lack of precision in contacting and leaving the paper surface, so there are "tails" to the lines, like an incomplete cursive approach to lettering.

Often the change in level of care and detail signals redundancy. People drawing a time line often draw a few time markers and then add a scattering of poorly executed slurred strokes at increasing intervals across the page, a sort of graphic "et cetera." This happens regularly with token detail: One or two bricks in a wall are neatly delineated, two or three others larger and more quickly and loosely drawn. Ties on a railway line start neatly, then lose their consistency in length, spacing, orientation, and firmness. The communicative value of this "tailing off" can be appreciated if one considers the alternative – a few neat lines coming to an abrupt halt. A female informant drew a dress from the front, carefully defining shoulder line, arm opening, and so on, then produced the back view very quickly to display a single feature. Again this is an economical strategy, but it also signals to the audience by its speed and looseness what level of attention is appropriate, saying in effect: "The back is like the front; don't try to read the details of these strokes." Then the tempo slows a little as the critical feature is drawn.

The informant who drew a ceiling that he was relining followed the standard structure of *theme* ("This is the room") and *rheme* ("Here is the problem"). In this case, this thematic order happens to coincide with the order prescribed by formal executive constraints of conformity (which touches on a regularity of objects and actions in the world and frames and elaborations in drawing that is probably not accidental). When the drawer drew the boards, he used a couple of wispy lines to indicate their sides and scribbled across them, the message of the actions and the product being: "Here we cannot be precise by virtue of the problem itself," or "There are several ways to do this."

In maps there are often oscillating lines that announce a lack of literal representation. Such a line representing a path, an embankment, the edge of a patch of water is representational in the sense that the physical feature is not rectilinear and the general orientation is meant to be read more or less faithfully, but the particular contour is not meant to be precise. When there is an audience present, speed is of course a very important signal in these matters. An oscillating line drawn slowly usually means something very different from a rapidly drawn one, whereas many features drawn as a straight line are meant to be straight irrespective of speed.

A woman drew a key ring she had lost. The identifying feature was a piece of polished stone that was drawn and then overdrawn, while the keys, which were unimportant as identifiers, were represented as a set of loosely organized single radiating lines. *Overdrawing* is an interesting case of the apparent ambiguity of single features. Overdrawing is often a way of simultaneously correcting and emphasizing the importance of an element in a drawing and registering the significance of the precision of contour, but occasionally it is just the reverse. Some informants conveyed the message "Don't take this too literally" by a scribble of overdrawing of boundaries. Here the key semiotic ingredient is again the speed combined with a lack of accuracy in each succeeding stroke. (Indeed it may be only because there are multiple strokes that one can detect the inaccuracy.)

Feathering, the process of building up a line from short ballistic fragments end to end or overlapping, shares with overdrawing a primary ambiguity, but in this case it is not necessarily because feathering indicates different things in different contexts, but because it seems to carry a double message: insecurity about competence and an intention to be painstaking. ("I can't do this well, but this is my best effort.") Since "feathering" is often habitual, it carries most weight as a sign of care and emphasis when it is used contrastively; that is, when it is embedded in the context of a continuous line.

These examples of curved lines, overdrawing, and feathering carry three important lessons: (1) It seems unlikely that one could draw up a simple "codebook" matching feature to meaning. (2) It is necessary sometimes to look at a *complex* of features and to recognize that they may not be simply additive. Speed may modulate the meaning of curved lines, but not straight lines. Overdrawing with precision indicates care and literalness, overdrawing without precision may signal the reverse. (3) Finally, if one is prepared to spend time teasing apart the geometric, the semantic, the pragmatic, and the issue of personal style, and if one has the patience to entertain such interactive models, one might indeed succeed in penetrating past initial ambiguity to quite a tight theory of graphic prosodics.

Let me finish simply by listing a few of the properties of action and of drawing features that are more obvious candidates as prosodic features. Most of them are dimensional, and I have selected the pole that corresponds to focus or emphasis where that applies: slow speed, large size, thickness of line (distinctness), precision, detail and repetition of detail, continuity (as opposed to interruption), smoothness (as opposed to tremor), precise overdrawing, and feathering as a contrastive device. To these we can add certain kinesic elements such as active reorientation of the body or the paper.

What do they convey? In most instances I have documented they indicate emphasis and importance, and they convey messages about literalness and certainty. These general functions may serve a variety of particular social purposes. There is not one of the actions or features that could not be used representationally. (Even speed of production could in theory carry information about speed of movement.) Likewise, all of them can be products of a stable style and so could be saying little in a local way. And, of course, ordinarily they are all integrated tightly into the thematics of production and may be supported or complemented by speech and gesture when, as so often happens, drawing is done for a present audience.

On the linguistic analogy

Since the preceding section of this chapter on prosodics and thematics in drawing production depended more heavily than any other part of this book on the analogy with language analysis, it is appropriate to conclude with some comment on the parallel and its generality.

To state my conclusions first: I believe that the most important feature shared by the two systems, graphics and language, is the variety of levels of structure within each. This is the "layering" to which I referred in the very beginning of the book. Second, I think that this layering is found in many human activities but is not always so rich. Third, I think that what makes the difference between a richly layered and a simple system of human action is its involvement in social signification. Once an action conveys social meaning, the potential for it to acquire layer upon layer of structure rises steeply.

I should like to elaborate this first by reference to fine art because it allows us to see how venerable the parallels are. The earliest reference I have come across to the use of an explicit analogy between language and the visual arts involves the Italian commentator Leon Baltista Alberti. Baxandall (1972), in his book on fifteenth-century Italian painting, describes Alberti as the author of the oldest surviving treatise on painting, and in this treatise published in 1435, Alberti utilizes a conception of literary structure that subdivides the sentence into clauses, clauses into phrases, phrases into words. Parallel to this, Alberti produces a painting hierarchy that descends from the picture to the (human) figures within it, to the members (limbs, and so on) of the figures, to the planes from which the members were built. The treatment reminds one of the so-called picture grammars developed in the 1960s for automatic scene analysis (Clowes, Langridge, and Zatorski, 1970). Picture grammar was an attempt to express drawings as feature hierarchies on the model of linguistic phrase markers. The aim was to produce a general strategy of analysis that treated all pictures in basically the same way, segmenting them and then unifying them by transformations like deletion, substitution, and so on. At about the same time, tree diagrams and transformations were being used to analyze handwritten scripts in terms of character identity and difference (Powers, 1973, Watt, 1975).

In one sense, this is exactly what Alberti and his contemporary Landino were out to do. They segmented paintings and reliefs down into successive levels of detail and compared one with another to bring out the degree of coordination of the design and the variety or diversity of the forms and treatments within it (Baxandall, 1972, pp. 133–137). Partly by virtue of the richness of the subject matter on which they worked, including the painting and sculpture of Masaccio, Filippo Lippi, and Donatello, and partly because of their breadth of view, these Italian analysts ranged over a very broad spectrum of qualities. Alberti himself referred to color and the reception of light, to size, proportion, balance, the attitude of figures, their posture, gestures, movement, emotional qualities, to symbolism in pictures, and to their narrative structure (Alberti, 1972).

Although the range of properties is considerably more esthetically oriented than the dimensions with which we have been dealing in this book, the approach I should like to cultivate has much more in common with Alberti (or Baxandall himself) than with picture grammars. The appeal of picture grammars was in their rigor and explicitness, but their aims were "contractionist" in that they sought to reduce structure to universal principles. I think it is a healthier aim to let the individual subject matter speak for itself, to try to unpack whatever multiplicity of levels of structure, conscious or unconscious, exist in graphic activity and to explore the variety of ways they are interrelated.

Whether such a heterogeneity of levels exists within any and all subject matter is an empirical question. Sometimes human action is very shallow. There are many practical actions we carry out that we can analyze in terms of simple skills that have short histories and direct purposes. What would we include in an inventory of such things? Cooking, eating, dressing, shopping, driving? The difficulty is that any one of these things can be converted into a social performance. Indeed, one could claim that an act like eating can hardly escape being a social performance. We are accustomed to defining it as practical action: transferring food to plate, cutting it and lifting it to the mouth. Yet if we look through a broader window at the behavior so that we consider the provenance of the food, its preparation, and its consumption in a social setting, we are immediately involved with systems of belief and significance.

The best way to dramatize this is to contemplate at how many points one could make oneself or others uncomfortable by failing to arrange eating conduct appropriately in timing, dress, seating, deportment, conversation, the use of implements, the sequence of action. Consider a person who came to the table when people had almost finished eating, stood up, and proceeded to eat with her fingers one food item after another from the plates: first all the bread, then all the potato, the butter, the green vegetables, before departing without looking at or speaking to anyone. It is not simply a question of "manners." The normal pattern of social eating in our society is highly constrained at many levels – esthetic, nutritional, hygienic. It involves the tacit acknowledgment of social debts and transactions both with respect to the food and the social intercourse that accompanies its preparation and consumption. I do not want to labor the point. Various aspects have been dealt with eloquently by writers like Lévi-Strauss (1970), Mary Douglas (1982), Barthes (1973), and most recently Goody (1982.) Furthermore, I have no doubt that if anyone were interested, they could unpack a good deal of structure even from the minimal physical manipulations of consigning food and drink to the stomach.

Perhaps what distinguishes topics like eating from the domains we have been considering is that the constraints are more dispersed over time. Although one couldn't claim that nutrition and esthetics are evident only at the planning stages of a meal, and selection and combination at another stage, there is nonetheless an uneven distribution along the syntagmatic series. So this is the first dimension of variation: dispersal *versus* compactness. The other dimension is that of vertical complexity, where each area or element of action can be defined in terms of *the upper and lower bounds to simultaneous complexity.*

There is a certain irreducible minimum of simultaneous structure involved in any skilled action, be it speech, drawing, eating, playing a musical instrument, or working a machine, and the level of this minimum complexity will vary across domains. Although I believe that the irreducible level of simultaneous (and horizontal) complexity of an ordinary drawing production is quite high, I do not believe it is as formidable as that of speech, largely because the sound signal carries a lot more information and language is enormously more codified.

The *upper* bound of simultaneous complexity depends heavily on whether we are dealing with a semiotic system – actions that carry meaning – and to what purpose the expression of meaning is put. To follow Halliday (1970), those purposes can be ideational, interpersonal, and textual (to which I might add ludic and esthetic). As we saw in the case of everyday drawings, they can be used to organize thought, to affect the actions of others, to comment on themselves, to please and to amuse.

I believe it is easy to underestimate the intricacy of action at all levels of organization, but especially those of meaning and social action. To take a final bizarre example: Wielding a mop and bucket is at its lower bound a simple practical act. Yet it plays a role in a network of obligations and transactions (try spilling something and not mopping it up), and occasionally it is carried out more as a message than as a necessary act of neatness or hygiene, as when the sight and especially the sound of mopping becomes a sign of domestic martyrdom to both men and women.

The upshot of this is that when we confront the question of what degree and type of complexity we can expect to find in human action, it is useful to think of its horizontal structure, across which constraints are dispersed more or less widely or compactly, and the vertical structure of its components, which rises from a minimum of essential structure in mechanism and skill through a rich set of layers that become more and more numerous as the action becomes more semiotic and more significantly embedded in wider social processes. The final point is that the performers of these actions may not be conscious of the structure and complexity of their own conduct, so that the investigator is obliged to adopt a great variety of analytic stratagems to uncover them.

References

Abend, W., Bizzi, E., & Morasso, P. (1982). Human arm trajectory formation. *Brain*, 105, 331–48.
Alberti, L. B. (1972). *On Painting and on Sculpture: the Latin Texts of De Pictura and De Statua*, trans. C. Grayson. London: Phaidon.
André-Leicknam, B. (1982). Le système cunéiforme en mésopotamie: graphisme, fonctionnement et évolution. In *Naissance de l'écriture: cunéiformes et hiéroglyphes*, ed. B. André-Leicknam & C. Ziegler, p. 75. Paris: Édition de la réunion des musées nationaux.
Arnheim, R. (1964). *Art and Visual Perception*. Berkeley: University of California Press.
Austin, J. L. (1962). *How to Do Things with Words*. London: Oxford University Press.
Barthes, R. (1973). *Mythologies*. London: Granada.
Baxandall, M. (1972). *Painting and Experience in Fifteenth Century Italy*. Oxford: Oxford University Press.
Bender, L. (1958). Problems in conceptualization and communication in children with developmental alexia. In *Psychopathology of Communication*, ed. P. H. Hoch & J. Zubin, pp. 155–76. New York: Grune and Stratton.
Bent, I. D., Hiley, D., Bent, M., & Chew, G. (1980). Notation. In *The New Grove Dictionary of Music and Musicians*, ed. S. Sadie, pp. 333–420. London: Macmillan.
Berger, J. (1972). *Ways of Seeing*. London: BBC and Penguin Books.
Blau, T. H. (1977). Torque and schizophrenic vulnerability: as the world turns. *American Psychologist*, 32, 997–1005.
Bolinger, D. (1972). Around the edge of language: intonation. In *Intonation*, ed. D. Bolinger, pp. 19–29. Harmondsworth, England: Penguin Books.
(1975). *Aspects of Language*, 2nd ed. New York: Harcourt Brace Jovanovich.
Bourdieu, P. (1979). *La Distinction: Critique sociale du jugement*. Paris: Les Éditions de Minuit.
Bowerman, M. (1982). Hidden meanings: the role of covert conceptual structures in children's development of language. Paper presented to the conference on the Acquisition of Cognitive Skills, University of Keele, Keele, England.
Brooks, L. R. (1968). Spatial and verbal components of the act of recall. *Canadian Journal of Psychology*, 22, 349–50.
Brown, P., & Levinson, S. (1978). Universals in language use: Politeness phenomena. In *Questions and Politeness: Strategies in Social Interaction*, ed. E. N. Goody, pp. 56–289. Cambridge: Cambridge University Press.
Bühler, K. (1934). *The Mental Development of the Child*. London: Kegan Paul.
Chang, J. J., & Carroll, J. D. (1968). *How to Use MDPREF, a Computer Program for Multidimensional Analysis of Preference Data*. Bell Telephone Laboratories Technical Report.
Clark, H. H. (1973). Space, time, semantics and the child. In *Cognitive Development and the Acquisition of Language*, ed. T. E. Moore, pp. 28–64. New York: Academic Press.
Clowes, M. B., Langridge, D. J., & Zatorski, R. J. (1970). Linguistic descriptions. In *Picture Language Machines*, ed. S. Kaneff, pp. 87–117. London: Academic Press.
Connolly, K., & Elliott, J. (1972). The evolution and ontogeny of hand function. In *Ethological Studies of Child Behaviour*, ed. N. B. Jones, pp. 329–83. Cambridge: Cambridge University Press.

Crystal, D. (1976). *Prosodic Systems and Intonation in English*. Cambridge: Cambridge University Press.

Diringer, D. (1968). *The Alphabet*. London: Hutchinson.

Douglas, M. (1982). *In the Active Voice*. London: Routledge and Kegan Paul.

Dreyfuss, H. (1972). *Symbol Source Book*. New York: McGraw Hill.

Duncker, K. (1945). On problem solving. *Psychological Monographs*, 58, whole number. (Translated by L. S. Lees).

Edgerton, S. Y., Jr. (1976). *The Renaissance Rediscovery of Linear Perspective*. New York: Icon Editions, Harper & Row.

Eng, H. (1954). *The Psychology of Children's Drawings*, 2nd ed. London: Routledge and Kegan Paul.

Fairbank, A. (1968). *A Handwriting Manual*. London: Faber.

Forge, A. (1971). Art and environment in the Sepik. In *Art and Aesthetics in Primitive Societies*, ed. C. F. Jopling, pp. 290–314. New York: Dutton.

Fraser, B. (1975). Hedged performatives. In *Syntax and Semantics, Vol. 3: Speech Acts*, ed. P. Cole & J. L. Morgan, pp. 187–210. New York: Academic Press.

Getzels, J. W., & Csizszentmihalyi, M. (1976). *The Creative Vision: A Longitudinal Study of Problem Solving in Art*. New York: Wiley.

Goffman, E. (1955). On face work: An analysis of ritual elements in social interaction. *Psychiatry*, 18, 213–31.

Gombrich, E. H. (1972). The visual image. *Scientific American*, 227, 82–96.

Goodnow, J. J. (1977). *Children's Drawings*. London: Open Books.

Goodnow, J. J., Friedman, S., Bernbaum, M., & Lehman, E. B. (1973). Direction and sequence in copying: The effect of learning to write in English and Hebrew. *Journal of Cross-Cultural Psychology*, 4, 263–82.

Goody, J. (1982). *Cooking, Cuisine and Class*. Cambridge: Cambridge University Press.

Grice, H. P. (1975). Logic and conversation. In *Syntax and Semantics, Vol. 3: Speech Acts*, ed. P. Cole & J. L. Morgan, pp. 41–58. New York: Academic Press.

Halliday, M. A. K. (1967). *Intonation and Grammar in British English*. The Hague: Mouton.

(1970). Language structure and language function. In *New Horizons in Linguistics*, ed. J. Lyons, pp. 140–65. Harmondsworth, England: Penguin Books.

Haworth, M. R. (1970). *The Primary Visual Motor Test*. New York: Grune and Stratton.

Helfman, E. S. (1967). *Signs and Symbols Around the World*. New York: Lothrop, Lee, and Shepard.

Herron, J. (1980). Two hands, two brains, two sexes. In *Neuropsychology of Left-Handedness*, ed. J. Herron, pp. 233–60. New York: Academic Press.

Hornung, C. P. (1946). *Handbook of Designs and Devices*. New York: Dover.

Howard, I. P., & Templeton, W. B. (1966). *Human Spatial Orientation*. London: Wiley.

Ilg, F. L., & Ames, L. B. (1964). *School Readiness*. New York: Harper & Row.

Ivins, W. M. Jr. (1958). *How Prints Look: Photographs with a Commentary*. Boston: Beacon Press.

James, H. (1982). Personal communication.

Jarvella, R. J. (1971). Syntactic processing of connected speech. *Journal of Verbal Learning and Verbal Behavior*, 10, 409–16.

(1973). Coreference and short-term memory for discourse. *Journal of Experimental Psychology*, 98, 426–8.

Johnson-Laird, P. N. (1981). Comprehension as the construction of mental models. *Philosophical Transactions of the Royal Society of London, B.*, 295, 353–74.

Jones, S. (1972). An investigation into the conservative nature of children's drawings. Unpublished honors thesis, University of New South Wales, Australia.

Kennedy, J. M. (1975). Drawing was discovered not invented. *New Scientist*, 67, 523–25.

Knuth, D. E. (1978). Mathematical typography. *Bulletin (New Series) of the American Mathematical Society*, 1, 337–72.

Lévi-Strauss, C. (1970). *The Raw and the Cooked: Introduction to a Science of Mythology, I*. London: Jonathan Cape.

Levy, J., & Reid, M. (1976). Variations in writing posture and cerebral organization. *Science*, 194, 337–9.

Lings, M. & Safadi, Y. H. (1976). *The Qur'an*. London: World of Islam Festival Publishing Company.

McWhinnie, H. J. (1971). Review of recent literature on figure drawing tests as related to research problems in art education. *Review of Educational Research*, 41, 131–42.

Massoudy, H. (1981). *Calligraphe Arabe Vivante*. Paris: Flammarion.

Möller, G. (1909). *Hieratische Palaographie*, Vol. I. Leipzig: J. C. Hinrichs'sche Buchhandlung.

Olson, D. R. (1975). On the relations between spatial and linguistic processes. In *Children's Spatial Development*, ed. J. Eliot & N. J. Salkind, pp. 67–110. Springfield, Ill.: Charles C. Thomas.

Porter, T. & Greenstreet, B. (1980). *Manual of Graphic Techniques*. New York: Scribners.

Powers, V. M. (1973). Pen direction sequences in character recognition. *Pattern Recognition*, 5, 291–302.

Ross, R. (1934). Optimal orders. *Journal of Educational Psychology*, 25, 375–82.

Sadler, N. A. (1971). An analysis of letter reversals in children's writing. Unpublished B.A. honours thesis, University of New South Wales, Kensington, N.S.W.

Saussure, F. (1974). *Course in General Linguistics*. London: Fontana.

Searle, J. R. (1969). *Speech Acts*. Cambridge: Cambridge University Press.

Slee, J. A. (1976). The perceptual nature of visual imagery. Ph.D. thesis, Australian National University.

Smith, W. (1975). *Flags*. Maidenhead: McGraw-Hill.

Stanton, R. (1973). A further investigation into the conservative nature of children's drawings. Unpublished B.A. honors thesis, Macquarie University, Australia.

Thomassen, A. J. W. M., & Teulings, H-L. H. M. (1979). The development of directional preference in writing movements. *Visible Language*, 13, 299–313.

Trabasso, T., & Bower, G. H. (1968). *Attention and Learning: Theory and Research*. New York: Wiley.

Tung Tso-pin (1948). Ten examples of early tortoise-shell inscriptions. *Harvard Journal of Asiatic Studies*, 11, 122–9.

Watt, W. C. (1975). What is the proper characterization of the alphabet? I: Desiderata. *Visible Language*, 9, 293–327.

Williams, R. (1981). *Culture*. London: Fontana.

Index

Abend, W., 93
accretion strategy, 41, 45
  by aggregation, 214
  vs. anchoring, 212
  by attachment, 212
  in children's drawing, 212–14
  by conformity, 213
  and object structure, 214
  by seriation, 213
  in stairway design, 44
Alberti, L.B., 268
Ames, L.B., 76
André-Leicknam, B., 27
anchoring, serial, 137
anchoring constraint, 36–51
  accuracy, 40
  in open regions, 38, 40
  planning, 42–51
  at points, 38, 40
  potency, 41
  radial line drawing, 37–41
  size of line, region, 38, 40
  solids drawing, 69–71
  at T-intersections, 38, 40, 49
  tree drawing, 13
anticipated embedding, 44, 45–7, 111–12
anticipation, *see* planning, graphic
Arabic script, 24–6
  calligraphy, 93
  circles, 93
  paper contact, 30
  Thuluth script, 93
arc drawing
  in child drawing, 209
  different from circles, 72, 92
  left-handed, 74–6
  related to other tasks, 74–6
  starting position, 74–6
  stroke preference, 74–6
Arnheim, R., 187
arm position manipulated, 61–4
  dot-cluster effects, 64
  methods, 61–2
  radial line effects, 62
  rectangle copying, 62–4
  starting position effects, 60–4
  stroke direction effects, 60–4
arm use in stroke making
  accuracy, 16–17
  frequency response, 16
  rehearsal, 16
arrows drawn
  geometric constraints, 95
  semantic constraints, 95, 103–5
articulatory stage in drawing, 100,
  see also linguistic analogy
    (''phonology'')
aspect of objects, 125–6
asymmetrical conformity, 48–51
  in face drawing, 50
  in representational drawing, 50
Austin, J.L., 233, 234
awareness in drawing, 39,
  see also unconscious action

ballistic movements, 40
Barthes, R., 269
Baxandall, M., 268
Bender, L., 76
Bent, I.D., 27, 93
Bent, M., 27
Berger, J., 244
Bizzi, E., 93
Blau, T.H., 76
''blocking'' tendency, 170
Bolinger, D., 1, 262, 264
boundary deletion, 44, 45

Bourdieu, P., 244
Bower, G.H., 170
Bowerman, M., 258
brain pathology
  cube test, 143–4
  star test, 143–4
  test designs, 142–4
Brooks, L.R., 135, 140
Brooks effect, *see* Brooks, L.R.
Brown, P., 61, 243
Bühler, K., 198, 237
Burmese script, circles, 93

calligraphy, 92, 93–4
  circle form, 92
canonical stroked directions, *see* stroke making
Carroll, J.D., 9
central control of movement
  affecting wrist-finger movements, 12
  paper contact, 32
Chang, J.J., 9
"Cheshire cat effect," 229
Chew, G., 27
children's drawing, 161–232
  contour development, 196
  controlled *vs*. ballistic movement, 185
  evolution, 161–73, 174
  executive constraints, 175, 223
  innovation by addition, 177–80
  innovation by substitution, 180–4
  innovations, 174
  microstructure variation, 222–3
  mosaic of features, 182, 219, 221
  occlusion, 196–200
  perceptual-motor difficulties, 191–4, 195
  reception *vs*. production, 161
  repeated drawings, 174–6, 204
  salience and order, 211–14, 216
  stereotypes, 161–3
  stylized motifs, 161, 187, 204
  summary of variables, 231–2
  units of analysis, 177–8
  see also particular forms
chimney, child's drawing, 170–1
Chinese brush
  difficulty of stroke making, 11
  grip, 11
Chinese script
  average stroke direction, 11, 24–6
  early script production, 24
  k'ou radical, 31
Chomsky, N., 4
circle production, 76–84, 86–94
  anchored circles, 84–5
  by children, 76, 86–8, 185
  concentric, 79
  and dot-cluster start in children, 88
  hand placement, 91–2
  left-handers, 76, 77, 78, 79–80, 81, 88–92
  letter copying, 84–5
  manipulating starting location, 80–1
  mechanism, 88–92
  nonfigurative rotation, 76, 79, 89–90
  opposite to line production, 80, 89–90
  size effect, 77, 79
  starting location, 77, 79
  start-rotate principle, 80–92
  trajectories, uneven, 92–3
circles
  faceted in music notation, 28
  see also circle production
circle start manipulated
  deliberate variation, 80–1
  dot start, 80–1
  gap start, 80–1
circular plots, *see* polar plots
Clark, H.H., 253, 254
Clowes, M., 268
cognitive difficulty in reading diagrams, 247–9
communicative efficiency
  speech *vs*. graphics, 235
competence in drawing, *see* difficult graphic tasks
connection diagram, *see* connection network
connection network, 215–22
  bicycle, 215
  core *vs*. periphery, 215–17
  dispenser, 217
  fixed order, 215–16
  lamp, 218, 221
  optional order, 215–16
  side-chains, 215–16
Connolly, K., 263
conservatism in child's drawing, 163–172, 173
  definition, 166
  effect of delay, 171–2

effect of graphic suggestions, 170
contextual support for detail, 123
contour, 185, 189, 190–6
complementary, 191
complementary anticipated, 191
definition, 3
developmental summarized, 195–6
multiple origins, 190–6
overinclusiveness, 193
primary, 191
contrastive identity, *see* representational contrast
conventions, ix, 4, 60–4
greetings and farewells, 60–1
politeness, 61
conversational agreements
analogues in graphics, 108, 109–10, 116
cooperative principle, *see* conversational agreements
coordination, graphic, 201–3
copying, *see* subject headings
as research method, 3
critical contrast, *see* representational contrast
crosses, *see* stroke making, intersecting lines
Crystal, D., 260, 263
cubes, *see* solids copied
cube test design
error consequences, 142–3, 144, 157
curvilinear forms, 72–94
see also arc drawing; circle production; ellipses
cylinder drawn, 69
Czikszentmihalyi, M., 244

detail, *see* profile of detail
detectability of graphic errors, 40, 49, 51
diagram interpretation, 247–9
difficult graphic tasks, 131–60
braid logo, 136, 137
chain, 135, 137
cube, unfolded, 135
figure-of-eight loop, 135, 137, 154–5, 157
gemini, 136, 137
good performers, 156, 158–9, 160
knot, overhand, 136, 137, 151–4, 155–6, 157
inspection time, 138
linear skeleton, 149
offset cross, 136, 159, 160
poor performers, 158–9,160
procedural knowledge, 155
scoring categories, 138–9
success rates, copying, 137–8
success rates, drawing, 136–8
summary of analysis, 156–7
swastika, 135, 137, 149–51, 157, 159
triceps, (Mitsubishi logo), 135, 136, 137, 145–7, 149, 157
trinacria, (three-armed swastika), 131, 136, 137, 138–40, 142–3, 157, 159, 160
triquetra, 136, 137, 146–9, 156–7
triskele, (Isle-of-Man symbol), 136, 137, 140–2
difficulty ratings, stroke making
normal surface, 7–9
vertical surface, 17–18
doodling, *see* everyday drawing
dot clusters, *see* starting location
Douglas, M., 269
Dreyfus, H., 135
Dunckner, K., 170

Edgerton, S.Y. Jr., 144
11 o'clock start, 19–20, 42–3, 54–5, 61–3, 64, 69, 70, 74, 78, 89, 91–2, 110, 253
11-to-5 axis, 5, 21, 22, 37, 64, 76, 80, 85, 88–9
Elliott, J., 263
ellipses, 77, 79, 85–6
with gaps, 80–3
rotation, 85–6
starting position, 79
embedding, 44–8, 111–12
definitions, 47–8
linguistic, 47–8
procedural *vs.* structural, 46–8
in real-world scenes, 45–7
see also anticipated embedding
enactive knowledge, in drawing knot, 151–2
end control, 37–41
see also anchoring
Eng, H., 204–5
everyday drawing, 233–70
doodling, 237, 239, 240, 241, 243, 244–6

expressive function, 237, 243
female activity listed, 240
male activity listed, 241
mental working space, 237
organizing thought, 236, 239, 243
personal style, 262–3
public *vs*. private, 235, 242–3
recreational drawing, 237–8
reflects sociology, 233, 242
role of audience, 238–9
role of literacy, 234
survey methods, 238–9
vs. art-work, 237–8, 243–4
see also thematics
excursion envelope of hand, 9–10
executive constraints, 1–51
anchoring, 36–51
asymmetrical conformity, 48–51
in child drawing, 209
collinearity, 33–5
geometry and order, 33–5
order, 22, 33–5
paper contact, 30–3
proximity, 33–7
similarity, 33–6
starting position, 18–21
stroke preferences, 3–19
symmetry, 33–5
expressive drawing, 237, 243
"off-record" communication, 243

face drawing, 50, 122
see also asymmetrical conformity
"facing" of objects, 120–2
Fairbank, A., 93
fanning action of hand
accuracy, 10, 16
in drafting, 13
in shading, 13–14
feature extraction
in knot drawing, 152, 156
feature hierarchies, 268
flags, orientation, 121–2
flexion–extension of fingers
and paper contact, 11
pronation and supination, 11–12
scope of movement, 11, 91–2
flowcharts
quadrilateral figures, 58
swastika drawing, 150
triangle production, 52–3
focus, linguistic, 107–8
defined, 107
foreground salience, 111, 114
foreshortening, 109–10
Forge, A., 106
formal constraints, *see* executive constraints
frame: topic organization, 41
Fraser, B., 234
functional fixedness, 170

generative rules, 61
geometric constraints, *see* executive constraints
gesture accompanying drawing, 260
Getzels, J.W., 244
given: new organization, 41
Goffman, E., 60
Gombrich, E.H., 247–8
Goodnow, J.J., 3, 76
Goody, J., 269
"grape clusters"
geometry, 42
order of production, 42–4
topology, 42
"graphic acts," 233, 234, 235, 236, 246
"graphic engine," 246
graphic "habits," 77
graphic prosodics, *see* prosodics
graphic schema, 175
Greenstreet, B., 13
Grice, H.P., 116, 197

Halliday, M.A.K., 262, 270
Haworth, M.R., 76
Hebrew script, 24–6
circles, 76, 93
paper contact, 30
Helfman, E.S., 135
Herron, J., 7
hierarchical forms
alternative strategies, 15, 35–6
human figure drawing, 35
hieratic script, curves, 93
Hiley, D., 27
hooking of hand, *see* inversion of hand; left-handers
horizontal lines
rules, 4
shakiness, 7
Hornung, C.P., 135

Howard, I.P., 110
human action, analysis of, 2, 269–70
semiotic content, 270
simultaneous complexity, 269–70
human figure, hierarchical organization, 35

iconic relations, 188–9, 247–9
ideal triangles, 55–8
effects on drawing, 55, 58
order of preference, 56–8
Ilg, F.L., 76
imagery, visual
basis for drawing, 106
and drawing competence, 135
drawing as extension, 237
limitations, 155–6
see also Visual Elaboration Scale
Impressionists, 111
intersection, mutual, *see* anchoring, serial
inversion of hand in tracing, 17
see also left-handers
Ivins, W.M. Jr., 203

James, H., 126
Japanese script, *kuchi*, 31
Jarvella, R.J., 227
Johnson-Laird, P.N., 227
Jones, S., 162, 170, 174
Jools, P., 32, 197

Kennedy, J.M., 187
knot and braid theory, 151, 156
knot drawn, *see* difficult graphic tasks
Knuth, D.E., 94
Koenig, S., 238

Langridge, D., 268
Latin script
anchoring, 42, 84–5
child letter production, 93
geometry of letters, 101
rotated alphabetical letters, 101–3, 105
stroke direction, 24–6
left-handers
arc drawing, 74–6
circle production, 76, 78, 88–92
copying broken figures, 80–3
copying line sets, 23
dot cluster tracing, 19
dot cluster tracing, children, 20–1
ellipse production, 79, 87
errors in copying, 13
free line drawing, 5–6
"grape-cluster" production, 43
hand inversion, 5–7, 23, 74
line tracing, 5–6
nonfigurative rotation, 89–90
order, 22
subjects, 6–7, 74
starting location, circles, 76, 79–80
starting positions, 19–20, 91–2
stroke making, children, 20–1
triangle copying, 54–5
letter production, *see* Latin script
level of detail, *see* profile of detail
levels of structure, in braid design, 137
Levinson, S., 243
Lévi-Strauss, C., 269
Levy, J., 5
lines, signification, 187-8, 201
boundary, 187
cavity boundary, 187
pigment boundary, 187
reflectivity, 188
regions subdivided, 187
slant, 188
terminator of surface, 187
texture, 188
Lings, M., 93
linguistic analogy
copying and imitation, 50
embedding, 47–8
equivalents to word, sentence, discourse, 262
grammar, 203
intonation, 264–5
"layered" system, 1, 267
limitations, 260
mimetic drawing, codified language, 96
"morphology," 187
paradigmatic organization, 1
"phonology," 94, 95–6
phrase markers, 268
picture grammars, 268
pragmatics, 115, 116, 233
prosodics, 95, 259–67
semantics, 115, 233, 259
speech acts *vs.* graphic acts, 233, 234, 235, 236
surface form forgotten, 227

syntagmatic series, 1, 269
thematics, 261–2
tree diagrams, 34, 268
types *vs.* tokens, 187
voice quality, 262
"locking" of fingers and wrist, *see* stroke making

McWhinnie, H.J., 170
map drawing, 234, 239, 240, 241, 246–7, 249–54, 259–60, 266
map orientation, 249–54
summary, 252–3
Massoudy, H., 93
mathematical analysis, *see* knot and braid theory
meaning, *see* semantics
medium, graphic, 197, 231
memory for executive process, 227
mental rotation, *see* rotation, mental
mirror-image reversal, in knot drawing, 156
Möller, G., 93
Morasso, P., 93
motif, graphic, 185, 187, 189
motion, transverse portrayal, 256–7
motion expressed in stroke making, 95, 103–4, 105
multistable figure, 132
musical notation
curves, 93
evolution, 27–9

neuropsychology, *see* brain pathology

object drawing, *see* representational drawing
occlusion of objects,
children's mechanisms, 197–200
concentric portrayal, 109–12
and embedding, 46
hybrid devices, 198–9
object separation, 197
omission of objects, 109, 197
shown by gaps, 137
solids, 69
strategies of representation, 108–14
transparency, 109–12, 197–200
vertical displacement, 109–11
Olson, D.R., 16
order of mention, 107–8, 112
order in stroke making
child drawing, 209, 215–16
connectivity, 36
collinearity effect, 33–5, 37, 39
11-to-5 axis, 22
geometric constraints, 33–5
hand inversion, 23
parallel lines, 59
proximity effect, 22, 33–5, 36, 37, 39
semantic effect, 33–5, 36
similarity effect, 33–5, 36
starting position effect, 22
symmetry effect, 33–5, 37, 39
orthoscopic viewpoint
adult, 259
child, 198–9, 201

painting order
foreground *vs.* background, 111
Impressionists, 111
paper contact constraint, 30–3
affects framing, 32
affects stroke order, 32–3
broken lines, 31–2, 55
closed figures, 52, 59
developmental data, 32
economy, 31–2
effect of angles, 31–2
repetition of figures, 31
size of figures, 31–2, 55
speed of production, 55
tracing *vs.* copying, 31
triskele, 141
paper rotation, basis in writing, 10
parallelograms, distortions in shape, 59–60
perceptual analysis, 131–60
affected by graphics, 121
competent drawers, 133–4, 156, 158–9, 160
defective analysis, 158–60
drawing failure, 131–60
easy topics, 133–4
memory storage, 131
perceptual effects, in copying solids, 64–9
personal style, 262–3
perspective, *see* reversed perspective
"phonological" constraints, 1, 94, *see also* executive constraints
picture grammars, 268

planning, graphic, 42–51
backward dependencies, 43
complex sequences of actions, 50
forward control, 43
individual differences, 50
overlapping figures, 59
see also asymmetrical conformity
planning in child drawing, conservative effect, 172
plans, 241, 246–7, 249–54
object plans, 253–4
play, graphic, 245
polar plots
children's free line drawing, 21
children's starting position, 21
explanation, 5, 25
free line drawing, 6
hand position variation, 8
line copying errors, 12
line set copying, 23
script production, 25–6
starting position, 19
stroke difficulty, 9
tracing lines, 6
tree branches, roots, 15
on vertical wall, 18
Porter, T., 13
Powers, V.M., 268
practical logic, 60
pragmatics, 1, 2, 233–70
"motive-free" drawing, 116, 223
primitive art, research strategy, 105–6
primitives, graphic, 1, 184–6, 189, 201
in object drawing, 127
in signification, 189
taxonomy, 185–6
principle of least effort, 123
prisms, *see* solids copied
procedural knowledge, *see* difficult graphic tasks
production sequence, guide to meaning, 105–6
profile, *see* face drawing
profile of detail, 116, 126–30
consistency, 125
definition, 129–30
discontinuous, 127
"leveling" of detail, 123
need for contrast, 123–4
revisions of basic strategy, 129
role of effort, 128
social factors, 122, 125
use of "samples," 129
prosodic devices
body language, 267
care, 265, 267
dimensionality of, 267
feathering, 266, 267
fragmented line, 259–60, 265, 267
intrinsic characteristics, 260
level of detail, 265, 267
line thickness, 267
looseness of style, 129
overdrawing, 266, 267
size, 267
speed, 265, 266, 267
"tailing off," 265–6
token detail, 265
prosodic messages
emphasis, 267
literalness, 267
prosodics, 95, 259–67
"code-book," 267
devices used, 265–7
inquiry strategies, 261–2
interaction between devices, 265–7
prototypicality, *see* representational drawing
proximity in space
effect on drawing, 108–14
foreground salience, 111, 114
psychological "facing," in map orientation, 252–4

radial line drawing
anchoring effect, 37–40
arm position change, 62
order of strokes, 37, 39
planning, 42
starting location, 37–40
stroke direction, 37–8
rationalism, ix, 138
reasoning, graphic, development, 47
recognition, visual
as evidence of visual analysis, 131–5
multistable figure, 132–3
rectangle construction
concentric, 59
extended sides, 59
long sides, 59
normal process, 62–4
overlapping, 59

paper contact, 31, 59
theoretically possible sequences, 59
rectilinear figures, 52–71
see also rectangle construction; triangle construction
recursiveness, in doodling, 245
Reid, M., 5
repeated drawings, children, 174–84
methods, 175–6
representation, *see* semantics
representational contrast, 122, 123–5, 188–9
in children's drawings, 190
contrast set, 124
contrastive isolation, 190
language effects, 124–5
level of familiarity, 124
minimal hallmarks, 124
in musical notation, 27
semiotic theory, 188–9
task sequence, 124–5
representational drawing, 115–30
aspect of objects, 126
executive constraints, 117–22
"graspability" of objects, 121
intrinsic right-handed objects, 120–1
oblique orientation, 117, 119–20
old-fashioned style, 126
prototypicality, 125–6
solidity, 127, 129
texture, 127
see also face drawing; "facing" of objects; semantics
research strategies
experimental approaches, 2
naturalistic observation, 2
reversed perspective, 144–5
room plans, 250–2, 258–9
two viewpoints, 252
Ross, R., 9
rotation
as geometric property, 137
as process in drawing, 137, 140
rotation, mental
in difficult drawing tasks, 146, 149, 153–5
rule
as convention, 4
discreteness, 4
grammatical analogy, 4
Sadler, N., 84–5
Safadi, Y.H., 93
salience, prism faces
angle size effect, 67
area effect, 67
method, 66–7
orientation effect, 67
Saussure, F., 188, 189
scene analysis, 268
schema, graphic, 36
school drawing
"artistic," 115–16
functional, 115
"recreational," 116
script, stroke direction, computer analysis, 25–6
script analysis, automatic, 268
script evolution
Arabic, 24–6
Chinese, 24–6
cuneiform, 27
cursive effect, 24–5, 27
Hebrew, 24–6
Latin script, 24–6
legibility factor, 25–6
starting position effect, 24
summary of influences, 26–7
Searle, J.R., 233
semantics, 95–114
affected by executive constraints, 114
compete with executive constraints, 95, 105
in contour, 99, 100
determine order, 100
overridden by geometry, 99
review of impact, 114
segmentation effect, 99–101, 105
stroke making, 105
suppressed by repetition, 105
Sepik River art, 105
serial action, cumulative effects, 246
shading, affected by stroke preference, 13
da Vinci, Leonardo, 16
shared knowledge
in everyday drawing, 259
in object drawing, 123
signification in graphics, 187, 188–9
signifier *vs.* signified, 188–9
skill, 1, 2, 231, 269, 270
Slee, J., 135

social context of drawing studies, 115–17, 122, 235
solids
  copied, 64–71
  copying strategies, 66–71
  drawn, 69
  generating stimulus set, 64–5
  salience of faces, 65–9
speech acts, 233, 234
  vs. "language acts," 235–6
  scope, 234
squares, with gaps, 80–3
stairway drawings, strategies, 44–7
Stanton, R., 170, 171, 172, 174
star, test design, 143–4, 157
starting location
  affected by order of letters, 103
  affected by stroke preference, 64
  in child drawing, 20–1, 209
  copying letters, 20
  dot-cluster drawing, 20
  dot-cluster tracing, 19–20
  dual start in left-handers, 89–90
  independence of arm position, 64
  independence of stroke preference, 17–20
  nongraphic tasks, 20
  on objects in space, 110–11, 122
  on page, 122
  in representational drawing, 117–18
  triangle copying, 53–5
  variety of tasks, 54
stereotypes, 161–3
stick figures, 201
straight line production, *see* stroke making
strategies, graphic
  backtracking, 154, 155
  "breaking off," 46
  coalescence of regions, 47
  frame plus detail, 99
  pathfinding, 154, 155
  substrate plus anchoring, 42
  see also difficult drawing tasks
stroke accuracy, *see* stroke making
stroke making, 3–19
  accuracy of copying, 12–13
  ballistic, 3
  basis of preferences, 7–12
  bias, 5
  canonical stroke directions, 16
  in child drawing, 20–1, 209
  difficulty, 7, 9
  drafting effects, 13
  "easiness," 7
  grouping of movements, 8–9
  intersecting lines, 13–14
  lines drawn from centers, 83
  "locking" of fingers and wrist, 16
  preferences, 4, 8
  semantic effects, 95, 103–4, 105
  shading, 13, 16
  straight line production, 4–7
  tracing lines, 4–5, 17
  triangle copying, 53–5
  see also fanning action of hand; flexion–extension of fingers
structural redundancy, in complex designs, 131–5
subjects
  class background, ix
  country of origin, ix, 74
  educational background, ix
subroutine, graphic, 36

templates, 17
Templeton, W.B., 110
Teulings, H-L.H.M., 76, 79, 90–1
Thai script, circles, 93
thematics, 261–2
theme-rheme, 266
Thomassen, A.J.W.M., 76, 79, 90–1
threading, *see* paper contact constraint
time in diagrams
  American Sign Language, 256
  lists, 255, 257–8
  "plan" of time, 256–7
  spatial analogues, 254, 255, 256–8
  time-line, 255–6, 265
  two metaphors, 254–5
  use in publications, 256
"top" and "bottom" of pages, 110
topology, "grape-clusters," 42
Trabasso, T., 170
tracing
  end control, 42
  gaps at intersections, 42
  reversal of stroke making, 17
  visibility, 17
transformations, 268
transparency, *see* occlusion of objects
triangle construction

by children, 209
distortions, 55–8
with gaps, 80–3
paper contact, 55
starting location, 53
stroke preferences, 53
theoretically possible sequences, 52
Tung Tso-pin, 24
typefaces, curves, 94

unconscious action, 39, 40, 269, 270

verbal description
impact on copying, 96–101
impact on drawing, 106–14
"vernacular" drawers, xii
vertical lines
confident stroke, 7
rules, 4
semantic origins, 4, 190
vertical surface, *see* stroke making
visibility in stroke making, *see* tracing
Visual Elaboration Scale, 135

Watt, W.C., 268
Williams, R., 244
wrist-hand configuration, 7–8
wrist movement, 7, 10
see also fanning action of hand

writing
arm orientation, 10
paper rotation, 10

Zatorski, R.J., 268